Essential Paediatric Orthopaedic Decision Making

Essential Paediatric Orthopaedic Decision Making

A Case-Based Approach

Edited by
Benjamin Joseph, Selvadurai Nayagam and
Randall T Loder

Content Editor
Anjali Benjamin Daniel

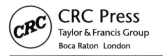

CRC Press
Taylor & Francis Group
Boca Raton London

CRC Press is an imprint of the
Taylor & Francis Group, an **informa** business

First edition published 2022
by CRC Press
6000 Broken Sound Parkway NW, Suite 300, Boca Raton, FL 33487–2742

and by CRC Press
2 Park Square, Milton Park, Abingdon, Oxon, OX14 4RN

© 2022 Taylor & Francis Group, LLC

CRC Press is an imprint of Taylor & Francis Group, LLC

Library of Congress Cataloging-in-Publication Data
Names: Joseph, Benjamin (Professor of orthopaedics) editor. | Nayagam, Selvadurai, editor. | Loder, Randall T., editor.
Title: Essential paediatric orthopaedic decision making : a case-based approach / edited by Benjamin Joseph,
 Selvadurai Nayagam, Randall Loder; content editor, Anjali Benjamin Daniel.
Description: First edition. | Boca Raton : CRC Press, 2022. | Includes bibliographical references and index.
Identifiers: LCCN 2021027435 (print) | LCCN 2021027436 (ebook) | ISBN 9780367553623 (pbk) |
 ISBN 9780367618773 (hbk) | ISBN 9781003106920 (enhanced ebk) | ISBN 9781003232308 (ebk)
Subjects: MESH: Musculoskeletal Diseases | Child | Orthopedic Procedures | Case Reports
Classification: LCC RD732.3.C48 (print) | LCC RD732.3.C48 (ebook) | NLM WS 275 | DDC 618.92/7—dc23
LC record available at https://lccn.loc.gov/2021027435
LC ebook record available at https://lccn.loc.gov/2021027436

ISBN: 978-0-367-61877-3 (hbk)
ISBN: 978-0-367-55362-3 (pbk)
ISBN: 978-1-003-10692-0 (enhanced ebk)
ISBN: 978-1-003-23230-8 (ebk)

DOI: 10.1201/9781003106920

Typeset in Minion
by Apex CoVantage, LLC

We dedicate this book to the children who trusted us to make the right decisions while treating them.

CONTENTS

Contents

DETAILS OF AUTHORS

Caroline M Blakey
Consultant Orthopedic Surgeon and Educational Lead
Department of Paediatric Orthopaedics
Trauma and Spinal Surgery
Sheffield Children's NHS Foundation Trust
Sheffield, UK

Leo Donnan
Associate Professor, University of Melbourne
Murdoch Children's Research Institute
Royal Children's Hospital
Melbourne, Australia

James A Fernandes
Consultant Orthopaedic Surgeon and Paediatric Limb Reconstruction Lead
Department of Paediatric Orthopaedics, Trauma and Spinal Surgery
Sheffield Children's NHS Foundation Trust
Sheffield, UK

Nick Green
Consultant Orthopaedic Surgeon
Department of Paediatric Orthopaedics, Trauma and Spinal Surgery
Sheffield Children's NHS Foundation Trust
Sheffield, UK

Benjamin Joseph
Retired Professor & Former Head of Paediatric Orthopaedic Service
Kasturba Medical College
Karnataka, India

Randall T Loder
Garceau Professor Emeritus of Orthopaedic Surgery
Riley Children's Hospital
Indianapolis, USA

Selvadurai Nayagam
Retired Consultant and Orthopaedic
Trauma and Limb Reconstruction Surgeon
Alder Hey Children's Hospital NHS Foundation Trust
Liverpool, UK

Nicholas Peterson
Consultant Orthopaedic Surgeon, Paediatric and Adult Limb Reconstruction Surgery
Alder Hey Children's Hospital NHS Foundation Trust
and

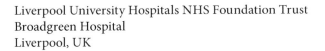

Liverpool University Hospitals NHS Foundation Trust
Broadgreen Hospital
Liverpool, UK

Christopher Prior
Consultant in Children's Orthopaedics and Limb Reconstruction Surgery
Alder Hey Children's Hospital NHS Foundation Trust
Liverpool, UK

Hitesh Shah
Professor & Head of the Department of Paediatric Orthopaedics
Kasturba Medical College
Manipal Academy of Higher Education
Karnataka, India

David A Spiegel
Division of Orthopaedic Surgery
Children's Hospital of Philadelphia
Professor of Orthopaedic Surgery
Perelman School of Medicine at the University of Pennsylvania
Philadelphia, USA

Binu Prathap Thomas
Professor & Head
Paul Brand Centre for Hand Surgery
Christian Medical College
Tamil Nadu, India

FOREWORD BY DR. CATTERALL

I am very pleased to be asked to provide a Foreword to this book, which I am sure has an important place in paediatric orthopaedic education. It is a follow-up presentation to *Paediatrics Orthopaedics*, published by the same authors and now in its second edition.

One of the problems in teaching this subject is that textbooks explain the clinical conditions and their treatment, but do not really help in the management of clinical problems encountered in an individual case, particularly when there are complications. This book is designed to help in this matter.

The authors state that the book is aimed at the orthopaedic trainee and clinical fellow. I think that there is a further and important group, who are the recently appointed consultants who by their training will be able to deal with the common problems, but are out of their depth with the more difficult problem and need a mentor. This book clearly addresses this issue.

The way that the text is presented is helpful. There is a history and examination, after which the problems are defined and then individually discussed. As a result, a method of management is evolved which the surgeon may consider. In some cases, the details of the surgical techniques are presented. They will then decide whether they can undertake the management or wish to seek help from other sources. The matter can then be discussed with the patient and their family, and decisions made. At the end of the case, a reference back to *Paediatric Orthopaedics*, second edition is provided.

I am sure that this book will find its place in helping children with orthopaedic problems, and identify better methods of management in these difficult cases.

I warmly recommend this book.

Dr. Anthony Catterall, FRCS
Consultant Orthopaedic Surgeon
Royal National Orthopaedic Hospital
Stanmore, UK

FOREWORD BY PROFESSOR GRAHAM

One of the many aphorisms of the late Dr Robert B. Salter was "decisions are more important than incisions". The timing of this book is inspired because in the era of COVID-19, traditional teaching of clinical surgery by apprenticeship, with unlimited access to patients and mentors, has been somewhat curtailed. The text book *Essential Paediatric Orthopaedic Decision Making* goes a long way to make up for limited access in these difficult times. Dr. Benjamin Joseph and his co-authors have compiled a practical, useful and unique text for trainees in paediatric orthopaedics. It will be especially useful for those at the Registrar/Resident level and for those undertaking Fellowship training. Sixty challenging clinical scenarios are presented, from malunion of a tibial fracture to pseudarthrosis of the tibia, after failed primary surgery. Each case is approached in a systematic manner with a background history, key features of physical examination and a series of questions. This is where the reader should stop and consider the questions without going to the answers! If the reader approaches the carefully designed material, in the spirit in which it has been compiled, there will be much to learn. The questions lead to the goals of surgery, followed by a list of options for the management of each case. The option chosen by the surgeon is then presented, usually with intraoperative, clinical and radiographic illustrations. The majority of cases have substantial follow-up to illustrate the wisdom of the surgical decision-making, the surgical skill employed and the diligent post-operative care and follow-up.

There is much to learn in the case material presented. In a busy Paediatric Orthopaedic Unit, Residents and Fellows could profitably absorb the contents of one or two cases per week, as they encounter them in the clinic, in the operating theatre or in post-operative follow-up. In this way, the context for surgical decision-making, for both rare and complex problems, would be more readily appreciated than in most of the specialist text books currently available. I anticipate that this will become a classic text, to be used in conjunction with the second edition of *Paediatric Orthopaedics—A System of Decision-Making*. Together these textbooks will unravel many of the mysteries and complexities of paediatric orthopaedic decision-making. I believe that this book will improve the outcomes for children under our care, those children recognised in the Dedication:

> *We dedicate this book to the children who trusted us to make the right decisions while treating them.*

Kerr Graham, MD, FRACS
Professor of Orthopaedic Surgery
University of Melbourne
Melbourne, Australia

FOREWORD BY PROFESSOR WILKINS

This textbook, *Essential Paediatric Orthopaedic Decision Making*, is predicted to become a very important resource for the process of educating orthopaedic surgeons on the basic principles of managing patients with challenging conditions in the paediatric age group.

One of the outstanding contributions this textbook is the wealth of knowledge the distinguished editors Benjamin Joseph, Selvadurai Nayagam and Randall T. Loder share with the reader from their many years of experience in managing challenging paediatric orthopaedic conditions. These esteemed paediatric orthopaedic surgeons are from different continents, which results in a world-wide fund of knowledge and experience.

The concepts of teaching the principles of challenging paediatric orthopaedic conditions in this textbook are unique in many ways.

Firstly, there is their innovative method of teaching the basic principles of managing the treatment of these paediatric orthopaedic conditions.

Most of the presently accepted paediatric orthopaedic texts present their material in a passive manner. The basic principles are presented, but there is truly little re-enforcement of the concepts presented. Often only one generic treatment process is proposed. The reader must learn to apply these treatment principles simply by passive memory or experience.

This textbook utilises the interactive approach in which various alternative procedures that are available for the treatment process are evaluated. Instead of suggesting only one preferred technique of the standard textbook's author or authors, the emphasis in this textbook is to force the treating surgeon to carefully stop and evaluate the pros and cons of the available treatment alternatives. Rather than rushing into a specific plan, this method of pre-evaluation increases the chance of a successful outcome. This technique of taking time to critically plan their treatment process leads to a deeper and more permanent retention of assimilating the basic principles of managing challenging paediatric orthopaedic conditions.

The most valuable lesson produced with this textbook is to stimulate the paediatric orthopaedic surgeon to evaluate the treatment alternatives critically in developing a well-thought-out treatment plan. Utilising this unique interactive teaching process will be extremely valuable for stimulating orthopaedic residents to develop an organisational approach to their patients following their training process.

Secondly, the cases presented represent complicated problems that require more than just applying the standard techniques for the common paediatric orthopaedic conditions. For example, the management of a virgin clubfoot usually responds to treatment with the Ponseti technique. The incomplete or poorly treated rigid equinovarus clubfoot requires critical evaluation of multiple rigid deformities that require a multiplicity of decisions and organisation of treatment alternatives. The authors have shared their vast experience with organising a treatment plan for these conditions that the average paediatric orthopaedic surgeon will rarely encounter.

The majority of conditions presented to the general paediatric orthopaedic surgeon have a standard, well-established treatment process. For example, treating displaced fractures of the distal radius and metaphyses or shafts can usually be managed appropriately with a standard reduction and immobilisation process. A late radial-ulnar malunion involves a more challenging treatment process that requires critical evaluation of the advantages and goals of several treatment alternatives. The use of the critical evaluation process presented in this textbook will serve as a valuable guide to managing paediatric orthopaedic conditions that have a combination of multiple deformities or sequelae of their traumatic or disease processes.

The authors of this textbook have had a vast experience of treating conditions such as residual deformities from non- or inadequate treatment that is rarely presented to the average paediatric orthopaedic surgeon. The value of this textbook is in organising a treatment plan that involves how to critically develop a treatment algorithm that can be used to approach the challenging paediatric orthopaedic conditions.

Many orthopaedic surgeons participate in orthopaedic outreach-activity in resource-poor areas. In these areas, they will be presented with many non- or poorly treated paediatric orthopaedic conditions with which they have had no experience and are not amenable to the standard simple orthopaedic treatment techniques seen in their home practices. The authors of this textbook have extensive experience with such challenging conditions and share their approaches in managing these complicated orthopaedic problems utilising the evaluation processes outlined in this textbook.

It is predicted that this critical approach in managing complicated paediatric orthopaedics will become a standard teaching process for orthopaedic surgeons in the future. We as paediatric orthopaedic surgeons will benefit greatly by incorporating this textbook's interactive and critical evaluation process in the management of the challenging paediatric orthopaedic problems.

The authors are to be congratulated for sharing their innovative approach to the management of challenging orthopaedic conditions in the paediatric age group in this textbook. The orthopaedic community will benefit immensely from having this unique educational resource.

Kaye E. Wilkins, DVM, MD
Professor Emeritus
Department of Orthopedics
University of Texas Health Science Center at San Antonio
San Antonio, Texas, USA

PREFACE

In the first and second editions of *Paediatric Orthopaedics—A System of Decision-Making*, the authors outlined a systematic approach to choosing treatment options based on factors relevant to each clinical situation. As we pondered on how best we could illustrate this approach, it became very clear that real-life examples of patients treated would convey the message.

In this collection of sixty illustrative cases, we have attempted to emphasise how a particular treatment was chosen for each case. We have used a common format throughout the book beginning with a brief case summary followed by a standard list of questions. We encourage the reader to answer these questions before proceeding to read the rest of the chapter.

In each chapter, the problems to be addressed and the aims of treatment are listed as are the various options for achieving the listed aims. The authors then list factors that influenced their choice of treatment in the form of a table. The details of treatment and the outcome are then described.

At the end of each case, a link to the corresponding chapter in the 2nd Edition of *Paediatric Orthopaedics—A System of Decision-Making* has been included to enable the reader to get some more insight into rational clinical decision-making.

We hope that the trainee and the Fellow in Paediatric Orthopaedics will find this book useful.

The Editors

DEFORMITIES

Christopher Prior, Nicholas Peterson, Selvadurai Nayagam

Case

An 11-year-old girl was referred with a marked equinus deformity of the right ankle. She had congenital talipes equinovarus (CTEV), which was treated in infancy by the Ponseti method with a percutaneous Achilles tenotomy. Due to compliance issues with boots and bars, the equinus recurred. A tibialis anterior tendon transfer and a gastroc-soleus lengthening were undertaken at age 3 years. A further relapse necessitated an open tenotomy a year later. The patient was lost to follow-up, but at age 7 years she presented with a 20-degree equinus deformity. The treating surgeon decided the deformity could not be managed with further soft tissue intervention and performed a distal tibial osteotomy in an attempt to bring the ankle into dorsiflexion.

Clinical examination at presentation now revealed a 30-degree equinus contracture, a 25-degree apex-posterior tibial deformity (recurvatum) (Figure 1.1) and a 25mm limb length difference with the right side shorter. The hindfoot was mobile and pain-free. The forefoot was plantarflexed but not adducted. She walked with compensatory hyperextension of the knee. The neurovascular examination was normal.

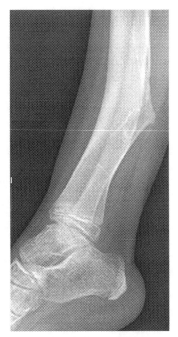

Figure 1.1 The distal tibial osteotomy has left a residual recurvatum deformity after five years.

Questions

- What are the problems that need to be addressed in this girl?
- What are the aims of treatment?
- What are the commonly available options for treatment?
- What are the factors that may influence your choice of treatment?
- What treatment would you recommend for this girl?
- How long would you follow-up this girl after treatment?

The Problems That Need to Be Addressed Are

- Equinus deformity causing functional and cosmetic problems
- Difficulty in fitting a shoe
- Risk of recurrence during growth due to underlying CTEV
- Limb length discrepancy (LLD)

The Aims of Treatment

- Correct the deformity in the tibia and at the ankle
- Restore a mobile, pain-free, plantigrade foot to allow stability and function
- Prevent recurrence

Options for Treatment

- Correction of equinus

  - Serial manipulation and casting
  - Soft tissue procedures

    - Revision of Achilles tendon lengthening
    - Posterior ankle release
    - Plantar fascia release

  - Gradual correction of ankle equinus

    - With a circular external fixator with or without foot osteotomies
    - Anterior distal tibial hemiepiphyseodesis

  - Arthrodesis

    - Triple arthrodesis (Lambrinudi)
    - Ankle arthrodesis

- Correction of recurvatum

  - Tibial osteotomy (closed wedge) with acute correction and internal fixation
  - Gradual correction by circular external fixation

- Correction of tibial shortening

  - Tibial lengthening
  - Contralateral epiphyseodesis

FACTORS THAT INFLUENCED THE CHOICE OF TREATMENT

- Results of previous treatment
- Residual effects of previous treatment
- Potential adverse effects of treatment options
- Age of the child

The choice of treatment based on these factors is outlined in Table 1.1.

Table 1.1 Factors Influencing the Choice of Treatment

Factors		Treatment Implications
Results of previous treatment	Serial casting was attempted previously but was unsuccessful	Further attempts at serial casting are unlikely to achieve correction of the deformity of the foot.
Residual effects of previous treatment	Repeated soft tissue releases	Further release or lengthening of scarred tissue is difficult, often ineffective and runs the risk of injury to the neurovascular bundle.
Age of the child	11 years	An ankle or triple fusion in a 11-year-old child with growth remaining will produce stunting of growth in the foot and add to a greater leg length difference. They may be considered as a salvage procedure for those near skeletal maturity if other options are not available.
Potential disadvantages of treatment options	Repeat Achilles tendon lengthening	Lengthening of the Achilles reduces plantarflexion power.[1]
	Closed wedge osteotomy to correct tibial recurvatum	Closed wedge osteotomy will increase the limb-length difference.
	Gradual deformity correction with an external fixator	The treatment is protracted and requires a great deal of co-operation from the family.
	Correction of tibial recurvatum	The degree of ankle equinus will be worsened by the correction of tibial recurvatum.
	Arthrodesis as a means of correcting equinus	Arthrodesis will result in stiffness of the foot.

How Was This Girl Treated?

Since the ability for gradual correction of severe and established contractures by the Ilizarov method is well established[2] and since the tibial deformity could also be corrected by this technique, we recommended this option to the parents, explaining in detail the protracted nature and complexity of treatment. The patient and family were willing to comply with their involvement in the treatment.

Treatment

The procedure was performed in two stages to lessen the possibility for confusion as the distraction protocol for correction of tibial recurvatum and ankle equinus would be in opposite directions.

Stage 1: Correction of the Tibial Deformity

An oblique osteotomy was performed with a sagittal saw at the junction of middle and distal third of the fibula. A four-ring Ilizarov frame was constructed with a proximal and a distal segment, each parallel to the corresponding tibial segment on either side of the CORA. Intraoperatively, the limb was rotated under fluoroscopy to reveal an oblique plane deformity (some minor valgus as well as the apex-posterior deformity). The hinges were positioned to subtend an axis in a plane orthogonal to that which, when the tibia was rotated, produced a straight-looking bone under fluoroscopy. The hinges were aligned slightly behind the posterior cortex so that a small amount of lengthening would occur during correction (Figure 1.2). A low-energy osteotomy was performed at the CORA and the fixator assembled with an anterior motor unit.

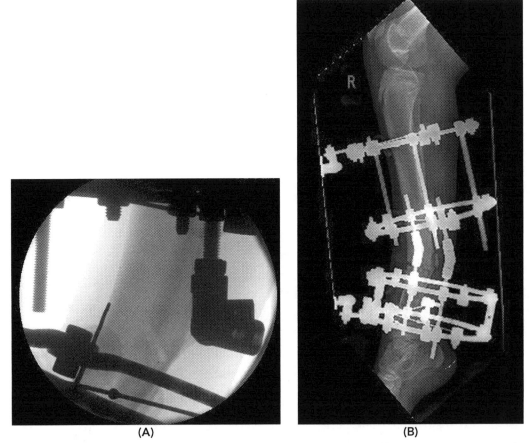

(A)   (B)

Figure 1.2 Hinges were placed just behind the posterior cortex. The osteotomy was made between the two tibial segments.

After a seven-day latency period, correction was commenced with the parents taught to perform a half-turn four times a day on the anterior motor unit.

Stage 2: Application of the Ankle and Forefoot Frame

The tibia straightened after four weeks. The patient was taken back to theatre the following week for a planned revision of the circular fixator for the second stage of treatment. The plantar fascia was divided through the plantar aspect of the foot under tourniquet control. Two olive wires were inserted across the calcaneum and attached and tensioned on a 5/8 ring to create a hindfoot segment. Two additional wires were passed across the distal metatarsals and attached and tensioned on a second 5/8 ring to make the forefoot segment. The hindfoot segment was attached to the distal most tibial ring with hinges medially and laterally in line with the intermalleolar (Inman's) axis. Posteriorly, a universal hinge construct was placed in line with the subtalar axis in the event correction of hindfoot varus was required. This hinge unit was connected to a distraction rod to enable correction of ankle equinus.

The hindfoot segment was attached to the forefoot segment with two motor units to distract the forefoot. The forefoot segment was attached to the tibial segment through two motor units attached to a T-shaped construct made from a long plate and dual-posts. These anterior motor units were to correct forefoot plantarflexion while the posterior motor units corrected the ankle equinus. The T-shaped construct was built far forward anteriorly so as to ensure the vector of force to correct forefoot plantarflexion was applied at a tangent to an arc with its centre of rotation at the intermalleolar axis. This minimised the risk of anterior subluxation of the ankle as correction progressed. Further details on the assembly of this equinovarus correction construct are available (Figure 1.3).[3]

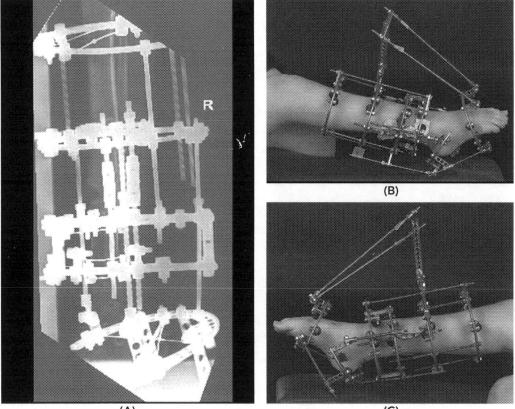

(A)   (B)   (C)

Figure 1.3 X-ray (A) and clinical pictures (B and C) of right lower limb after application of the hindfoot and forefoot rings and before correcting the equinus deformity.

Postoperative Management

The ankle joint was distracted first and the presence of an increased joint space checked on x-ray. This ensured that the cartilage of the talus was not crushed against the tibial plafond in the process of correction (Figure 1.4).

Simultaneous correction of the ankle equinus and forefoot plantarflexion followed, and to this was added some forefoot distraction. A prescription was used to instruct the parents on how to perform the nut turns on the distraction rods and monitor compliance and progress. The rate and rhythm of corrections were titrated depending on the patient's reported tolerance at weekly clinic reviews. X-rays of the tibia were taken intermittently to ensure that the distal tibial epiphysis did not separate from the metaphysis during treatment and that the earlier tibial shaft

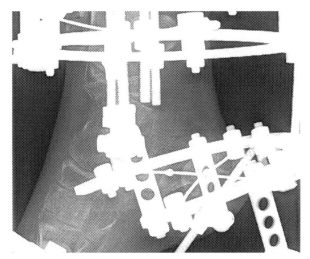

Figure 1.4 X-ray to demonstrate ankle distraction prior to ankle correction.

osteotomy was uniting. Weekly clinic visits for review were arranged to coincide with meticulous pin-site care and regular physiotherapy. Attention was paid to prevent contractures of the toes and knee as correction progressed.[4]

A correction to 10 degrees of dorsiflexion was accomplished with the patient tolerating the process of treatment. A small amount of residual hindfoot varus was also corrected. The improved position was held for four weeks to ensure adaptation of the soft tissues occurred to reduce the risk of relapse. X-rays confirmed that the tibial osteotomy had united before the fixator was removed at just over five months (Figure 1.5).

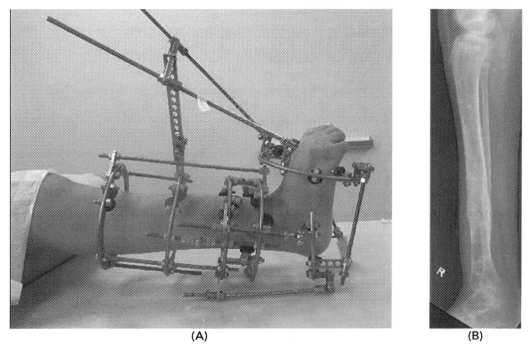

(A)   (B)

Figure 1.5 Clinical picture of the foot position post correction (A), with x-rays (B, C, D) to confirm satisfactory union and alignment of the tibial osteotomy.

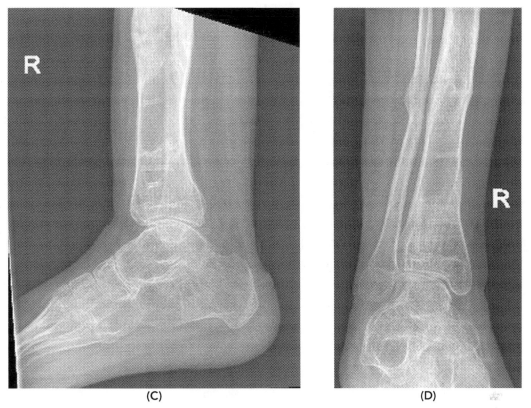

(C)   (D)

Figure 1.5 (Continued)

Under general anaesthesia, the fixator was removed and the foot placed over-corrected in a moulded below-knee cast for four weeks. Neutral ankle-foot orthoses (AFOs) were used in the day to maintain the position, and at night-time, custom-casted AFOs in overcorrection were substituted. Regular physiotherapy was undertaken to re-establish a normal gait and to reactivate tibialis anterior action. After four months, a narrow posterior leaf AFO was made to prevent equinus contracture but allow ankle dorsiflexion during the second rocker. Regular removal was encouraged to allow tibialis anterior activation and range-of-movement rehabilitation.

Prolonged splint usage (for 12 months full-time, and night-time until post-pubertal growth spurt) was recommended after completion of successful treatment. At the final follow-up, the girl had 12mm limb length discrepancy that is well tolerated and is partly compensated for by the use of an AFO. The girl needs to be followed up till she is skeletally mature.

Comment

This case draws two important pointers in CTEV incalcitrant to Ponseti treatment. There can be different reasons for failure in Ponseti treatment, and a return to this may not always be feasible. Classic open surgery with soft tissue releases and tendon lengthenings have a small role to play but must not be repeated if unsuccessful or faced with rapid relapses. The scarring induced through repeated surgery adds stiffness to a recurrent deformity. Gradual correction by Ilizarov treatment is useful for such cases and even for those cases of severe deformities untreated previously but predicted to be cast-resistant.[5]

The second feature is the use of osteotomy to correct for ankle equinus. This is not a good early option for children with resistant equinus (the osteotomy remodels quickly) but may have a role in the skeletally mature. If chosen as a treatment option, the osteotomy is located in the supra-malleolar region with appropriate posterior translation of the distal segment to follow osteotomy principles, Rule 2.

References

1. Firth GB, McMullan M, Chin T, Ma F, Selber P, Eizenberg N, Wolfe R, Graham HK. Lengthening of the gastrocnemius-soleus complex: An anatomical and biomechanical study in human cadavers. *J Bone Joint Surg Am*. 2013 Aug 21;95(16):1489–96. doi: 10.2106/JBJS.K.01638. PMID: 23965699.
2. Malizos KN, Gougoulias NE, Dailiana ZH, Rigopoulos N, Moraitis T. Relapsed clubfoot correction with soft-tissue release and selective application of Ilizarov technique. *Strategies Trauma Limb Reconstr*. 2008 Dec;3(3):109–17. doi: 10.1007/s11751-008-0049-5. Epub 2008 Dec 5. PMID: 19057984; PMCID: PMC2599798.
3. Peterson N, Prior C. Correction of the neglected clubfoot in the adolescent and adult patient. *Foot Ankle Clin*. 2020 Jun;25(2):205–20. doi: 10.1016/j.fcl.2020.02.008. PMID: 32381310.
4. Davies R, Holt N, Nayagam S. The care of pin sites with external fixation. *J Bone Joint Surg Br*. 2005 May;87(5):716–19. doi: 10.1302/0301-620X.87B5.15623. PMID: 15855378.
5. Nunn TR, Etsub M, Tilahun T, Gardner ROE, Allgar V, Wainwright AM, Lavy CBD. Development and validation of a delayed presenting clubfoot score to predict the response to Ponseti casting for children aged 2–10. *Strategies Trauma Limb Reconstr*. 2018;13(3):171–7.

Nicholas Peterson, Christopher Prior, Selvadurai Nayagam

Case

A 14-year-old boy with ataxia telangiectasia (a life-limiting condition associated with sensitivity to radiation)[1] presented with a progressive deformity of the right foot (Figure 2.1). The deformity had deteriorated to the point that it was difficult to accommodate his foot in an ankle-foot orthosis (AFO), rendering the orthosis ineffective in controlling the deformity. The patient used a powered wheelchair for mobility but was able to stand for transfers and use a Kaye walker and walk for therapy. He did not have any pain in the foot.

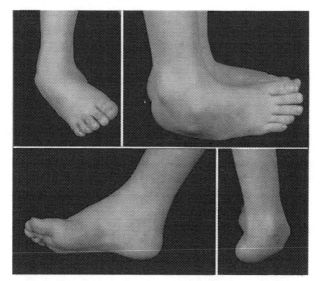

Figure 2.1 The patient's right foot was in a position of severe equinovarus and was only partially correctable.

On examination, he had an equinovarus deformity of the right foot. The ankle was in 15 degrees of plantarflexion with the knee flexed; when checked with the knee in extension, the equinus deformity increased to 30 degrees. Forefoot adduction and hindfoot varus could be only partially corrected passively.

During formal gait analysis and foot assessment, motor power of plantarflexion and inversion was found to be MRC grade 4, whereas dorsiflexion and eversion were MRC grade 3.

Gait analysis with the aid of a Kaye walker showed that initial foot contact on the right side was on the lateral border of the forefoot which then rolled over the ankle for progression.

The boy was keen to have the deformity corrected but was averse to having to use an orthosis.

Questions
- What are the problems related to his right foot that need to be addressed in this boy?
- What are the aims of treatment?
- What are the available options for treatment?
- What are the factors that may influence your choice of treatment?
- What treatment would you recommend for this boy?
- How long would you follow-up this boy after treatment?

The Problems That Need to Be Addressed

- Deformity of the right foot
- Risk of recurrence after treatment due to an incurable, progressive neuromuscular condition

The Aims of Treatment

- Correct the deformity and achieve a pain-free, plantigrade foot
- Minimise the risk of recurrence of the deformity
- Reduce a dependence on orthotics

Options for Treatment

- Correcting the deformity

  o Serial manipulation and casting
  o Soft tissue procedures and orthoses

    □ Soft tissue release
    □ Tendon transfer

  o Gradual correction with circular frame
  o Extra-articular osteotomies (e.g., mid-tarsal osteotomies)
  o Triple arthrodesis

- Minimising risk of recurrence

  o Muscle re-balancing by weakening the invertor and plantarflexor

    □ Tenotomy
    □ Tendon lengthening
    □ Tendon transfer

FACTORS THAT INFLUENCED THE CHOICE OF TREATMENT

- Natural history of the underlying condition
- Severity of the deformity
- The patient's wish to discard orthoses
- Age of the patient

The choice of treatment based on these factors is outlined in Table 2.1.

Table 2.1 Factors That Influenced the Choice of Treatment

Factors		Treatment Implications
Natural history of underlying condition	Progressive disorder	High risk of recurrence of deformity. Even if correction of the deformity is achieved by serial casting or the Ilizarov technique, recurrence is highly probable as the muscle imbalance is not addressed.

(Continued)

Table 2.1 (Continued)

Factors		Treatment Implications
Severity of deformity	Moderately severe deformity that cannot be completely corrected passively	It is unlikely that serial casting would achieve complete correction. Even if the deformity is corrected, an orthosis would need to be worn indefinitely.
The patient's wish to discard orthoses	He was adamant that he did not wish to continue with his AFOs	Treatment that entails the use of orthotics is unacceptable.
Age of the patient	14 years	A triple arthrodesis is considered acceptable at this age as the growth of the foot is almost complete.

How Was the Boy Treated?

Decision-making was influenced by the desire to achieve the stated aims with one operation and limit the need for further surgery in the event of recurrence.[2] In spite of the usual practice of using joint-preserving procedures in Paediatric Orthopaedics, a triple arthrodesis was chosen as complete acute correction of the deformity is possible with this option.[3] Lengthening of the Achilles tendon and the tibialis posterior were chosen as the method of re-balancing muscle forces to reduce the risk of recurrence of deformity. Tendon transfers and tenotomy were not considered as the results of tendon transfers are unpredictable in progressive neurologic conditions and a tenotomy could result in overcorrection if some power is present in the opposing muscle group.

The procedures were performed under general anaesthesia with regional blocks. Through a postero-medial approach, z-lengthening of the Achilles tendon and the tibialis posterior was performed, but the tendons were not sutured at this stage. A modified Ollier's[4] curvilinear incision was used to perform the triple arthrodesis (Figure 2.2). Care was taken to protect the sural and superficial peroneal nerves. The extensor digitorum brevis (EDB) was elevated with sharp dissection from proximal to distal, and the fat was removed from the sinus tarsi (Figure 2.3). The anterior process of the calcaneum was osteotomised (Figure 2.4). The anterior facet of the subtalar joint, head of the talus and the talonavicular joint were identified. An elevator was passed deep to the peroneal tendons and the tendons retracted posteriorly, exposing the capsule over the posterior facet of the subtalar joint. The capsule was removed using a rongeur. The calcaneocuboid joint and the talonavicular joint were exposed and their capsules excised (Figure 2.5).

The articular cartilage of the three joints were denuded to expose bleeding subchondral bone (Figure 2.6). After resecting of appropriate bone wedges, the foot was manipulated to a corrected neutral position. The subtalar joint was fixed with a single 6.5 mm partially threaded cannulated screw inserted through the talar neck. The talonavicular and calcaneocuboid joints were held in the desired position with K-wires temporarily and later fixed definitively with locking plates (Figure 2.7). The Achilles and tibialis posterior tendons were repaired at the appropriate tension using non-absorbable sutures. A plaster back-slab was applied to protect the wounds for the first two weeks.

Post-Operative Management

Weight-bearing was avoided for the first six weeks. An AFO mould was cast at the time of wound review two weeks post-operatively. At six weeks, these new orthoses were used to maintain the correction of equinus and prevent contractures in the tibialis posterior or Achilles tendon during

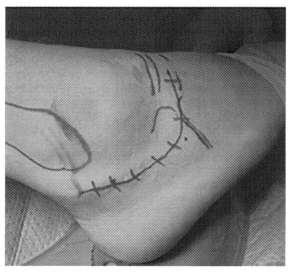

Figure 2.2 The modified Ollier's incision incorporates the middle of the calcaneocuboid joint in order to facilitate plate fixation after joint preparation and coaptation.

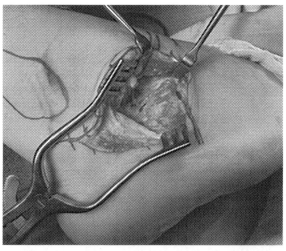

Figure 2.3 The EDB is elevated sharply and lifted anteriorly to expose the sinus tarsi.

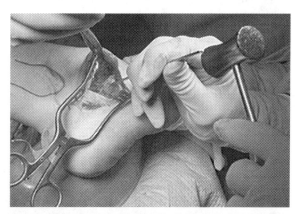

Figure 2.4 The anterior process of the calcaneum is removed to facilitate joint preparation.

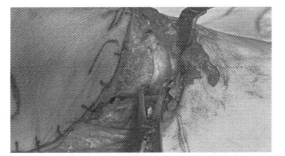

Figure 2.5 The talonavicular joint is prepared by patient and sequential removal of the exposed articular cartilage until, eventually, the medial side of the joint can be visualised.

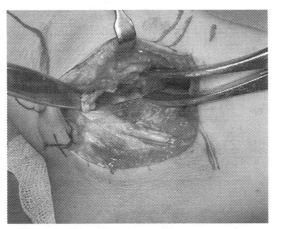

Figure 2.6 The posterior facet of the subtalar joint is exposed and prepared. The flexor hallucis longus tendon can be seen in the depths of the wound on the medial side of the joint, indicating adequate exposure.

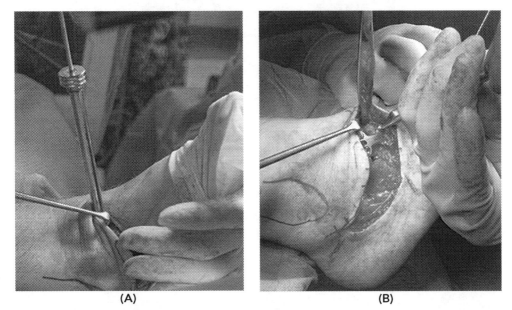

(A)   (B)

Figure 2.7 The corrected position is held using (A) a cannulated screw placed through the dorsal wound which holds the subtalar joint and (B) utility plates across talonavicular and calca-neocuboid joints

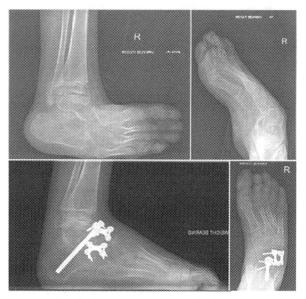

Figure 2.8 The pre-operative and post-operative radiographic appearances are shown.

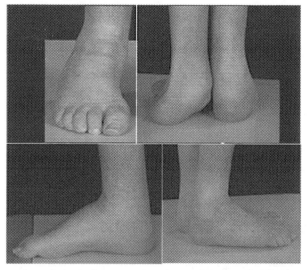

Figure 2.9 Post-operative clinical photographs demonstrating the final corrected position of the right foot.

healing. The AFO was used continually for three months and then recommended for night-time use for another 12 months to avoid a recurrence of deformity.

The pre-operative and current radiographic and clinical images are shown in Figures 2.8 and 2.9.

The patient is able to stand with a plantigrade foot both in and out of his orthoses. He and his family are satisfied that the aims of surgery have been met.

Comment

The triple arthrodesis is often referred to as a salvage procedure. Whilst this is true for most problems of hindfoot and midfoot deformity, it remains an assured method for restoring a well-aligned foot that is stable and pain-free. The boy should be followed up into adulthood to see the long-term effects of arthrodesis.

References

1. van Os NJH, Haaxma CA, van der Flier M, Merkus PJFM, van Deuren M, de Groot IJM, et al. Ataxia-telangiectasia: Recommendations for multidisciplinary treatment. *Dev Med Child Neurol*. 2017 Jul;59(7): 680–9.
2. Lee MC, Sucato DJ. Pediatric Issues with cavovarus foot deformities. *Foot Ankle Clin*. 2008 Jun;13(2): 199–219.
3. Saltzman CL, Fehrle MJ, Cooper RR, Spencer EC, Ponseti IV. Triple arthrodesis: Twenty-five and forty-four-year average follow-up of the same patients. *J Bone Joint Surg Am*. 1999 Oct;81(10):1391–402.
4. Steindler A. A text-book of Operative Orthopedics. *Br J Surg*. 1926 Jan;13(51):594.

Christopher Prior, Nicholas Peterson, Selvadurai Nayagam

Case

A skeletally mature adolescent male was referred with a deformity of the left foot that developed following posteromedial soft tissue release for congenital talipes equinovarus (CTEV) as an infant.

Clinical examination showed excessive dorsiflexion of the ankle joint (Figure 3.1) with no plantarflexion beyond the neutral position of the ankle. He stood with a calcaneus posture of the hindfoot with the forefoot barely able to reach the ground. His gait pattern was distinctly abnormal; in the stance phase, only the first of the three rockers of foot progression (i.e., heel strike) was present. He attempted to achieve foot flat by excessively plantarflexing his toes, and push-off was absent. The power of ankle plantarflexion was Grade 3+ on the MRC scale. The power of all other muscles around the foot and ankle were normal. Lateral weight-bearing radiographs of the foot showed that the calcaneal pitch was abnormally high (43 degrees) and that there was a cavus deformity (Figure 3.2).

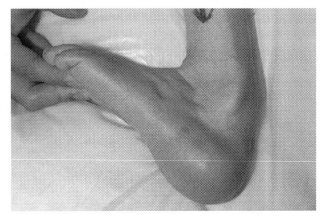

Figure 3.1 Excessive passive dorsiflexion from continued weakness of gastrocnemius-soleus after excessive lengthening of the Achilles tendon in a posteromedial release for CTEV.

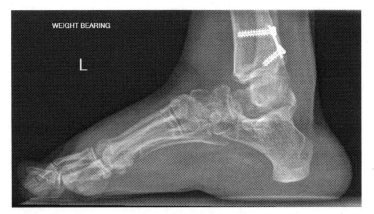

Figure 3.2 The reversed articular slope of the distal tibia achieved by guided growth has failed to reduce the impact of the weak plantarflexion in gait. The os calcis is in calcaneus.

Previous treatment attempted to improve the situation by guided growth. An 8-plate was positioned across the distal tibial physis posteriorly to reverse the sagittal slope of the ankle joint, thereby changing the arc of dorsiflexion and plantarflexion.[1] However, this did not improve the push off significantly although excessive ankle dorsiflexion had been reduced.

Questions

- What are the problems that need to be addressed in this adolescent?
- What are the aims of treatment?
- What are the commonly available options for treatment?
- What are the factors that may influence your choice of treatment?
- What treatment would you recommend for this boy?

The Problems to Be Addressed
- Weakness of ankle plantarflexion
- Calcaneus position of the hindfoot

The Aims of Treatment
- Improve strength of ankle plantarflexion
- Prevent excessive dorsiflexion of the ankle
- Improve calcaneus posture of hindfoot and the cavus

Options for Treatment
- Increasing strength of ankle plantarflexion
  - Tendon transfer
    - Tibialis anterior transfer to Achilles tendon (Peabody)[2]
    - Flexor digitorum longus (FDL) to Achilles tendon
  - Plication of the over-lengthened Achilles tendon
  - Increase the lever arm of the gastroc-soleus by a calcaneal proximal displacement osteotomy
- Preventing excessive dorsiflexion of the ankle
  - Guided growth of distal tibial growth plate
  - Plication of the Achilles tendon
- Improving the calcaneus posture of the hindfoot
  - Calcaneal displacement osteotomy (proximal shift)[3,4]

FACTORS THAT INFLUENCED THE CHOICE OF TREATMENT

- The age of the patient and status of skeletal maturity
- Previous surgery
- Effects of tendon transfer for augmenting the power of plantarflexion
- Effects of calcaneal displacement osteotomy

The choice of treatment based on these factors is shown in Table 3.1.

Table 3.1 Factors Influencing the Choice of Treatment

Factors		Treatment Implications
Age of the patient and the status of skeletal maturation	Skeletally mature adolescent	Options involving modulation of growth are not feasible as the growth plate is fused.
Previous surgery	Guided growth of the distal growth plate	This procedure cannot be repeated as the growth plate is fused.

(Continued)

Table 3.1 (Continued)

Factors		Treatment Implications
Effects of tendon transfer	Tibialis anterior transfer	Transfer of the tibialis anterior will cause the first ray to drop, and this will accentuate the cavus deformity. Furthermore, this is a non-phasic transfer.
	Flexor digitorum longus (FDL) transfer	This is a phasic transfer, but the muscle is not as strong as the tibialis anterior.
Effects of calcaneal displacement osteotomy	Proximal shift of tuberosity of the calcaneum	The osteotomy reduces both the calcaneal pitch and the cavus deformity and increases the lever arm of the gastroc-soleus muscle.

How Was This Boy Treated?

Based on the various factors that needed to be considered, a decision was made to perform a proximal displacement osteotomy of the calcaneum and a plication of the Achilles tendon, and to augment the gastroc-soleus by transferring the FDL to the Achilles tendon. Templates of the hind foot bones were prepared from calibrated lateral x-ray images, and simulations of the planned osteotomy were done (Figure 3.3a, 3.3b).

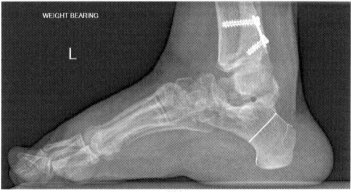

(A)

Figure 3.3a–3.3b Analysis of the deformity and correction using software-based image manipulation allows simulation to guide surgery. Here an oblique osteotomy through the os calcis would need to be rotated through an axis of rotation based around the centre of the ankle to reposition the arc of dorsiflexion-plantarflexion. The simulation indicates proximal shift and angulation would achieve the desired effect.

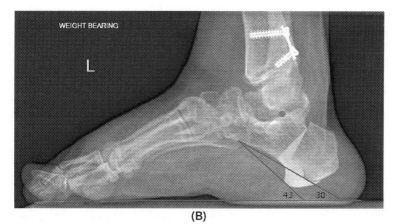

(B)

Figure 3.3a–3.3b (Continued)

Through a postero-lateral incision parallel to the lateral border of the Achilles tendon, the sural nerve and short saphenous vein were protected, and a Z-plasty of the Achilles tendon was performed. The interval between peroneus longus and flexor hallucis longus (FHL) was developed, and the FHL and the posterior tibial neurovascular bundle were retracted medially, exposing the posterior ankle, subtalar joint and dorsal surface of the calcaneum (Figure 3.4a). K-wires were inserted into the calcaneum under x-ray guidance—to define a closing wedge with its base on the dorsal surface of the calcaneum (Figure 3.4b). The size of this wedge was determined from the pre-operative simulations shown in Figures 3.3a and 3.3b. The wedge was excised using broad osteotomes following the guide wires (Figures 3.4c, 3.4d). The wedge of bone was removed and the osteotomy closed, and the tuberosity was shifted proximally to improve the calcaneal pitch further. The osteotomy was fixed with cannulated lag screws and two-hole plates applied across the osteotomy (Figures 3.4e, 3.4f).

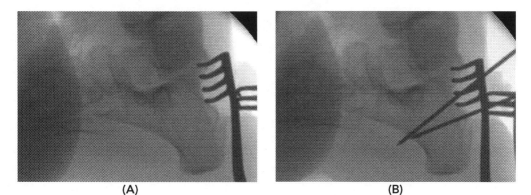

(A)	(B)

Figures 3.4a–3.4f A sequence of intraoperative x-ray images showing how the size of wedge—as determined through preoperative planning and simulation of correction—is created at surgery and removed and the osteotomised fragment shifted proximally before internal fixation with a pair of two-hole plates and screws.

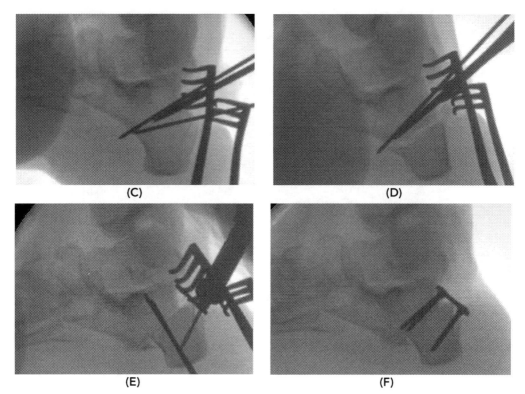

(C)

(D)

(E)

(F)

Figures 3.4a–3.4f (Continued)

The FDL tendon was harvested with the ankle plantarflexed to allow a generous length to be retrieved. The tendon was sectioned as far distally as possible, and the distal stump was attached to the FHL. The ankle was then held in a position of about 15 degrees of plantarflexion, and the Z-plasty of the Achilles tendon was repaired under tension in this position so as to achieve some shortening of the tendon. The shortened Achilles tendon was augmented by weaving the proximal stump of the FDL through the Achilles tendon under tension. The tourniquet was deflated and haemostasis assured prior to wound closure. A below-knee plaster slab was applied to hold the ankle in plantarflexion.

Post-Operative Management

A scheduled wound check at around two weeks was followed with a change of the plaster slab support to a full cast holding the ankle at 15 degrees plantarflexion. The cast was removed at eight weeks and a hinged ankle foot orthosis (AFO) set in plantarflexion was used for a further four weeks. Physiotherapy sessions to reinforce active plantarflexion activity were begun, and dorsiflexion beyond neutral was prevented. The AFO was set to plantigrade at 12 weeks, and physiotherapy continued for active strengthening of the gastrocnemius and soleus muscles (Figure 3.5). The AFO was discontinued at six months.

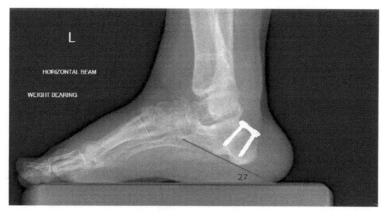

Figure 3.5 The post-operative weight-bearing lateral x-ray with an improved calcaneal pitch and reduction of the high-arched foot deformity. The patient's gait had also improved.

An inspection of gait at the final follow-up revealed the second rocker of foot progression (stance phase) had been restored. There was an improved push-off, although it was still evident that the patient was using his toes to assist in this action. Formal assessment of the gastroc-soleus action showed power at MRC grade 4. The appearance of the foot when standing had improved markedly (Figure 3.2, Figure 3.5), and the overall clinical result was pleasing to both the patient and his parents.

Comment

Different techniques of calcaneal osteotomy to reduce calcaneal pitch have been described.[3,4] The authors use an osteotomy and displacement method that attempts to achieve deformity correction around a CORA that is the centre of rotation of the ankle. The simulations in Figures 3.3a and 3.3b show that for this correction to be achieved, a proximal displacement and angulation of the calcaneal tuberosity fragment is needed. This was replicated during surgery but using a closing wedge method instead of opening wedge.

References

1. Sinha A, Selvan D, Sinha A, James LA. Guided growth of the distal posterior tibial physis and short term results: A potential treatment option for children with calcaneus deformity. *J Pediatr Orthop.* 2016;36(1):84–8.
2. Peabody CW. Tendon transposition: An end result study. *Journal of Bone & Joint Surgery—American Volume.* 1938;20(1):193–205.
3. Hansen ST. Osteotomy techniques. In: Hansen ST, editor. *Functional reconstruction of the foot and ankle.* Philadelphia: Lippincott Williams & Wilkins; 2000. pp. 372–3.
4. Samilson RL, Dillin W. Cavus, cavovarus, and calcaneocavus: An update. *Clin Orthop Relat Res.* 1983(177):125–32.

CASE 4: CAVOVARUS DEFORMITY

David A Spiegel

Case

A 13-year-old female with a history of Charcot-Marie-Tooth 1a secondary to *PMP22* duplication presented for the evaluation of her feet.

She had bilateral progressive foot deformities, more severe on the left. She had been treated with physical therapy, stretching and serial casting and had worn shoe inserts in the past but refused to wear an AFO. She had been able to run and jump in the past, although her participation in sports had been limited in comparison to her peers. Recently her function had deteriorated and the deformity worsened on the left side. She frequently tripped and fell. She complained of pain on the lateral side of her ankles and medially near the origin of the plantar fascia. She also complained that she was easily fatigued and that she had trouble with clearing her left foot when she walked.

On clinical examination, she had bilateral cavovarus deformities; the left side was considerably more severe than the right (Figure 4.1a–c). Her right foot dorsiflexed 10° beyond neutral while the left side dorsiflexed only to neutral. The power of dorsiflexion and eversion on the right was Grade 4 (MRC Grade) and Grade 4 on the left. Her tibialis posterior was Grade 4. She had decreased sensation to vibration and pinprick extending up to the middle of her leg. There was fixed plantar flexion of the left first metatarsal with contracture of the plantar fascia. On the right side her plantar fascia was also tight, though the cavus was passively correctable. Her heel could be moved into 5° of valgus on the prone hind-foot flexibility test on the left. She ambulated independently with a mild foot drop on the left, and her left foot remained supinated in both swing and stance phases. Weight-bearing radiographs were obtained (Figure 4.2a, b), and the alignment was consistent with the typical changes seen in a cavovarus foot.[1]

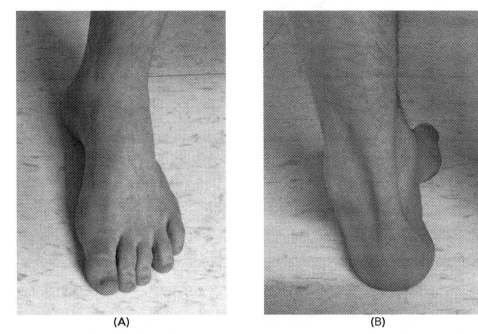

(A) (B)

Figure 4.1a–c Clinical photos of the left cavovarus foot.

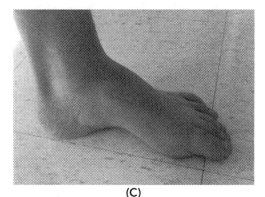

(C)

Figure 4.1a–c (Continued)

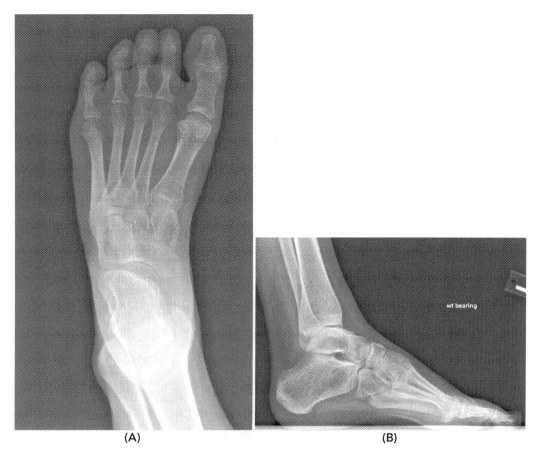

(A)   (B)

Figure 4.2a, b On the standing AP radiograph, there is a parallel relationship between the long axes of the talus and the calcaneus consistent with hindfoot varus. "Over-reduction" of the navicular on the talar head (talo-navicular coverage angle 26°) is present. The first metatarsal is adducted relative to the talus (AP talo-first metatarsal angle: −30°; normal range: +10 to −7°). Recognizing that the tibia is not completely vertical on the weight-bearing lateral radiograph, there is plantarflexion of the first metatarsal with talo-first metatarsal angle (Meary angle) of 26°. Both the tibio-calcaneal angle (76°) and the calcaneal pitch angle (28°) are within normal ranges, suggesting that the ankle is not in equinus.

Questions

- What are the problems that need to be addressed?
- What are the aims of treatment?
- What are the commonly available options for treatment?
- What are the factors that may influence your choice of treatment?
- What treatment would you recommend for this girl?
- How long would you follow-up this girl after treatment?

The Problems That Need to Be Addressed with Reference to the Left Foot Are

- Progressive deformity of the foot
- Foot pain
- Poor foot clearance during swing phase due to weakness of pretibial muscles
- Poor stability in stance phase due to muscle imbalance and fixed skeletal deformity

The Aims of Treatment in This Girl Are to

- Correct deformity and achieve a plantigrade foot
- Balance muscle forces around the ankle and foot
- Relieve pain
- Enable ambulation without the need for an orthosis, if possible

Options for Treatment

Since all non-operative measures have been tried in this girl, surgical options only were considered.

- Options for correcting the deformity and achieving a plantigrade foot
  - Soft tissue release/lengthening of structures contributing to the deformity[2-7]
    - Tendon release/lengthening or transfer
      - Heel cord lengthening
      - Tibialis posterior release/transfer
      - Peroneus longus release/transfer
    - Plantar fascia release
  - Osteotomies[8,9]
    - Extension osteotomy of the medial column
      - Basal metatarsal osteotomy
      - Cuneiform osteotomy
    - Mid-tarsal osteotomy
    - Calcaneal osteotomy
  - Arthrodesis[10]
    - Triple arthrodesis
- Options for rebalancing muscle forces around the ankle and foot[2-7]
  - Tibialis posterior transfer to the dorsum of the foot lateral to the axis of the subtalar joint
  - Peroneus longus transfer to the peroneus brevis

FACTORS THAT INFLUENCED THE CHOICE OF TREATMENT

- Age of the child
- Severity of symptoms
- Severity and flexibility of the deformity
- Power of muscles acting on the ankle and foot

The factors taken into consideration in the choice of treatment are shown in Table 4.1.

Table 4.1 Factors Affecting the Choice of Treatment

Factors		Treatment Implications
Age of the child	13 years	Deformities in the younger child are supple to begin with; by the age of 13 the deformities tend to become more rigid.
Severity of symptoms	The girl has significant symptoms related to her feet that are affecting her gait	Surgical intervention to alleviate her symptoms is indicated as non-operative measures have failed.
Severity and flexibility of each deformity	Cavus deformity is only partially correctable	Release of the plantar fascia alone may not suffice; an osteotomy to dorsiflex the first ray or the forefoot may be required.
	Forefoot deformity primarily involves the first ray which is plantarflexed; the lateral rays are not affected	If an osteotomy is considered necessary after release of the plantar fascia, it may be limited to the first ray.
	Hindfoot varus is supple and can be passively corrected	Correction of the forefoot pronation and release of the tibialis posterior is likely to improve the hindfoot varus without having to resort to a calcaneal osteotomy.
Power of muscles acting on the foot and ankle	Ankle dorsiflexors: Tibialis anterior—Grade 3 (L), Grade 4 (R) Toe dorsiflexors—Grade 3 (L), 4 (R) Ankle plantarflexor: Gastroc-soleus—Grade 5	Ankle dorsiflexors power needs to be augmented by a tendon transfer to improve foot clearance in the swing phase. Improving the muscle balance at the ankle can reduce the chances of an equinus deformity developing.
	Invertors: Tibialis posterior—Grade 4 Tibialis anterior—Grade 3 Evertors: Peroneus longus—Grade 4 Peroneus brevis—Grade 3	Ideally, tendons of muscles with Grade 5 power only should be considered for transfer if the aim is to restore function. However, muscles with Grade 4 power may be transferred to improve muscle balance to correct deformity and to minimise chances of recurrence of deformity by removing a deforming force.[2-7] Thus, tibialis posterior may be transferred to correct the hindfoot varus and improve muscle balance at the subtalar joint, and peroneus longus may be transferred to correct the first metatarsal drop and restore muscle balance at the first ray.

Since cavovarus deformity develops due to an underlying neurologic condition in the vast majority of instances, it is important that the diagnosis is made before embarking on treatment of the deformity. The diagnoses include those involving the central nervous system (cerebral palsy, traumatic brain injury, Friedrich's ataxia), spinal cord (polio, tethered cord, myelodysplasia), or peripheral nervous system (hereditary motor and sensory neuropathy).[2,3] Less common causes may include residual clubfoot deformity, post-traumatic deformity (compartment syndrome, pilon or talar neck fractures), and idiopathic.[2,3] The commonest cause is a hereditary sensory and motor neuropathy (HSMN), especially Charcot-Marie-Tooth disease (CMT), as in this girl.

Treatment strategies and the anticipated outcomes should be based on the natural history of the underlying disease (static versus progressive). Since in this child the natural history is one of progression, we cautioned her and her parents that it is possible that the intervention may not relieve her pain completely, that she might need to use orthoses in the future to address muscle weakness or relapse of her deformity due to her progressive weakness and that further surgical intervention might be required in the future.

How Was This Child Treated?

The patient underwent a left plantar fascia release, followed by a dorsiflexion osteotomy of the base of the first metatarsal, transfer of the peroneus longus to the peroneus brevis, and transfer of the tibialis posterior to the lateral cuneiform. Intra-operatively, she achieved 10° of passive ankle dorsiflexion, and a simulated weight-bearing view continued to demonstrate a normal tibio-calcaneal angle and a normal calcaneal pitch angle, so lengthening of the gastroc-soleus was not required. The peroneus longus was transected at the level of the distal calcaneus and attached to the peroneus brevis using a Pulvertaft weave. An interference screw was used for fixation of the transferred tibialis posterior tendon. Though the right foot was asymptomatic, we performed a plantar fascia release.

Post-Operative Management

The patient was placed in a weight-bearing short leg cast on the right side, and on the left a short leg splint to allow for swelling. A short-leg cast was placed on post-operative day 10. At six weeks, she was transitioned to an AFO and was started on physical therapy. The right side was placed in a CAM boot, and she was allowed to bear weight as tolerated.

At three months, she was ambulating in her AFO without discomfort, and her goal was to develop sufficient strength to become brace-free (Figure 4.3). While her hindfoot did tilt into some valgus on the hindfoot flexibility test, she had a few degrees of residual varus when

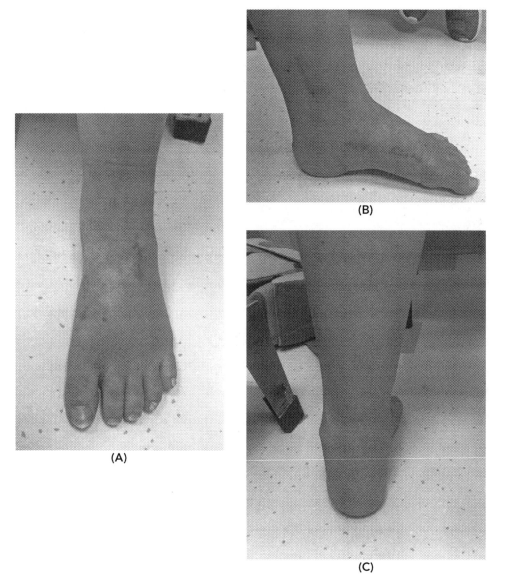

Figure 4.3a–c Standing post-operative images of the left foot from the front (A), side (B) and back (c).

standing which will need to be followed; she may potentially benefit from a calcaneal osteotomy if this does not remain stable.

Comment

The principles of surgical treatment of cavovarus are:

- to restore range of motion through soft tissue release and osteotomy,
- to balance muscle forces by tendon transfer.

Arthrodesis a salvage procedure for severe, rigid deformities and arthritic changes. The menu of surgical options is extensive and must be tailored to the individual patient. The optimal timing of surgery has yet to be established, and it seems reasonable to take a reactive stance and treat only those with persistent symptoms or functional problems despite non-operative measures, though some may argue that early soft tissue interventions may possibly delay or alleviate the need for more extensive procedures such as triple arthrodesis later on.

References

1. Davids JR, Gibson TW, Pugh LI. Quantitative segmental analysis of weight-bearing radiographs of the foot and ankle for children: Normal alignment. *J Pediatr Ortho.* 2005;25:769–76.
2. Ziebarth K, Krause F. Updates in pediatric cavovarus deformity. *Foot Ankle Clin.* 2019;24:205–17.
3. Georgiadis AG, Spiegel DA, Baldwin KD. The cavovarus foot in hereditary motor and sensory neuropathies. *JBJS Rev.* 2015;3:01874474-201512000-00003.
4. Pfeffer GB, Gonzalez T, Brodsky J, Campbell J, Coetzee C, Conti S, Guyton G, Herrmann DN, Hunt K, Johnson J, McGarvey W, Pinzur M, Raikin S, Sangeorzan B, Younger A, Michalski M, An T, Noori N. A consensus statement on the surgical treatment of Charcot-Marie-Tooth disease. *Foot Ankle Int.* 2020;41:870–80.
5. Ward CM, Dolan LA, Bennett DL, Morcuende JA, Cooper RR. Long-term results of reconstruction for treatment of a flexible cavovarus foot in Charcot-Marie-Tooth disease. *J Bone Joint Surg Am.* 2008;90:2631–4262.
6. Dreher T, Wolf SI, Heitzmann D, Fremd C, Klotz MC, Wenz W. Tibialis posterior tendon transfer corrects the foot drop component of cavovarus foot deformity in Charcot-Marie-Tooth disease. *J Bone Joint Surg Am.* 2014;96:456–62.
7. Ortiz C, Wagner E. Tendon transfers in cavovarus foot. *Foot Ankle Clin.* 2014;19:49–58.
8. Mubarak SJ, Van Valin SE. Osteotomies of the foot for cavus deformities in children. *J Pediatr Orthop.* 2009;29:294–99.
9. Wicart P, Seringe R. Plantar opening-wedge osteotomy of cuneiform bones combined with selective plantar release and Dwyer osteotomy for pes cavovarus in children. *J Pediatr Orthop.* 2006;26:100–8.
10. Wetmore RS, Drennan JC. Long-term results of triple arthrodesis in Charcot-Marie-Tooth disease. *J Bone Joint Surg Am.* 1989;71:417–22.

Christopher Prior, Nicholas Peterson, Selvadurai Nayagam

Case

A 6-week-old boy presented with congenital rocker-bottom deformities of both feet. He was otherwise a healthy baby born at full term after an uncomplicated pregnancy and a birth weight of 3.35 kg. On examination, both hindfeet were in fixed equinovalgus. The forefeet were dorsiflexed and abducted (Figure 5.1). The head of the talus was palpable in the plantar aspect of both feet. The upper limbs, knees, hips and spine were normal with no features of arthrogryposis or spinal dysraphism. There was no facial dysmorphism suggesting that this was part of a syndrome and genetic analysis excluded chromosomal abnormalities associated with this deformity. An ultrasound showed normal hips.

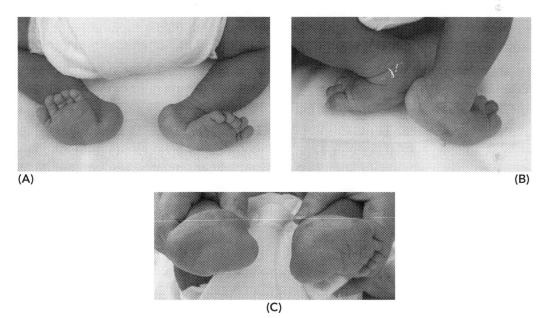

(A)
(B)
(C)

Figure 5.1 Clinical pictures of bilateral foot deformities in an infant. The forefeet are so abducted that when the baby is prone (A) the feet appear to be pointing backwards.

A lateral radiograph of the foot in maximum plantarflexion revealed that the forefoot was unable to plantarflex owing to irreducible subluxation at the talonavicular joint. The talus was severely plantarflexed, and its long axis was not colinear to the axis of the first metatarsal (Figure 5.2), distinguishing congenital rocker bottom deformity or congenital vertical talus (CVT) from a positional calcaneovalgus deformity and severe planovalgus.

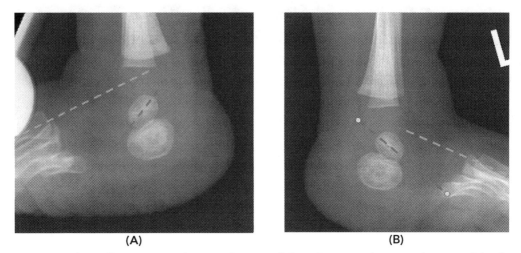

(A) (B)

Figure 5.2 Plantarflexion views showing the axis of the talus not colinear to the axis of the first metatarsal.

Questions

- What are the problems that need to be addressed in this infant?
- What are the aims of treatment?
- What are the commonly available options for treatment?
- What are the factors that may influence your choice of treatment?
- What treatment would you recommend for this infant?
- How long would you follow-up this child after completion of treatment?

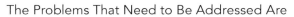

The Problems That Need to Be Addressed Are

- Complex deformity involving the forefoot and the hindfoot

  o Ankle equinus
  o Hindfoot valgus
  o Forefoot dorsiflexion
  o Forefoot abduction
  o Talo-navicular dislocation

- Soft tissue contractures

  o Joint capsules and ligaments

    □ Ankle joint—posterior capsule
    □ Talo-navicular joint—dorsal capsule

  o Tendons

    □ Achilles tendon
    □ Tibialis anterior
    □ Extensor digitorum & extensor hallucis
    □ Peroneus longus and brevis

The Aims of Treatment Are to

- Establish a pain-free, mobile, plantigrade foot by

  o Reducing the talonavicular joint
  o Correcting the forefoot deformity
  o Correcting the hindfoot deformity

- Prevent recurrence of deformity

Options of Treatment to Fulfil Each Aim

Reducing the talonavicular joint and correcting hindfoot and forefoot deformities

- Serial manipulation and casting
- Serial manipulation and minimally invasive surgery
- Open reduction of talonavicular dislocation and soft tissue release
- Open reduction of talonavicular dislocation and soft tissue release with tendon transfers
- Salvage surgery

  o Navicular excision
  o Subtalar fusion

Preventing recurrence of deformity

- Bracing
- Tendon transfer (Tibialis anterior to the neck of the talus)

FACTORS THAT INFLUENCED THE CHOICE OF TREATMENT

- Age of the child
- Underlying condition
- Risk of stiffness of the foot
- Response to treatment

The choice of treatment based on the factors that influenced treatment are outlined in Table 5.1.

Table 5.1 Factors Influencing the Choice of Treatment

Factors		Treatment Implications
Age of the child	Infant	The chances of achieving correction by serial manipulation and casting are best in the young infant.[1,2] Salvage surgeries such as navicular excision and joint fusion are only resorted to in older children.
Underlying condition	Idiopathic CVT	The chances of achieving correction by serial manipulation and casting are best in children who do not have arthrogryposis or spina bifida.
Risk of stiffness following treatment	Soft tissue release	Treatment by extensive open soft tissue releases and open reduction of the dislocation is often associated with skin healing issues and stiffness of the foot.[3]
Response to treatment	Good response to serial manipulation	In an infant, treatment should begin with serial manipulation. If satisfactory correction of all components of the deformity is achieved, no further intervention apart from maintaining the correction is warranted.
	Partial correction of deformity with serial manipulation	Limited soft tissue release with talonavicular joint reduction is justified.
	Poor response to serial manipulation	More extensive soft tissue release and talonavicular joint reduction may be required.
	Recurrence of deformity following satisfactory correction	Tibialis anterior tendon transfer to the neck of talus is a good option.
	Recalcitrant deformity in the older child	Salvage procedures are to be considered only if prior treatment attempts are unsuccessful and the child is old enough.

How Was This Child Treated?

Social circumstances surrounding the child incurred a delay in treatment. Consequently, serial manipulations and casting were carried out in the clinic on both feet simultaneously at the age of 8 months.

The first step was to bring the forefoot into plantar flexion and inversion while maintaining the position of the talus with pressure from the plantar aspect of the foot. The foot position was maintained in an above-knee cast. The manipulations were repeated every week. An x-ray was taken at five weeks to ensure the alignment of the talonavicular joint (as seen from the axis of the talus and first metatarsal—Figure 5.3) was satisfactory.[4,5]

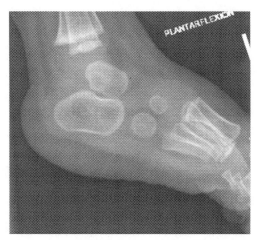

Figure 5.3 Lateral plantarflexion view of the left foot taken five weeks after serial manipulation and casting.

When the alignment was confirmed, the final cast was removed a week later under general anaesthesia and the talonavicular fixation performed. The right foot was found to be stiffer and required an open reduction of the talonavicular joint. A 2 cm incision was made over the joint medially; a capsulotomy was performed and the joint visualised. The subtalar joint was freed partly by dissection to allow the talus to be elevated and thus the talonavicular joint reduced. The reduction was held with a 2 mm Kirschner wire passed retrograde. On the left side, a small incision exposing the joint confirmed a satisfactory reduction, and this was then held with a 2 mm wire (Figure 5.4). Both sides had a percutaneous Achilles tenotomy to allow correction of the hindfoot equinus. After closure of wounds, above-knee plaster-of-Paris casts were applied with the foot in neutral and the ankle in 5 degrees of dorsiflexion.

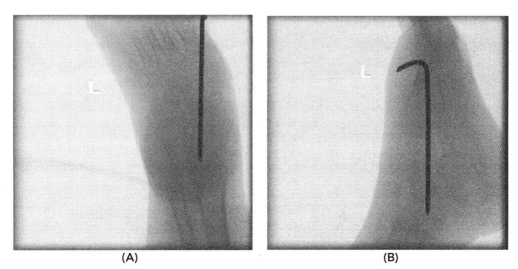

(A)   (B)

Figure 5.4 Intraoperative fluoroscopy showing reduction and K-wiring of the talonavicular joint of the left foot.

Post-Operative Management

The wires were removed in the clinic at five weeks and new casts applied for a further two weeks in a more dorsiflexed position at the ankle. The baby was then fitted with a 'boots and bars' bracing system to keep the feet pointing forwards. This was worn for 23 hours a day for the first three months, and thereafter only during sleep until the age of 18 months. A solid AFO was made then to hold the forefoot in 30 degrees of plantarflexion. The parents were encouraged to perform regular stretches of the forefoot. At 17 months, the child was walking with pain-free plantigrade feet (Figure 5.5). Follow-up for recurrence of contractures and muscle imbalance will continue until skeletal maturity.

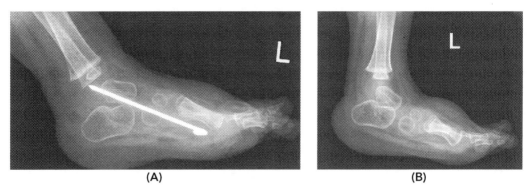

(A)   (B)

Figure 5.5 Lateral radiographs taken (A) five weeks post-procedure and (B) three months post-procedure demonstrating satisfactory alignment of the axis of the talus and the first ray.

Comment

The Dobbs method of treating congenital vertical talus has evolved to become a first-line treatment. It is minimally invasive, induces little scarring but requires careful interpretation of serial x-rays to know if the technique is achieving the desired effect of reducing the talonavicular dislocation.[5] Relapse continues to be a significant problem, and follow-up studies to skeletal maturity have yet to be published.[1,6]

References

1. Yang JS, Dobbs MB. Treatment of congenital vertical talus: Comparison of minimally invasive and extensive soft-tissue release procedures at minimum five-year follow-up. *J Bone Joint Surg Am.* 2015;97(16):1354–65.
2. Chan Y, Selvaratnam V, Garg N. A comparison of the Dobbs method for correction of idiopathic and teratological congenital vertical talus. *J Child Orthop.* 2016;10(2):93–9.
3. Ramanoudjame M, Loriaut P, Seringe R, Glorion C, Wicart P. The surgical treatment of children with congenital convex foot (vertical talus): Evaluation of midtarsal surgical release and open reduction. *The Bone & Joint Journal.* 2014;96-b(6):837–44.
4. Merrill LJ, Gurnett CA, Connolly AM, Pestronk A, Dobbs MB. Skeletal muscle abnormalities and genetic factors related to vertical talus. *Clin Orthop Relat Res.* 2011;469(4):1167–74.
5. Eberhardt O, Fernandez FF, Wirth T. The talar axis-first metatarsal base angle in CVT treatment: A comparison of idiopathic and non-idiopathic cases treated with the Dobbs method. *J Child Orthop.* 2012;6(6):491–6.
6. Wright J, Coggings D, Maizen C, Ramachandran M. Reverse Ponseti-type treatment for children with congenital vertical talus: Comparison between idiopathic and teratological patients. *The Bone & Joint Journal.* 2014;96-b(2):274–8.

CASE 6: PLANOVALGUS DEFORMITY

Leo Donnan

Case

A 12-year-old boy presented with increasing symmetric deformities of both feet. He complained of an ache along the medial aspect of his feet which was related to physical activity. The pain in his feet was severe enough to make him withdraw from playing sport. His parents also noted that his shoes were getting wrecked in a very short period.

When viewed from behind while standing, the "too many toes sign" (Figure 6.1a) was positive (lateral four toes were visible). He walked awkwardly with an external foot progression angle of 25 degrees, complete collapse of the medial arch (Figure 6.1b) with significant hind foot valgus, forefoot abduction and a poor push-off.

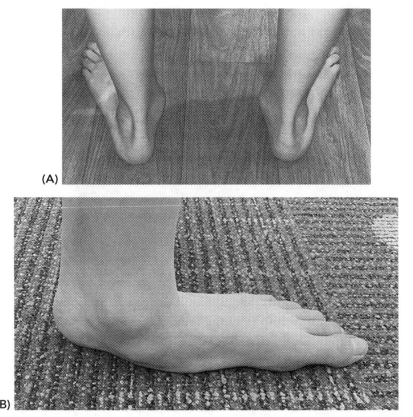

Figure 6.1 Appearance of the feet while weight-bearing. Forefoot abduction with a positive "too many toes sign" (A) and complete collapse of the medial arch (B) are clearly seen.

Passive elevation of the great toe did not restore the medial longitudinal arch, but on tip-toe standing the contour of the arch did improve and the heel valgus came to neutral but not into varus. The gastrocnemius and soleus were contracted. The forefoot was supinated, and when the hind foot was stabilised in the neutral position the first ray was grossly elevated. The power of plantarflexion was Grade 4 (MRC grade). He had moderate generalised ligament laxity. The ranges of motion of the subtalar and mid-tarsal joints were limited by the respective deformities, but there was no pain on passive movement.

Weight-bearing anteroposterior and lateral radiographs of the feet confirmed the forefoot abduction with uncovering of the medial part of the talar head[1] (Figure 6.2a), the collapsed arch with reduction of the calcaneal pitch and plantarflexion of the talus (Figure 6.2b). There were no arthritic changes in the subtalar and mid-tarsal joints.

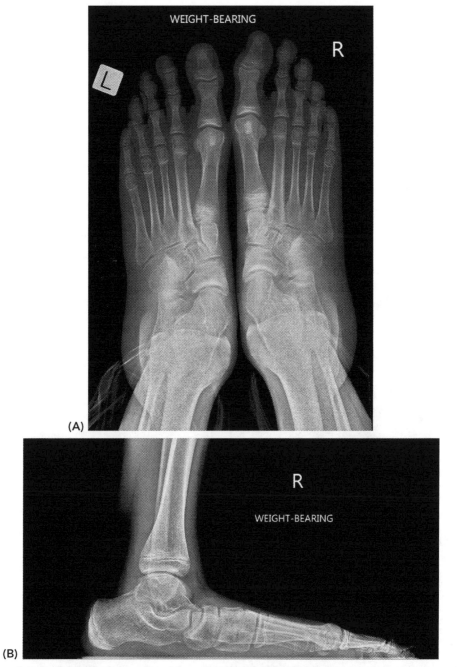

Figure 6.2 Standing radiographs of feet showing forefoot abduction with uncovering of talar head (A) and reduced calcaneal pitch with plantar flexion of talus (B).

Questions

- What are the problems that need to be addressed in this boy?
- What are the aims of treatment?
- What are the available treatment options to fulfil these aims?
- What are the factors that may influence your choice of treatment?
- Based on these points, what treatment would you recommend for this child?
- How long would you follow-up this boy after treatment?

The Problems That Need to Be Addressed Are

- Progressive hind foot valgus, forefoot abduction and collapse of the medial longitudinal arch
- External rotation of the foot and lever arm dysfunction with weak push-off
- Pain in the foot

The Aims of Treatment in This Boy Are to

- Correct the hind foot valgus and forefoot abduction
- Restore the normal medial longitudinal arch
- Improve the gait pattern
- Relieve foot pain and improve shoe wear

Options for Treatment

- Correcting the hind foot valgus

    - Medial displacement calcaneal osteotomy[2]
    - Calcaneo-stop procedure (arthroereisis)[3]
    - Subtalar fusion and triple fusion

- Correcting forefoot abduction

    - Lateral column lengthening

        - Calcaneal lengthening (opening wedge)[4]
        - Cuboid osteotomy (opening wedge)

    - Medial column shortening

        - Medial cuneiform osteotomy (closing wedge)

- Restoring the medial longitudinal arch

    - Orthotic management
    - Reefing the spring ligament and the tibialis posterior along with the bony surgery (soft tissue procedures alone have no role in the management of the planovalgus foot deformity)
    - Lengthening the triceps surae
    - Plantar flexion of first ray
    - Correcting the hindfoot valgus and forefoot abduction as outlined previously

- Improving the gait pattern

    - Correct the out-toeing gait
    - Improve the lever arm of the triceps surae and improve the push-off

        - Correct the hind foot valgus
        - Increase ankle range of motion

- Relieving pain and reduce wearing down of shoes by correcting the deformity

FACTORS THAT INFLUENCED THE CHOICE OF TREATMENT

- The presence of pain
- The age of the boy
- The severity of the deformity
- Presence of ligament laxity
- Presence of arthritic changes

The choice of treatment based on these factors is outlined in Table 6.1.

Table 6.1 Factors that influenced the choice of treatment

Factors		Treatment Implications
Presence of pain in the feet	Pain severe enough to be forced to limit physical activity	This justifies intervention (asymptomatic planovalgus often does not require any treatment).
Age of the boy	12 years	No scope for spontaneous resolution (planovalgus deformity may resolve in young children).
Severity and rigidity of the deformity	The planovalgus deformity is severe	Treatment in an orthosis is not justified (may be considered in mild cases).
	The deformity is moderately rigid—the hind foot valgus can be passively corrected only to the neutral position	Release of contracted triceps surae is indicated to facilitate correction of the hind foot valgus.
		Calcaneo-stop procedure or arthroereisis is more suited for a flexible foot.
Presence of generalised ligament laxity	Moderate laxity present	Relying on soft tissue surgery alone is inappropriate as the propensity for recurrence is very high.
Presence of arthritic changes	No clinical or radiologic features of arthritis	Options that avoid stiffening of joints are preferred in the absence of arthritis (no justification for performing subtalar or triple arthrodesis).

Mild deformities, without a significant calf contracture, can be managed with an appropriate orthosis or the calcaneo-stop procedure, which is a form of arthroereisis that helps correct the hind foot valgus. More significant deformities, as in this boy, require bony correction to restore the normal alignment of the foot. The spring ligament and the tibialis posterior that have been excessively stretched need to be plicated, and the contracted triceps surae must be lengthened. Those with significant secondary joint changes may need a triple fusion.

The final options for bony surgery in this boy include:

- Calcaneal displacement osteotomy
- Lateral column lengthening
- Medial column shortening

How Was This Child Treated?

A calcaneal lengthening osteotomy, with K-wire stabilisation of calcaneocuboid joint, was performed to correct the talar plantar flexion and forefoot abduction (Figure 6.3a and b). The spring ligament was plicated and tibialis posterior tendon advanced to correct the medial laxity (Figure 6.4a, 6.4b). A dorsal opening wedge osteotomy of the medial cuneiform (Cotton) corrected the abnormal dorsiflexion of the first ray and finally, the calf contracture was released by performing lengthening in Zone 1 (Strayers).

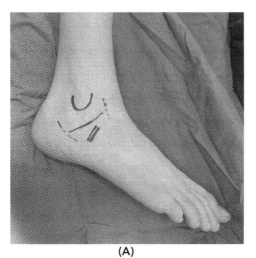

(A)

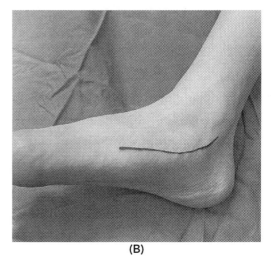

(B)

Figure 6.3 Marking of surgical incisions.

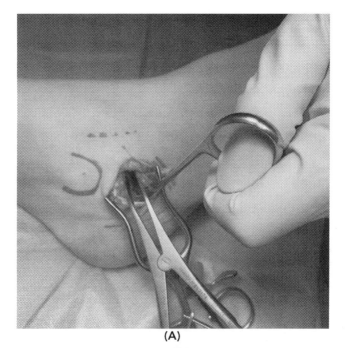

(A)

Figure 6.4 Calcaneal lengthening and medial capsular plication with tibialis posterior re-tensioning.

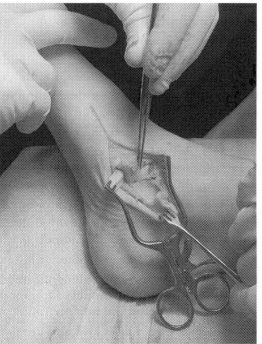

(B)

Figure 6.4 (Continued)

Lateral column lengthening provides a powerful correction at the site of deformity (calcane-opedal unit) whilst maintaining foot mobility and suppleness. Healing is rapid with few complications, returning patients to independent ambulation expediently.

In this case, small titanium implants were used to illustrate positioning. In most cases, autograft is completely satisfactory.

Post-Operative Management

A well-padded, split below-knee cast was applied and retained for six weeks with a cast change at two weeks for wound check and to permit K-wire removal. Weight-bearing was avoided till the cast was removed and check radiographs showed adequate healing of the osteotomies.

Moulded insoles for the shoes were used to support the corrected foot posture, and exercises to strengthen the tibialis posterior and calf muscles were begun.

Follow-Up

At six months after surgery, the feet were stable and pain-free, so a graduated return to sports was allowed (Figure 6.5a and b) and (Figure 6.6). He needs to be followed up to see if he remains free of symptoms in the long term.

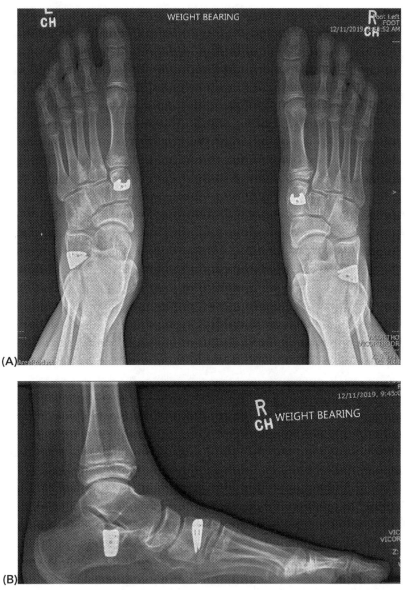

Figure 6.5 Standing radiographs of feet showing correction of forefoot abduction with restoration of calcaneal pitch and longitudinal arch.

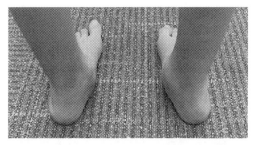

Figure 6.6 Appearance of the feet showing correction of deformities.

Comment

Successful correction of the planovalgus foot relies on a careful analysis of the deformity and application of considered bony and soft tissue corrections to achieve a lifelong stable result.[5]

References

1. Ghanem I, Massaad A, Assi A, Rizkallah M, Bizdikian AJ, Abiad RE, et al. Understanding the foot's functional anatomy in physiological and pathological conditions: The calcaneopedal unit concept. *J Child Orthop.* 2019;13(2):134–46.
2. Moraleda L, Salcedo M, Bastrom TP, Wenger DR, Albiñana J, Mubarak SJ. Comparison of the calcaneo-cuboid-cuneiform osteotomies and the calcaneal lengthening osteotomy in the surgical treatment of symptomatic flexible flatfoot. *J Pediatr Orthoped.* 2012;32(8):821–9.
3. Pavone V, Vescio A, Silvestri CAD, Andreacchio A, Sessa G, Testa G. Outcomes of the calcaneo-stop procedure for the treatment of juvenile flatfoot in young athletes. *J Child Orthop.* 2018;12(6):582–9.
4. Mosca VS. Calcaneal lengthening for valgus deformity of the hindfoot: Results in children who had severe, symptomatic flatfoot and skewfoot. *J Bone Jt Surg Am Volume.* 1995;77(4):500–12.
5. Nejib K, Delpont M. Medium-term results of calcaneus lengthening in idiopathic symptomatic flat foot in children and adolescents. *J Child Orthop.* 2020;14(4):286–92.

Hitesh Shah and Benjamin Joseph

Case

A 7-year-old boy presented with complaints of a deformity of the right foot first noted at birth (Figure 7.1). In early childhood, release of soft tissues in the lateral aspect of the leg and ankle had been done (exact details of the surgery are not known), but the deformity persisted.

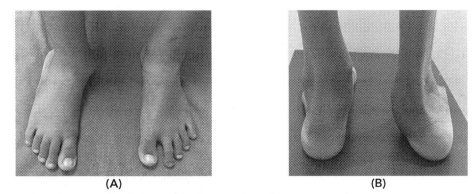

(A)   (B)

Figure 7.1 Severe valgus deformity of the right hindfoot.

On examination, apart from severe valgus deformity of the right hindfoot, there were no other deformities of the extremities. The normal proportions of body segments were maintained apart from a 3.0 cm shortening of the right lower limb which was mainly in the foot (Figure 7.2). Passive dorsiflexion of the ankle was 15 degrees more than that of the normal limb, and plantar flexion was reduced by 30 degrees. The peroneal tendons stood out prominently, and no passive inversion of the hindfoot was possible. Mid-tarsal movements were normal. The gait was awkward with a poor push-off.

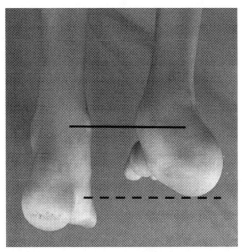

Figure 7.2 There was 3.0 cm shortening of the limb which was predominantly in the foot (broken line). The tibia was only 0.5 cm shorter (solid black line).

Plain radiographs of the foot and ankle were difficult to interpret on account of the severe valgus deformity (Figure 7.3). The ankle mortise was not grossly tilted in valgus, the distal tibial epiphysis was not wedge-shaped, and the lateral malleolus was not situated proximally. The absence of these features indicated that the deformity was not at the ankle. Since the subtalar joint could not be visualised clearly on the plain radiographs, CT scans were done. The CT scan clearly showed that the ankle joint was almost horizontal but the subtalar joint was abnormally inclined at about 65 degrees from the horizontal. On account of this, the calcaneum was not under the tibia but was laterally displaced (Figure 7.4a, b).

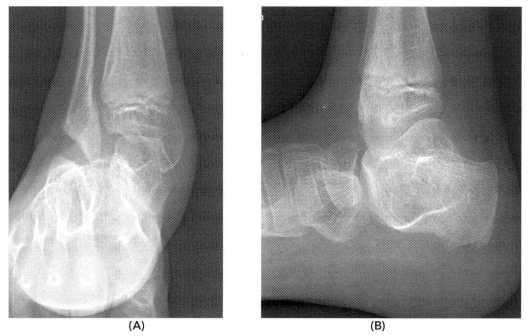

(A) (B)

Figure 7.3 Plain radiographs of the ankle. The antero-posterior view (A) shows that the distal tibial growth plate is almost horizontal, and the distal tibial epiphysis is not wedge-shaped. In the lateral view (B), the subtalar joint cannot be seen as the calcaneum overlies the talus.

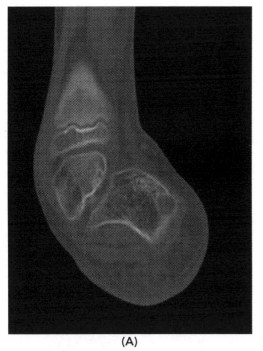
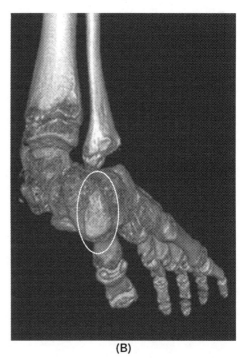

(A)   (B)

Figure 7.4 (A) CT scan section through the ankle and subtalar joints shows that the ankle joint is almost horizontal but the plane of the subtalar joint is 65 degrees from the horizontal. (B) Three-dimensional reconstruction of the CT scan shows that the calcaneum is displaced laterally (white circle outlines the calcaneal tuberosity).

Questions

- What are the problems that need to be addressed in this boy?
- What are the aims of treatment?
- What are the available treatment options?
- What are the factors that may influence your choice of treatment?
- What treatment would you recommend for this boy?
- How long would you follow-up this boy after treatment?

The Problems to Be Addressed in This Boy Include

- An unacceptable valgus deformity of the hindfoot
- Lateral displacement of the heel with lever arm dysfunction resulting in a weak push-off
- Limb length inequality mainly confined to the foot

The Aims of Treatment in This Boy Are to

- Correct the deformity and restore the normal alignment of the calcaneum in relation to the tibia
- Equalise limb length or minimise limb length inequality

Options for Treatment

- Medial displacement osteotomy of the calcaneum
- Subtalar fusion
- Subtalar fusion after wedge resection
- Limb length equalising procedure on the tibia

FACTORS THAT INFLUENCED THE CHOICE OF TREATMENT

- Site of the deformity
- Severity of the deformity
- Suppleness of the foot
- Site of shortening

The choice of treatment based on these factors is shown in Table 7.1.

Table 7.1 Factors that influenced the choice of treatment

Factors		Treatment Implications
Site of the deformity	Subtalar joint	Since the deformity is at the subtalar joint (and not at the ankle), surgery should be centred on the subtalar joint.
Severity of deformity	Severe	The valgus deformity is too severe to get sufficient correction by a displacement osteotomy of the calcaneum.[1] A liberal wedge resection followed by fusion is needed in this boy. In the presence of such a severe valgus deformity, a medial approach to the subtalar joint is safer than the standard lateral approach while a wedge resection of this magnitude is performed.[2,3]
Suppleness of the foot	The foot cannot be passively brought to the neutral position	Classical techniques of fusion of the subtalar joint like the Dennyson and Fulford technique[4] cannot be employed as the heel cannot be passively inverted. Furthermore, correction of the lateral displacement of the heel will not be possible by performing a classical subtalar fusion.

(Continued)

Table 7.1 (Continued)

Factors		Treatment Implications
Site of shortening	Shortening is mainly confined to the foot	Since the shortening is in the foot, lengthening of the tibia should be deferred till the length gained by surgery on the foot becomes clear.

How Was This Boy Treated?

Through a curved lateral incision, the peroneal tendons were lengthened, and through a horizontal medial incision the sustentaculum tali was identified and a medial-based wedge of bone was excised from the talus and calcaneum astride the subtalar joint (Figure 7.5a). The wedge was closed; this enabled the heel valgus to be corrected and the calcaneum to be aligned under the tibia. The talus and calcaneum were fixed with a single Blount staple. A Kirschner wire was passed from the heel into the distal tibia (Figure 7.5b). At the end of the operation, the foot was plantigrade; the medial longitudinal arch was restored, and appearance of the foot was normal (Figure 7.6a, 7.6b, 7.6c).

Post-Operative Management

The foot and ankle were immobilised in a below-knee cast for six weeks, after which the Kirschner wire was removed and full weight-bearing was permitted.

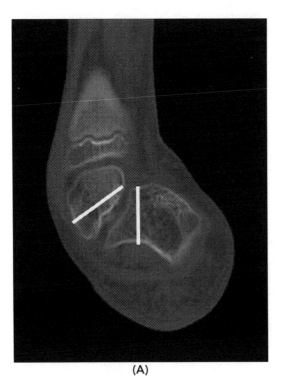
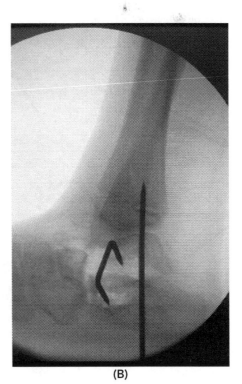

(A) (B)

Figure 7.5a (A) The planned osteotomy lines in the talus and calcaneum are shown in white. (B) Intra-operative radiograph shows that talo-calcaneal relationship is restored and the calcaneum lies under the tibia.

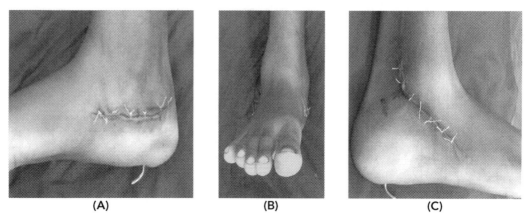

| (A) | (B) | (C) |

Figure 7.6a, 7.6b, 7.6c Post-operative appearance of the foot.

Follow-Up

The boy was followed up for 2.5 years. At the last follow-up, the deformity remained well corrected (Figure 7.7). The limb length inequality was 1.3 cm, and the gait pattern had improved significantly.

Comment

The boy had a very unusual deformity with abnormal inclination of the subtalar joint. He needs to be followed up till skeletal maturity to monitor the limb lengths and to see if the correction is maintained.

This case is ideal to illustrate the extent to which shortening of the foot can contribute to lower limb length discrepancy.[5]

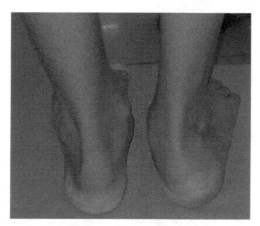

Figure 7.7 Appearance of the right heel at the last follow-up visit; the valgus deformity has been corrected to a very large extent, and the height of the heel has improved.

References

1. Koman LA, Mooney JF 3rd, Goodman A. Management of valgus hindfoot deformity in pediatric cerebral palsy patients by medial displacement osteotomy. *J Pediatr Orthop*. 1993;13:180–3.
2. Widnall J, Mason L, Molloy A. Medial approach to the subtalar joint. *Foot Ankle Clin*. 2018 Sep;23(3):451–60. doi: 10.1016/j.fcl.2018.04.006. PMID: 30097084.
3. Knupp M, Zwicky L, Lang TH, Röhm J, Hintermann B. Medial approach to the subtalar joint: Anatomy, indications, technique tips. *Foot Ankle Clin*. 2015;20(2):311–18. doi: 10.1016/j.fcl.2015.02.006.
4. Hadley N, Rahm M, Cain TE. Dennyson-Fulford subtalar arthrodesis. *J Pediatr Orthop*. 1994;14(3):363–8. doi: 10.1097/01241398-199405000-00017.
5. Lane G. A novel technique to determine foot contribution to limb-length discrepancy. *J Am Podiatr Med Assoc*. 2017;107(4):340–341. doi: 10.7547/16-062.

Benjamin Joseph and Hitesh Shah

Case

An 8-year-old boy, the son of a gardener from a city in south India, presented with anterior bowing of the right leg. He had undergone surgery for this on two previous occasions without success. He had features of neurofibromatosis type I with café-au-lait spots. There was frank abnormal mobility at the junction of the middle and lower thirds of the leg and shortening of two centimetres. Antero-posterior and lateral radiographs of the leg are shown in Figure 8.1.

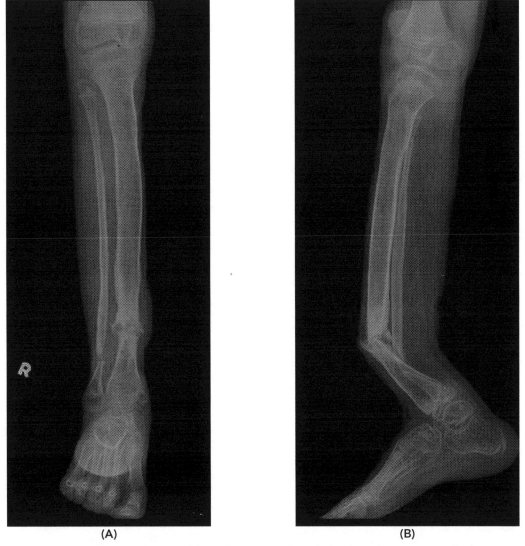

(A)   (B)

Figure 8.1 Antero-posterior and lateral radiographs of the leg showing Crawford type IV pseudarthrosis of the tibia and fibula.

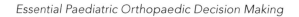

Questions

- What are the problems that need to be addressed?
- What are the aims of treatment?
- What are the commonly available options for treatment?
- What are the factors that may influence your choice of treatment?
- What treatment would you recommend for this boy?
- How long would you follow-up this boy after treatment?

The Problems That Need to Be Addressed Are

- Obtain union in this boy in whom two previous attempts have failed
- Even after obtaining union, there is significant risk of re-fracture[1]
- Limb-length inequality

The Aims of Treatment in This Boy Are to

- Obtain union of the pseudarthrosis
- Minimise the risk of a re-fracture
- Equalise limb lengths by skeletal maturity

Options for Treatment

Currently, there are three options for obtaining union of a pseudarthrosis; they are:

- Excision of the pseudarthrosis and intra-medullary rodding and bone grafting[2–5]
- Excision of the pseudarthrosis and Ilizarov fixator application and bone grafting[6,7]
- Excision of the pseudarthrosis and vascularised free fibular transfer.[8]

The results of these three methods of treatment are comparable.[9,10]
The treatment options for minimising the risk of re-fracture include:

- Retaining an intra-medullary rod in the tibia till skeletal maturity and
- Bracing of the leg with a protective orthosis.

FACTORS THAT INFLUENCED THE CHOICE OF TREATMENT

- Presence of additional deformities of the tibia (e.g. proximal tibial bowing) and ankle valgus
- Extent of shortening
- Availability of technical expertise
- Cost considerations

The choice of treatment based on these factors is shown in Table 8.1.

Table 8.1 Choice of treatment based on factors influencing decision-making

Factors		Treatment Implications
Presence of additional deformities of the tibia (e.g. proximal tibial bowing) and ankle valgus	There were no additional deformities of the tibia and ankle	The Ilizarov technique would have been preferred if in addition to dealing with the antero-lateral bowing there was significant shortening and posterior bowing of the proximal tibia. Since these additional deformities were not present, the Ilizarov technique was not chosen.
Extent of shortening	2 cm shortening in an 8-year-old boy	Since this extent of shortening could be managed by contralateral proximal tibial epiphyseodesis a couple of years later, concomitant limb lengthening was not considered.

(Continued)

Table 8.1 (Continued)

Factors		Treatment Implications
Availability of technical expertise	No one trained in microvascular techniques was available	Free fibular transfer was not feasible for this reason.
Cost considerations	The family had limited financial resources	A simple and cheap method of treatment, namely intra-medullary rodding and bone grafting, was the preferred choice.

How Was This Child Treated?

The boy was treated by excision of the pseudarthrosis, which entailed:

- Resection of about 5mm of the sclerotic bone from the tip of each fragment of the tibia till some fresh bleeding from the bone ends was seen,
- Meticulous excision of fibrous tissue between the fragments of the tibia and
- Circumferential excision of about 2 cm of thickened periosteum around the pseudar-throsis site.

The angulation was corrected, and it was ensured that the fragments of the tibia were in good contact (no gap between the fragments and no overlap of the fragments).

The tibia was fixed with an intramedullary Rush rod of 4 mm thickness inserted from the heel, through the calcaneum and talus into the distal tibia and across the pseudarthrosis site.

A long cortical strut of bone was harvested from the subcutaneous surface of the opposite tibia, divided into three pieces and placed around the site of the pseudarthrosis (Figure 8.2a–8.2d).

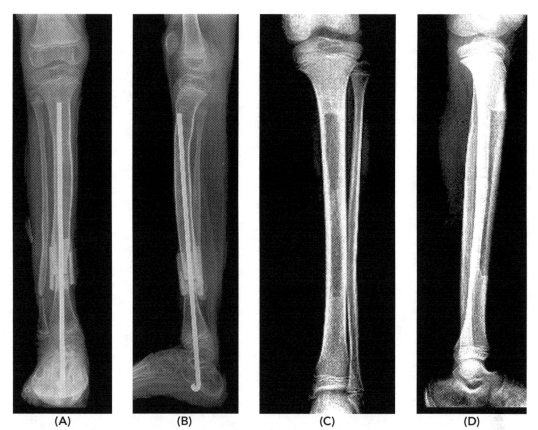

(A)   (B)   (C)   (D)

Figure 8.2 The pseudarthrosis was excised, and the tibia has been fixed with a Rush rod passed from the heel into the proximal tibial metaphysis (A, B). The tibial fragments are in good contact. A long strut of cortical bone has been harvested from the subcutaneous surface of the opposite tibia (C, D) and divided into three pieces and placed around the pseudarthrosis site (A, B).

No attempt was made to fix or graft the fibula or to obtain cross-union of the tibia and fibula.

Post-Operative Management

A groin-to-toe cast was applied after the operation and retained till union of the tibia was noted on the radiograph; weight-bearing on this limb was not permitted till the cast was removed. Thereafter, a thermoplastic clam-shell orthosis was used whenever he was ambulant.

The opposite limb (graft donor limb) was encased in a groin-to-toe cast, and weight-bearing was not permitted for six weeks.

Sequential radiographs were obtained every six weeks till union of the pseudarthrosis was confirmed (Figure 8.3, 8.4). Following sound union, the boy was followed-up annually till skeletal maturity. The intra-medullary rod was retained and bracing was continued till skeletal maturity.

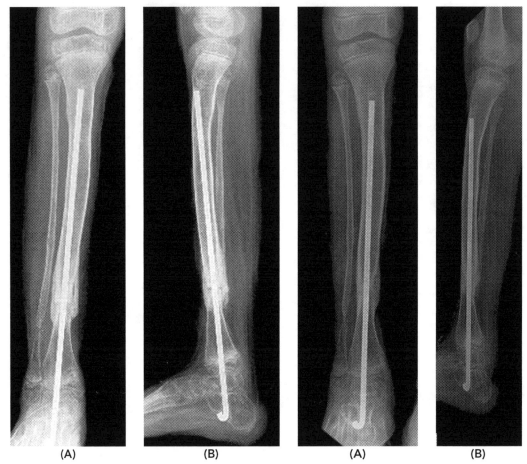

(A)   **(B)**   **(A)**   **(B)**

Figures 8.3 and **8.4** The radiographic appearance six weeks following surgery (8.3A, B) and eight months following surgery (8.4A, B); early union is noted at six weeks. At eight months, sound union with continuity of four cortices (anterior, posterior, medial and lateral) is evident.

The tibia remained soundly united till skeletal maturity (Figures 8.5, 8.6). The Rush rod remained intact, and at skeletal maturity the tip of the rod had receded towards the middle third of the tibia but was still supporting the pseudarthrosis site (Figure 8.6).

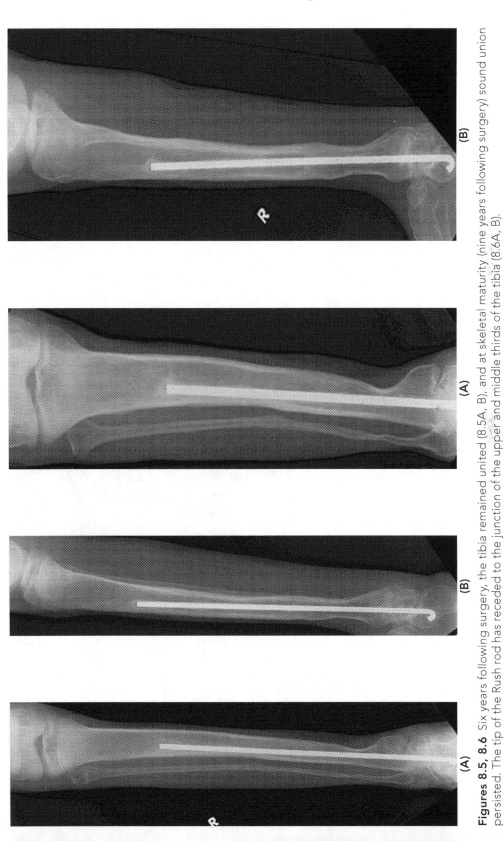

Figures 8.5, 8.6 Six years following surgery, the tibia remained united (8.5A, B), and at skeletal maturity (nine years following surgery) sound union persisted. The tip of the Rush rod has receded to the junction of the upper and middle thirds of the tibia (8.6A, B).

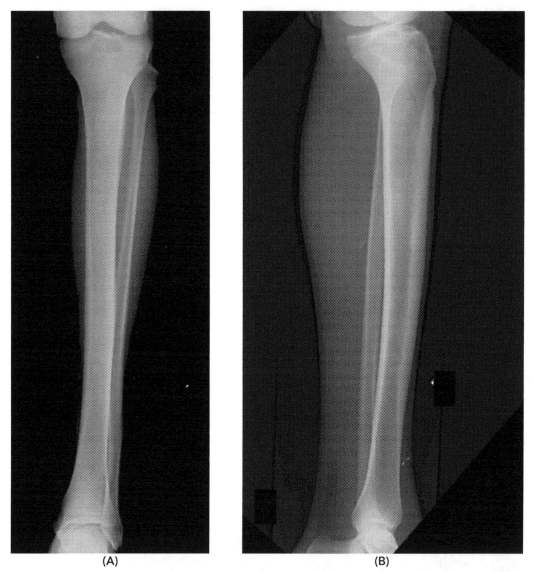

(A) (B)

Figure 8.7 The opposite tibia from where bone graft was harvested appears normal (8.7).

At skeletal maturity, there is 4 cm shortening of the tibia which needs to be addressed. Limb length equalisation by contralateral epiphyseodesis had been offered earlier, but the parents preferred to avoid surgery again on the normal limb. The ankle and sub-talar joints remain stiff on account of the rod crossing the ankle and subtalar joints. The donor site on the normal tibia has healed with no apparent ill effect; at skeletal maturity, the tibia appears normal (Figure 8.7).

Comment

Some studies have suggested that in addition to using one of the methods mentioned here, use of periosteal grafts, administering bisphosphonates or the use of bone morphogenetic protein improves the union rate. However, none of these studies are Level I studies, and none have followed the patients till skeletal maturity.

References

1. Khan T, Joseph B. Controversies in the management of congenital pseudarthrosis of the tibia and fibula. *Bone Joint J.* 2013;95-B:1027–34.
2. Joseph B, Mathew G. Management of congenital pseudarthrosis of the tibia by excision of the pseudarthrosis, onlay grafting and intramedullary nailing. *J Pediatr Orthop B.* 2000;9:16–23.
3. Shah H, Doddabasappa SN, Joseph B. Congenital pseudarthrosis of the tibia treated with intramedullary rodding and cortical bone grafting: A follow-up study at skeletal maturity. *J Pediatr Orthop.* 2011;31(1):79–88.
4. Dobbs MB, Rich MM, Gordon JE, Szymanski DA, Schoenecker PL. Use of an intramedullary rod for treatment of congenital pseudarthrosis of the tibia: A long-term follow-up study. *J Bone Joint Surg Am.* 2004 Jun;86-A(6):1186–97.
5. Johnston CE II. Congenital pseudarthrosis of the tibia: Results of technical variations in the Charnley-Williams procedures. *J Bone Joint Surg Am.* 2002;84:1799–810.
6. Cho T-J, Choi IH, Lee SM, Chung CY, Yoo WJ, Lee DY, Lee JW. Refracture after Ilizarov osteosynthesis in atrophic-type congenital pseudarthrosis of the tibia. *J Bone Joint Surg [Br].* 2008;90-B:488–93.
7. Choi IH, Lee SJ, Moon HJ, Cho TJ, Yoo WJ, Chung CY, Park MS. "4-in-1 osteosynthesis" for atrophic-type congenital pseudarthrosis of the tibia. *J Pediatr Orthop.* 2011 Sep;31(6):697–704.
8. Sakamoto A, Yoshida T, Uchida Y, Kojima T, Kubota H, Iwamoto Y. Long-term follow-up on the use of vascularised fibular graft for the treatment of congenital pseudarthrosis of the tibia. *J Orthop Surg.* 2008;6:13.
9. Inan M, El Rassi G, Riddle EC, Kumar SJ. Residual deformities following successful initial bone union in congenital pseudarthrosis of the tibia. *J Pediatr Orthop.* 2006;26:393–9.
10. Tudisco C, Bollini G, Dungl P, Fixsen J, Grill F, Hefti F, Romanus B, Wientroub S. Functional results at the end of skeletal growth in 30 patients affected by congenital pseudarthrosis of the tibia. *J Pediatr Orthop B.* 2000;9:94–102.

Nick Green and James A Fernandes

Case

A 7-year-old girl born with posteromedial bowing of the left tibia was referred for persistent deformity of the tibia and shortening (Figure 9.1a). She had calcaneovalgus at birth that was treated with stretches; later orthotics were used for the limb length discrepancy.

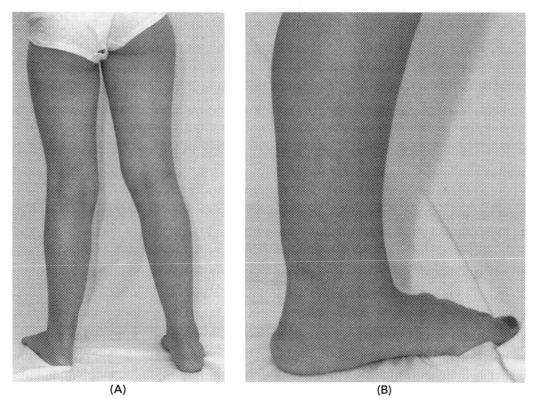

| (A) | (B) |

Figure 9.1 (A) Shows pelvic obliquity and knee joint creases at different heights, indicating that most or all the discrepancy is below the knee. (B) Shows a posteromedial pucker sign which might indicate a field defect.

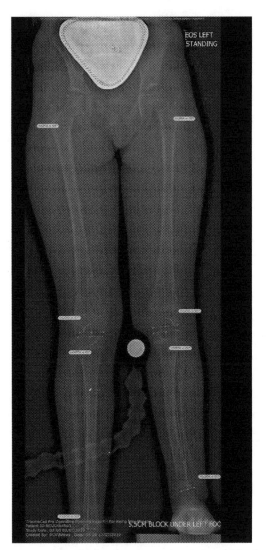

Figure 9.1 (C) Demonstrates mechanical axis view with a 5.5 cm block slightly over-correcting the pelvis and annotations of joint line angles and mechanical axes.

Examination revealed posteromedial bowing of the tibia and a pucker sign at the apex of the bow (Figure 9.1b).[1] The shortening that was entirely in the tibial segment measured 5.5 cm both with the block test and on calibrated mechanical axis–view x-rays (Figure 9.1c). Predicted height and leg length discrepancy at maturity were 166 cm and 6.7 cm respectively.[2,3]

Questions

- What are the problems that need to be addressed?
- What are the aims of treatment?
- What are the options to treat each aim?
- What are the factors that influence choice of treatment?
- Based on these points, what treatment would you recommend for this child?
- How long would you follow-up this child?

The Problems That Need to Be Addressed Are

- 6.7 cm of tibial shortening at maturity
- Posteromedial angulation deformity of the tibia

The Aims of Treatment in This Girl Are to

- Equalise or compensate for limb length discrepancy
- Correct tibial angular deformity

Options for Treatment to Fulfil Each Aim[4]

- Equalising or compensating for left-sided short tibia

  - Orthotic: combination of heel and shoe raise
  - Planned epiphyseodesis of contralateral tibia
  - Lengthening with external fixator
  - Correction with lengthening nail (older child)
  - Combination of the previous

- Apex posteromedial deformity correction

  - Partial correction by creation of secondary deformity using guided growth
  - Acute correction with internal fixation
  - Gradual correction with external fixation

Summary of Options for Lower Limb Treatment

- **Orthotic/guided growth/epiphyseodesis approach:** In situations where prolonged treatment in a frame is either not wanted, or ill advised due to social or patient factors, the LLD can be managed with an orthotic until such an age where a well-timed contralateral epiphyseodesis can be performed. In the interim, guided growth at the knee and/or ankle can augment natural modelling out of the deformity, albeit away from the CORA and thus creating a secondary translational deformity.
- **External Fixator:** Optimal deformity correction can be achieved with a bi-focal tibial osteotomy which can be staged or simultaneous. The proximal metaphyseal osteotomy is used for lengthening, and the distal osteotomy at the CORA is for angulation correction and minor lengthening.

FACTORS THAT INFLUENCED THE CHOICE OF TREATMENT
• Age of the child • Severity of limb length inequality • Associated angulation deformity • Parents' acceptance or rejection of treatment option

The choice of treatment based on these factors is shown in Table 9.1.

Table 9.1 Choice of Treatment Based on the Factors That Influenced the Decision

Factors		Treatment Implications
Age of the child	7 years	This primary school age is an optimal time for lengthening techniques as the child is better at understanding the goal, and demands of treatment. The consequences of interruptions in schooling are also arguably low.
Severity of limb length inequality	Severe shortening	An entirely tibial segment severe shortening of 6 to 7 cm cannot reliably or accurately be treated with an all-tibial epiphyseodesis. The resulting short segment might also result in a poor cosmetic outcome. Patient predicted height also weighs into the decision on whether to maintain or sacrifice leg length.
Associated angulation deformity	Posteromedial bowing	The presence of angulation as well as shortening perhaps tips the balance towards a frame technique which addresses both problems in the same episode. Guided growth will not achieve anatomic alignment since the CORA is in the diaphysis.
Parents' acceptance or rejection of frame option	Accepted	This is based on psychological, social and economic factors, as well as a proper understanding of what treatment entails.

How Was This Girl Treated?

The LLD was proving difficult to compensate in an orthosis, and so the family elected to go ahead with lengthening surgery using an external fixator.[5,6] The surgical tactic was a 4-ring construct (including a heel ring), a 2-stage bifocal tibial osteotomy with angular correction and some length gain from a distal osteotomy at the CORA (first stage) and later a second proximal metaphyseal osteotomy for most of the lengthening (second stage).

> **Stage 1**: The joint lines, growth plates and tibial anatomic axes were marked under fluoroscopy. Percutaneous fibular osteotomy was performed. The proximal 2-ring construct was made and aligned with the proximal tibial anatomic axis. This proximal 2-ring block was connected via 4 double hinges, in the plane of the deformity to a third ring distally which was aligned with the distal tibial anatomic axis. A final half ring was used at the heel with cross olive wires and connected with rods to the distal tibial ring, and the ankle joint was distracted by 3 mm to off-load the joint. A percutaneous low-energy distal tibial osteotomy was performed at the level of the deformity.

Post-Operative Care

She was allowed to weight-bear as tolerated. After a latency period of five days, distraction was commenced at 1 mm per day between the second and third rings to create enough clearance for angular correction (Figure 9.2). Differential distraction was then performed to correct the deformity. The amount of lengthening at this osteotomy was limited to 20 mm as the regenerate at this location is not as exuberant, partly due to the lack of muscle anterior and medially and some degree of congenital soft tissue dysplasia.

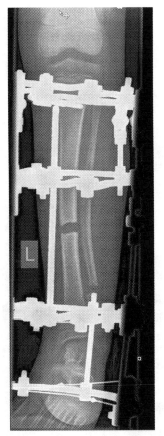

Figure 9.2 AP radiograph demonstrates the 4-ring frame construct with the proximal ring block intentionally slightly open anteromedially. The stage 1 tibial and fibular osteotomies are distracting, and some angular correction has occurred.

Stage 2: A proximal tibial osteotomy was performed four weeks later. After a latency of five days, distraction was performed at 1 mm per day till a total of 60 mm lengthening was achieved (Figure 9.3). Regular physiotherapy helped to maintain knee range of motion throughout lengthening. At three months, the metaphyseal osteotomy site was consolidating well (Figure 9.4a), but the original diaphyseal osteotomy site showed poor regenerate with a wide fibrous interzone (Figure 9.4b). To stimulate this site, an "accordion" program of cyclical compression and distraction was initiated. Despite this, the distal regenerate was poor, and she underwent debridement of fibrous tissue and autologous iliac crest grafting. At six months, the grafted regenerate site looked satisfactory (Figure 9.4c), and the frame was removed and a hinged cast-brace was applied. Due to a communication failure, lack of pain in the cast and six months of frustrated mobility, the child was too enthusiastic in mobilisation, which included activities such as trampolining. This led to bending of the regenerate, diagnosed two months later when the cast-brace was discarded (Figure 9.5 and 9.6). We expect some remodelling to occur, but further surgery is likely.

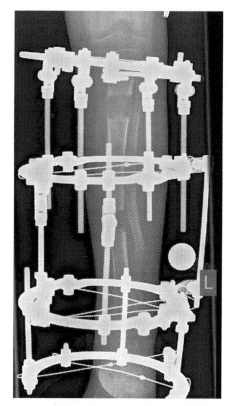

Figure 9.3 AP radiograph demonstrates the stage 2 proximal osteotomy which is distracting and forming optimal regenerate. Note that the ankle and knee joints are nearly parallel but the regenerate at the stage 1 osteotomy sites are lagging behind the proximal regenerate. This might further suggest that there is a field defect at the deformity site.

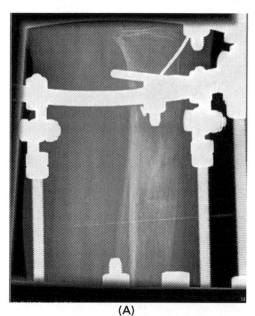
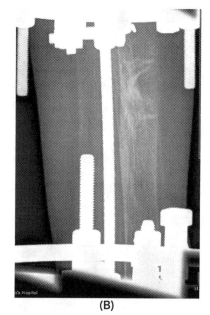

| (A) | (B) |

Figure 9.4 (A) Spot lateral radiograph of proximal tibial regenerate shows progressive consolidation. (B) Spot lateral radiograph of distal tibial regenerate shows poor regenerate anteriorly.

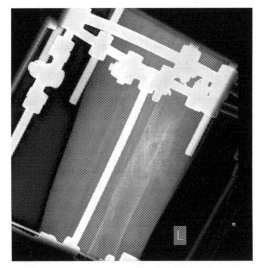

Figure 9.4 (C) Spot lateral radiograph shows the site after grafting and healing.

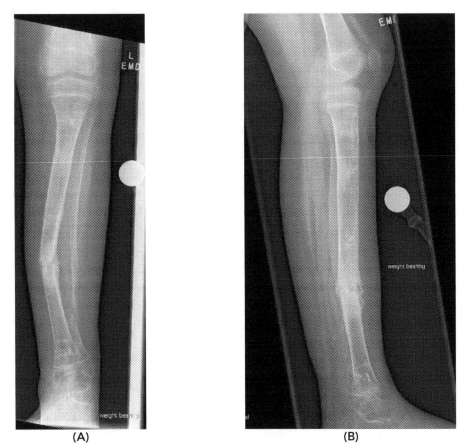

(A) (B)

Figure 9.5 (A) AP radiograph shows some medial angulation of the distal regenerate site and therefore a valgus distal segment. Despite this, the leg looks quite straight. (B) Lateral radiograph shows reasonable sagittal mechanical axis restoration. The distal regenerate is still consolidating.

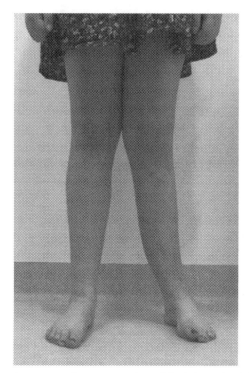

Figure 9.6 Clinical photo demonstrating restoration of limb length with knees at similar heights and the apex medial tibial deformity. Also note the pre-existent cavovarus deformity of the left foot, which needs to be considered when contemplating further surgery.

Comment

The senior author pre-sets the proximal rings with slight divergence with more opening antero-medially. At stage 2 when lengthening is performed through a proximal osteotomy between these rings, the expected deformity due to differential muscle tension will be procurvatum and valgus. When this anteromedial opening is corrected through differential lengthening, it will achieve a straight regenerate.

Although the patient is functioning well, partial loss of correction at the last hurdle was disappointing and is a lesson of the complexity of this treatment modality throughout all stages.[7]

References

1. Nogami H, Oohira A, Kuroyanagi M, Mizutani A. Congenital bowing of long bones: Clinical and experimental study. *Teratol.* 1986;33(1):1–7.
2. Hoffmann A, Wenger DR. Posteromedial bowing of the tibia: Progression of discrepancy in limb lengths. *J Bone Joint Surg Am.* 1981;63:3847.
3. Kaufman SD, Fagg JA, Jones S, Bell MJ, Saleh M, Fernandes JA. Limb lengthening in congenital posteromedial bow of the tibia. *Strategies Trauma Limb Reconstruction.* 2012 Nov;7(3):147–53.
4. Pappas AM. Congenital posteromedial bowing of the tibia and fibula. *J Paediatr Orthop.* 1984;4:525–31.
5. Saleh M, Goonatillake HD. Management of congenital leg length inequality: Value of early axis correction. *J Paediatr Orthop.* 1995;4:150–8.
6. Johari AN, Dhawale AA, Salaskar A, Aroojis AJ. Congenital postero-medial bowing of the tibia and fibula: Is early surgery worthwhile? *J Pediatr Orthop Br.* 2010;19(6):479–86.
7. Saleh M, Scott BW. Pitfalls and complications in leg lengthening: The Sheffield experience. *Semin Orthop.* 1992;7:207–22.

Nicholas Peterson, Christopher Prior, Selvadurai Nayagam

Case

A 9-year-old girl presented three months following a tibial fracture managed conservatively in another institution (Figure 10.1). At the time of cast removal, the girl and her family became concerned about the appearance of her leg. They described her foot turned out to the side when she walked, and, when trying to correct this, her knee would turn in.

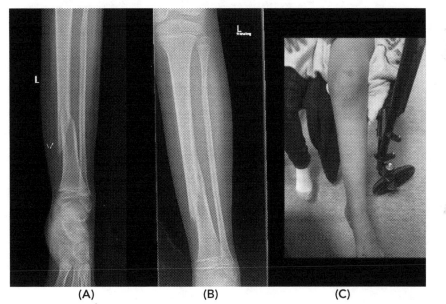

Figure 10.1 (A) Left tibial fracture with proximal fibula fracture at time of injury. (B) Left tibial fracture three months following injury demonstrating malunion in valgus. (C) A clinical photograph of the leg following cast removal, demonstrating external tibial torsion of the tibia.

Clinical examination revealed an out-toeing gait from a tibial fracture malunion in valgus and external rotation (Figure 10.2). The 'sudden' appearance of this acquired torsional deformity caused distress to the patient and her family. Clinical assessment of the rotational profile revealed 35 degrees external torsion to the tibia as compared to 5 degrees of external torsion on the contralateral side.[1] Sagittal plane alignment revealed mild translation without angular deformity, and there was a 7-degree valgus deformity in the coronal plane.

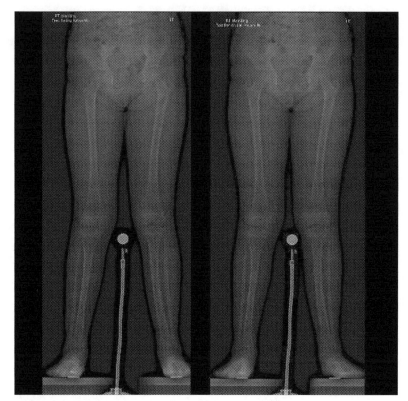

Figure 10.2 Low-dose EOS long leg radiographs taken eight months following the injury. With the feet facing forward (A) the left patella is in an internally rotated position and the valgus deformity of the tibia is evident. With patellae facing forwards (B) the left foot is externally rotated relative to the right.

Questions

- What are the problems that need to be addressed in this girl?
- What are the aims of treatment?
- What are the commonly available options for treatment?
- What are the factors that may influence your choice of treatment?
- What treatment would you recommend for this girl?
- How long would you follow-up this girl after treatment?

The Problems That Need to Be Addressed

- The cosmetic impact of the torsional malunion, producing significant concern for the patient and her family.
- Potential for torsional deformity adversely affecting the child's ability to run and participate in sports.
- The lateral mechanical axis deviation caused by the valgus tibial deformity.

The Aims of Treatment

- Correct torsional deformity
- Restore the normal mechanical axis

Options for Treatment

- Correction of torsional abnormality
  - Acute derotation osteotomy
  - Gradual derotation osteotomy
- Correction of valgus deformity
  - No intervention—wait for spontaneous remodelling.
  - Corrective osteotomy simultaneously with torsional correction.

FACTORS THAT INFLUENCED THE CHOICE OF TREATMENT

- Age of the patient
- Remodelling potential of deformity
- Level of osteotomy
- Acute versus gradual correction

The choice of treatment based on these factors is shown in Table 10.1.

Table 10.1 Choice of Treatment Based on the Influencing Factors

Factors		Treatment Implications
Age of the child	9 years	Remodelling may improve the valgus deformity as the patient is under 10 years of age.
Remodelling potential of deformity	30-degree torsional deformity	At age 9 years, the likelihood of significant remodelling of a rotational deformity of this magnitude is very small.
Level of osteotomy	Supra-malleolar osteotomy	Tibial derotation osteotomies for correcting foot progression are usually performed in the supra-malleolar region. In this child, if a supra-malleolar osteotomy was done with valgus correction, an 'S' shape deformity would be created. The alternative would be to correct rotation alone at the supra-malleolar level and allow the valgus deformity to remodel.[2]
	Osteotomy at the site of deformity	The CORA of the valgus deformity resolved to the junction of the middle and distal thirds of the tibia. An osteotomy at this level would allow the valgus to be corrected without translation and facilitate a derotation at the same level.

(Continued)

Table 10.1 (Continued)

Factors		Treatment Implications
Acute versus gradual correction	Gradual correction	Gradual derotation using an external fixator is an option for large deformities and makes injury to the common peroneal nerve less likely. This technique also allows the adjustment to be tailored until the patient and family are satisfied that the correction is optimal.
	Acute correction	Acute derotation from external rotation to internal rotation of 30 degrees may risk a stretch injury to the common peroneal nerve.
		Acute derotation over 20 degrees should be combined with common peroneal nerve decompression.[3]

How Was the Girl Treated?

In view of the cosmetic and potential functional issues the deformity was causing, with little scope for spontaneous resolution, it was decided to proceed with operative intervention.[4]

Fixation chosen was a locking plate inserted submuscularly.[5] An external fixator-assisted technique was used to facilitate an accurate acute correction.

Both lower limbs were prepped and draped to permit intraoperative comparison with the normal contralateral side during surgery.

A common peroneal nerve neurolysis was performed under tourniquet through an incision over the interval between the lateral head of the gastrocnemius and the peroneus longus (PL) muscle bodies. In this interval, using loupe magnification, the motor nerve to PL and the superficial peroneal nerve were identified and followed proximally. The attachment of PL to the head of the fibula was released, and the deep peroneal nerve was released as it traversed across the intermuscular septum into the anterior compartment (Figure 10.3). The tourniquet was released and haemostasis ensured.

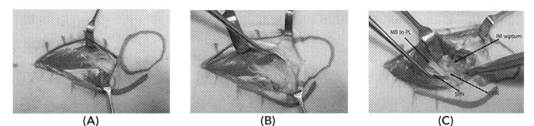

(A)   (B)   (C)

Figure 10.3 (A) The common peroneal nerve (CPN) is identified entering peroneus longus (PL) in the plane between that muscle and the lateral head of gastrocnemius (seen posterior to the nerve). (B) By tracing of the edge of PL lying over the nerve, the origin of PL from the head of the fibula is identified and can be detached sharply. This allows retraction of PL and visualisation of the branches of the CPN. (C) Careful dissection will reveal the motor branch to PL (MB to PL), superficial peroneal nerve (SPN), deep peroneal nerve (DPN) and the septum between peroneal and anterior muscle compartments (IM septum).

Image intensifier guidance was used to identify the planned position for the osteotomy. A mono-lateral rail external fixator system (LRS Advanced, Orthofix SRL, Bussolengo, Italy) with a derotation arc was used to achieve accurate derotation and simultaneous correction of the valgus deformity (Figure 10.4).

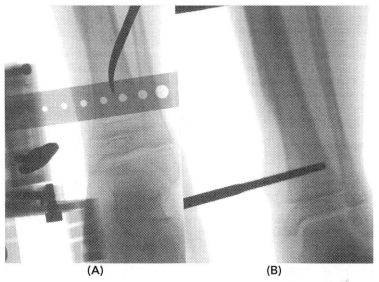

(A)   (B)

Figure 10.4 (A) A derotation arc of radius 100 mm is set to correct 30 degrees of external rotation. A ruler is used to position the arc 100 mm from the centre of the bone so that the derotation does not produce unwanted translation. (B) Half pins are inserted above and below the planned osteotomy level in order to allow correction of the external tibial torsion as well as the valgus of the distal tibia following osteotomy.

A low-energy, De Bastiani–type osteotomy was created through saline-cooled drilling and division of the bone using Hibbs osteotomes. The derotation was completed and the valgus deformity corrected. The image intensifier was used to check the mechanical axis of the limb and clinical examination used to confirm that the rotational profile of the limb was equal to the opposite side. Full correction was achieved without the need for an osteotomy of the fibula. The proximal and distal tibio-fibular joints were screened to ensure no subluxation or abnormality. The monolateral fixator was used to compress the osteotomy site, and the position of correction was rechecked before definitive fixation. A submuscular plane beneath the anterior compartment muscles was created through proximal and distal incisions, with great care taken to avoid injury to the neurovascular bundle in the anterior compartment. A large fragment plate was contoured and positioned with locking screws before the external fixator was removed (Figure 10.5).

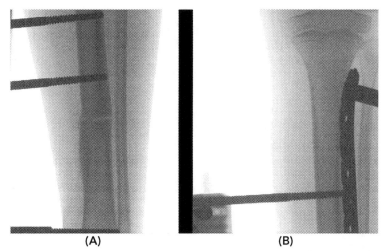

Figure 10.5 (A) The osteotomy is made, the derotation is performed, and then compression is applied using the rail system. (B) A submuscular plane is developed and a custom-contoured plate is used to secure the corrected position using locking screws prior to fixator removal.

Post-Operative Management

Postoperatively, the patient was allowed to partially weight-bear 50% of body weight using crutches and was followed up in the elective clinic. Physiotherapy was commenced to optimise knee and ankle range of motion, and full weight-bearing was permitted at six weeks. By three months, she was able to participate fully in sports (Figure 10.6).

Twelve months after surgery, the plate was removed. The patient and her family commented that the leg was back to 'normal' immediately after surgery and that the stated aims of improving the appearance of the leg as well as her ability to participate in sports had been achieved. Clinical images taken at the most recent follow-up appointment are shown in Figure 10.7.

Comment

In clinical practice, the problem resulting from torsional malalignment is one of either foot progression or patellar progression. Clinical assessment will need to include an observation of gait and static examination of both femoral and tibial profiles. The presence of angular malalignment may interfere with the reliability of clinical examination for assessing torsion.

CT imaging may not show the influence of dynamic elements resulting from the torsional problem. Over-reliance on these images for making quantitative decisions on the amount of derotation is not advised. A potential solution is the use of gait analysis where the asymmetry in behaviour of the two sides may be compared easily and measured.

In most cases of tibial torsion, a supra-malleolar osteotomy may be performed. This case demonstrates the principle of using an external fixator-assisted technique in order to achieve the planned amount of correction accurately. Deformities of up to 20 degrees would usually not require decompression of the common peroneal nerve before correcting from external to internal rotation. Derotation from internal to external rotation does not require neurolysis.

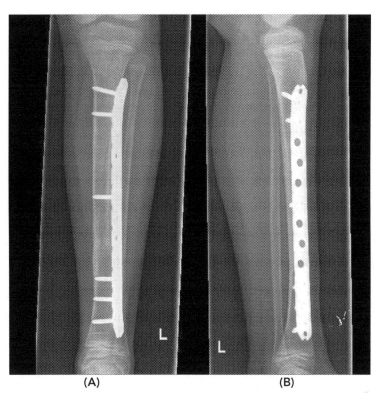

(A)   (B)

Figure 10.6 Postoperative appearance at five months following surgery showing consolidation of the osteotomy site and realignment of the tibia with a submuscular tibial plate.

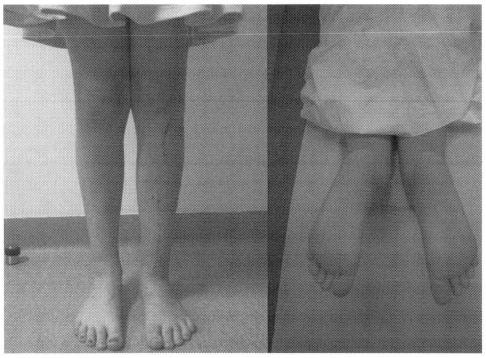

Figure 10.7 Clinical photographs demonstrating equalisation of the torsional profile of the lower limb following surgery.

References

1. Shih YC, Chau MM, Arendt EA, Novacheck TF. Measuring lower extremity rotational alignment: A review of methods and case studies of clinical applications. *J Bone Joint Surg Am*. 2020;102(4):343–56.
2. Krengel WF, 3rd, Staheli LT. Tibial rotational osteotomy for idiopathic torsion: A comparison of the proximal and distal osteotomy levels. *Clin Orthop Relat Res*. 1992;283:285–9.
3. Nogueira MP, Paley D. Prophylactic and therapeutic peroneal nerve decompression for deformity correction and lengthening. *Oper Tech Orthop*. 2011;21(2):180–3.
4. Staheli LT, Corbett M, Wyss C, King H. Lower-extremity rotational problems in children. Normal values to guide management. *J Bone Joint Surg Am*. 1985;67(1):39–47.
5. Paley D. *Principles of deformity correction*. 1st ed. Berlin (Heidelberg): Springer-Verlag; 2002. 806 p.

Hitesh Shah and Benjamin Joseph

Case

A 14-year-old girl presented with inability to walk on her feet. She had multiple symmetric deformities of the upper and lower limbs since birth. The deformities included flexion deformity of the knees, equinovarus deformities of the feet and flexion of the elbows and wrists (Figures 11.1, 11.2). A diagnosis of arthrogryposis multiplex congenita had been made when she was a young child, but no corrective surgery had been done because of severe financial constraints.

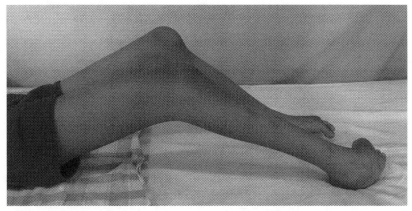

Figure 11.1 Bilateral fixed flexion deformities of the knee with severe equinovarus deformities.

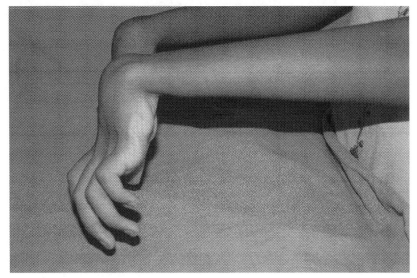

Figure 11.2 Bilateral symmetrical flexion deformities of the wrist.

She was a cheerful and intelligent girl who stood and walked on her knees (Figure 11.3) and was remarkably independent in spite of the deformities of the extremities.

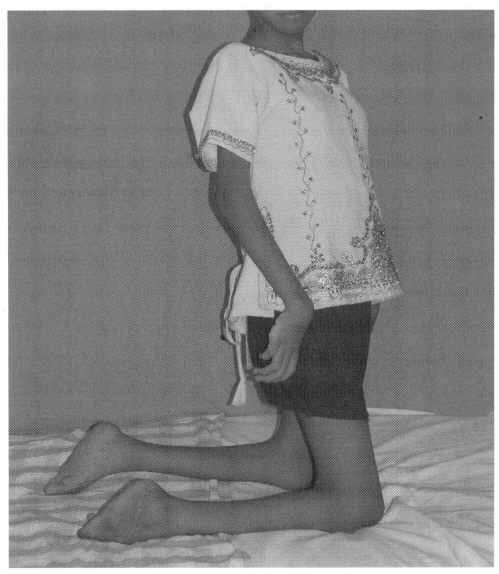

Figure 11.3 Kneel standing with good balance.

Examination of the Knees

Both knees had a fixed flexion deformity of 40 degrees. The quadriceps muscle was exceedingly weak (MRC Grade 2). Full flexion of the knees could be achieved both passively and actively with normal power (MRC Grade 5) of the hamstring muscles.

Questions

- What are the problems that need to be addressed?
- What are the aims of treatment?
- What are the available treatment options to fulfil these aims?
- What are the factors that may influence your choice of treatment?
- Based on these points, what treatment would you recommend for this child?
- How long would you follow-up this child after treatment?

The Problems Related to the Knees That Need to Be Addressed Are

- Fixed flexion deformities
- Weak quadriceps muscle and muscle imbalance
- Risk of damage to neuro-vascular structures while correcting the knee deformities

The Aims of Treatment in This Child Are to

- Correct knee flexion deformity without causing damage to the neuro-vascular structures
- Deal with quadriceps weakness

  o Restore power of active knee extension
  o Prevent knee from buckling during the stance phase of gait

- Prevent recurrence of the deformity

Options for Treatment to Fulfil Each Aim

- Correction of knee flexion deformity

  o Traction and serial plaster casts[1]
  o Posterior soft tissue release[2]
  o Anterior epiphyseodesis of the distal femur[3,4]
  o Supracondylar femur extension osteotomy[5]
  o Femoral shortening with or without extension of the distal fragment[6,7]
  o Gradual correction of knee deformity with an external fixator[8,9]

- Dealing with quadriceps weakness

  o Dynamic correction—Hamstring transfer to quadriceps
  o Static correction—Knee-ankle-foot orthosis

- Prevention of recurrence of the deformity by correcting muscle imbalance

  o Hamstring transfer to quadriceps
  o Orthosis

FACTORS THAT INFLUENCED THE CHOICE OF TREATMENT

The factors that influenced the choice of treatment of the knee deformity were:

- The underlying disease and its natural history
- The age of the child
- The severity of knee deformity
- Muscle power of the quadriceps and the hamstrings
- The side involved

The choice of treatment based on these factors is shown in Table 11.1.

Table 11.1 Factors Influencing the Choice of Treatment

Factors		Treatment Implications
The underlying disease and its natural history	Arthrogryposis multiplex congenita Non-progressive disease Normal intelligence	Good candidate for tendon transfer as the power of the transferred tendon will not deteriorate over time due to the non-progressive nature of the disease. The child should be able to co-operate with rehabilitation as her intelligence is good.

(Continued)

Table 11.1 (Continued)

Factors		Treatment Implications
The age of the child	14 years	Pubertal age—growth modulation by epiphyseodesis not feasible.[3,4]
The severity of knee deformity	40 degrees	Acute correction runs the risk of neuro-vascular stretch. Gradual correction with traction or external fixator may be considered. Alternatively, femoral shortening may be done.[6,7]
Muscle power of the quadriceps and the hamstrings	Quadriceps: Grade 2 Hamstrings: Grade 5	Muscle imbalance needs to be corrected to prevent recurrence of deformity. Tendon transfer (hamstring to quadriceps) could restore muscle balance and also the power of active knee extension.[10]
The side involved	Bilateral symmetric deformities	Bilateral femoral shortening will not result in limb length inequality.

How Was This Girl Treated?

The girl was treated with bilateral supracondylar femoral shortening and hamstring to quadriceps transfer. Once the osteotomy was performed, the fragments were allowed to overlap (Figure 11.4a, 11.4b). The flexion deformity could be corrected completely by merely shortening the femur, and hence the distal fragment was not extended. A segment of the femur of the same length as the extent of overlap of the fragment was excised (Figure 11.4c), and the fragments were fixed with contoured plates and screws. Bilateral triple arthrodesis was also done in the same sitting.

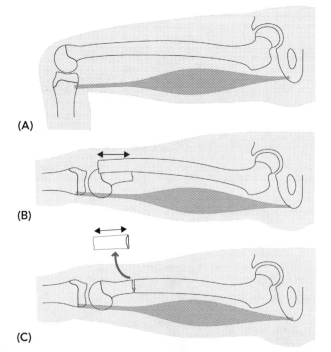

(A)

(B)

(C)

Figure 11.4 (A), (B), (C) The extent of overlap of the fragments and length of bone excised (double sided arrow)

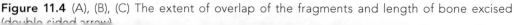

Post-Operative Management

Both lower limbs were protected in groin-to-toe casts for six weeks. Weight-bearing was permitted after three months when sound union of the femoral osteotomy was seen on radiographs (Figure 11.5a, 11.5b).

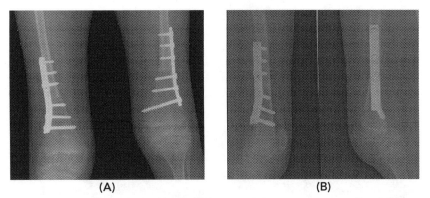

(A) (B)

Figure 11.5 Anteroposterior (A) and lateral (B) views show sound union of both femurs that were shortened.

Follow-Up

Active knee extension was restored, and deformities of the knees and feet were adequately corrected (Figure 11.6a, 11.6b). The girl began walking on her feet initially with ankle-foot orthoses and the support of a walker (Figure 11.7). The orthosis was discarded after a year. She gradually began walking independently and was walking well without the walker when last seen four years after the surgery, by which time she was skeletally mature.

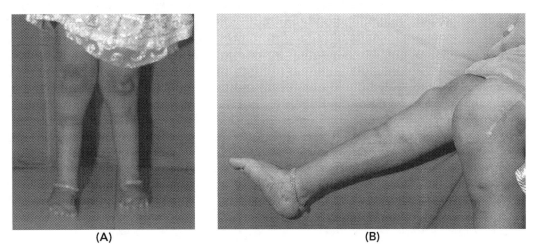

(A) (B)

Figure 11.6 Active knee extension has been restored (A), and the deformities are well corrected (B).

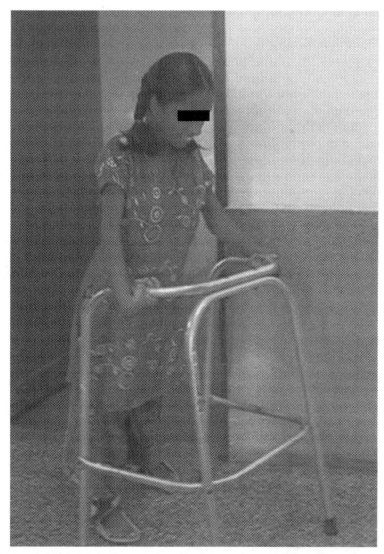

Figure 11.7 The child began walking with ankle-foot orthoses and a walker.

Comment

Later dorsal carpal wedge osteotomies were also performed to improve hand function.

References

1. Westberry DE, Davids JR, Jacobs JN, Pugh LI, Tanner SL. Effectiveness of serial stretch casting for resistant or recurrent flexion contractures following hamstring lengthening in children with cerebral palsy. *J Pediatr Orthop.* 2006;26:109–14.
2. Lampasi M, Antonioli D, Donzelli O. Management of knee deformities in children with arthrogryposis. *Musculoskelet Surg.* 2012;96(3):161–9. doi: 10.1007/s12306-012-0218-z.
3. Stiel N, Babin K, Vettorazzi E, et al. Anterior distal femoral hemiepiphysiodesis can reduce fixed flexion deformity of the knee: A retrospective study of 83 knees. *Acta Orthop.* 2018;89(5):555–9. doi: 10.1080/17453674.2018.1485418.

4. Klatt J, Stevens PM. Guided growth for fixed knee flexion deformity. *J Pediatr Orthop.* 2008;28(6):626–31. doi: 10.1097/BPO.0b013e318183d573.

5. Asirvatham R, Mukherjee A, Agarwal S, et al. Supracondylar femoral extension osteotomy: Its complications. *J Pediatr Orthop.* 1993;13:642–5.

6. Saleh M, Gibson MF, Sharrard WJ. Femoral shortening in correction of congenital knee flexion deformity with popliteal webbing. *J Pediatr Orthop.* 1989;9(5):609–11. doi: 10.1097/01241398-198909010-00020.

7. Joseph B, Reddy K, Varghese RA, Shah H, Doddabasappa SN. Management of severe crouch gait in children and adolescents with cerebral palsy. *J Pediatr Orthop.* 2010;30(8):832–9. doi: 10.1097/BPO.0b013e3181fbfd0e.

8. van Bosse HJ, Feldman DS, Anavian J, Sala DA. Treatment of knee flexion contractures in patients with arthrogryposis. *J Pediatr Orthop.* 2007;27(8):930–7. doi: 10.1097/bpo.0b013e3181594cd0.

9. Yang SS, Dahan-Oliel N, Montpetit K, Hamdy RC. Ambulation gains after knee surgery in children with arthrogryposis. *J Pediatr Orthop.* 2010;30(8):863–9. doi: 10.1097/BPO.0b013e3181f5a0c8.

10. Shahcheraghi GH, Javid M, Zeighami B. Hamstring tendon transfer for quadriceps femoris paralysis. *J Pediatr Orthop.* 1996;16(6):765–8. doi: 10.1097/00004694-199611000-00012.

Hitesh Shah

Case

A 17-year-old boy presented with a deformity of the right knee and shortening of the limb that had developed gradually and progressed over the course of five years following a traffic accident. The details of the exact nature of injury and treatment were not available apart from the fact that he was treated in a plaster cast for six weeks.

On examination, there was genu recurvatum of 30 degrees, and the normal prominence of the tibial tuberosity was not present (Figure 12.1a, 12.1b).

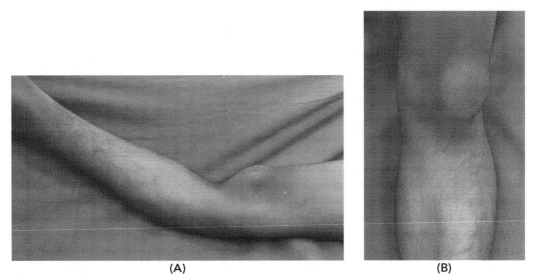

(A)　　　　　　　　　　　　　　　　　(B)

Figure 12.1 (A) Genu recurvatum (30 degrees) on the right side. (B) Normal prominence of the tibial tuberosity is absent.

Knee flexion was limited to 75 degrees. There was no coronal plane deformity at the knee. Shortening of 3 cm of the tibia was present. The lateral radiograph of the knee showed an abnormal forward inclination of the tibial articular surface (Figure 12.2a). The proximal tibial growth plate was completely fused, while the femoral and fibular growth plates were almost fused.

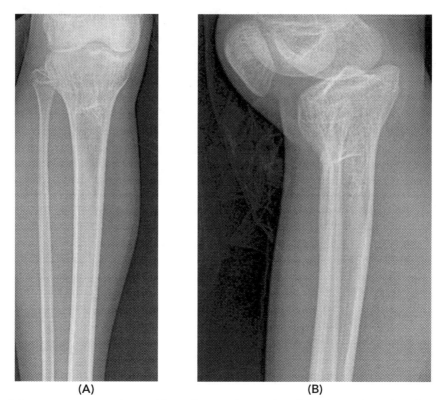

(A) (B)

Figure 12.2 Anteroposterior (A) and lateral (B) radiographs of the knee show that the growth plates of the femur and the fibula are almost fused, while the proximal tibial growth plate is completely fused.

Questions

- What are the problems that need to be addressed?
- What are the aims of treatment?
- What are the available treatment options to fulfil these aims?
- What are the factors that may influence your choice of treatment?
- Based on these points, what treatment would you recommend for this patient?

The Problems That Need to Be Addressed Are

- Genu recurvatum
- Limitation of knee flexion
- Shortening of the tibia

The Aims of Treatment in This Boy Are to

- Correct the genu recurvatum deformity
- Equalise limb lengths

Options for Treatment to Fulfil Each Aim

- Correction of the knee recurvatum deformity

    o Acute flexion osteotomy of the proximal tibia with an anterior open wedge[1]
    o Acute flexion osteotomy of the proximal tibia with a posterior closed wedge[2]
    o Gradual correction of the deformity with an external fixator[3,4,5]

- Equalising limb lengths

    o Lengthening of the short tibia
    o Shortening the opposite tibia

FACTORS THAT INFLUENCED THE CHOICE OF TREATMENT WERE

- The age of the boy and the degree of skeletal maturation
- The severity of deformity
- The presence of associated shortening of the tibia
- The amount of shortening

The choice of treatment based on these factors is shown in Table 12.1.

Table 12.1 Factors Influencing the Choice of Treatment

Factors		Treatment Implications
The age of the boy and the degree of skeletal maturation	17 years of age and virtually skeletally mature	Further progression of the deformity will not occur as the tibial growth plate is completely fused. Consequently, there is no risk of recurrence of deformity following correction. Options that entail growth modulation are not feasible since the growth plate is fused.

(Continued)

Table 12.1 (Continued)

Factors		Treatment Implications
The severity of deformity	30 degrees	Acute correction with an anterior open wedge runs the risk of excessive stretching of the skin over the proximal tibia and wound dehiscence. This complication can be avoided either by gradual correction with an external fixator or acute correction with a posterior closing wedge.
The presence of associated shortening of the tibia and severity of shortening	3 cm of shortening at skeletal maturity	Since limb length equalisation and deformity correction are required, a single procedure that can tackle both should be the preferred option. Though limb length inequality of 3 cm at skeletal maturity may be corrected by shortening of the contralateral tibia, it entails surgery on both the limbs since the deformity also needs correction. Gradual deformity correction combined with limb lengthening with the aid of an external fixator is the most acceptable option.[5]

How Was This Boy Treated?

The boy was treated with an osteotomy of the proximal tibia, gradual correction of the deformity and lengthening of the proximal tibia. An Orthofix Garches clamp was used to facilitate precise correction of the abnormal inclination of the tibial articular surface (Figure 12.3a, 12.3b). The clamp was applied parallel to the tibial articular surface and as the deformity was corrected, the clamp tilted the articular surface backwards and restored the normal alignment (Figure 12.4a, 12.4b).

Post-Operative Management

Distraction was begun 10 days after the osteotomy was performed and proceeded at the rate of 1 mm per day. After gaining 1 cm, the sagittal plane correction was done gradually. Once the sagittal deformity was corrected, another 2 cm lengthening was done. Excellent regenerate formed in the osteotomy gap (Figure 12.5a–12.5d). The external fixator was removed after the regenerate consolidated (Figure 12.5d).

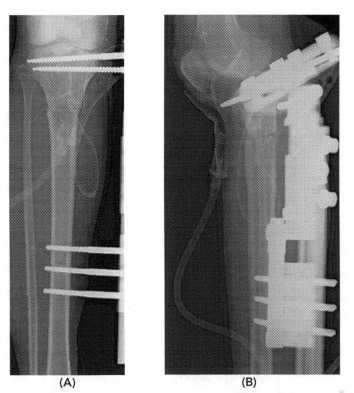

(A)   (B)

Figure 12.3 Post-operative anteroposterior (A) and lateral (B) radiographs show the proximal tibial osteotomy.

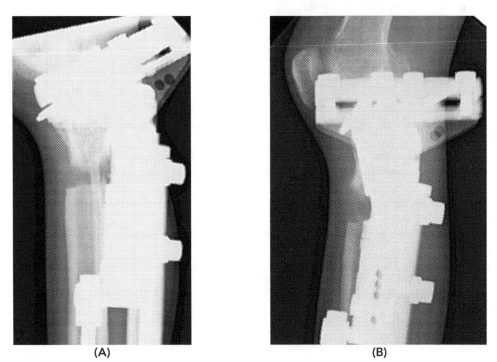

(A)   (B)

Figure 12.4 (A) The lateral radiograph shows straight distraction in progress. (B) Correction of the sagittal plane deformity was achieved after initial straight distraction.

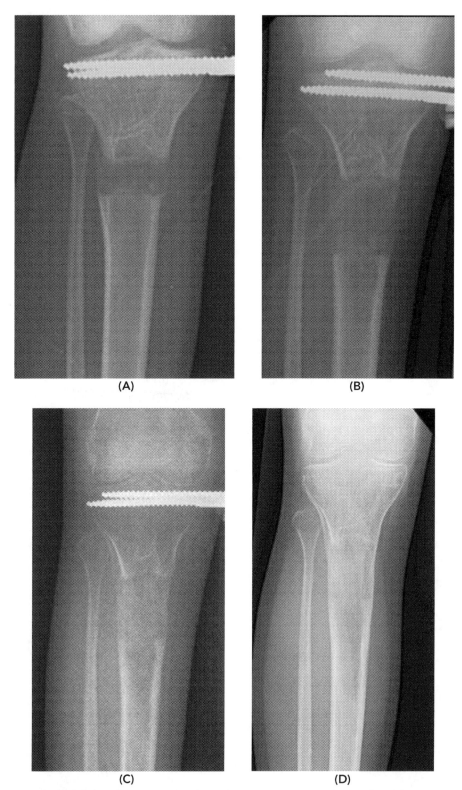

(A)

(B)

(C)

(D)

Figure 12.5a–12.5d Serial radiographs show distraction osteogenesis at the proximal tibia with good regenerate formation.

Follow-Up

One year later, the genu recurvatum and the shortening were corrected, and 120 degrees of knee flexion was possible (Figure 12.6). He had normal function of the limb.

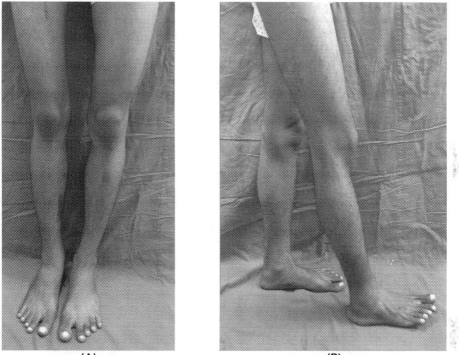

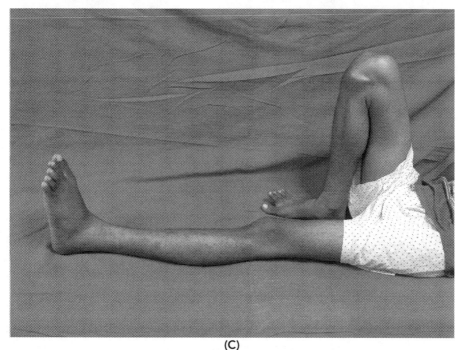

Figure 12.6 Full extension and flexion of the knee were present at skeletal maturity.

References

1. Moroni A, Pezzuto V, Pompili M, Zinghi G. Proximal osteotomy of the tibia for treatment of genu recurvatum in adults. *J Bone Joint Surg Am*. 1992;74:577–86.
2. Bowen JR, Morley DC, McInerny Y, MacEwen GD. Treatment of genu recurvatum by proximal tibial closing wedge/anterior displacement osteotomy. *Clin Orthop Relat Res*. 1983;179:194–9.
3. O'Dwyer KJ, MacEachern AG, Pennig D. Corrective tibial osteotomy for genu recurvatum by callus distraction using an external fixator. *Chir Organi Mov*. 1991;76(4):355–8.
4. Choi IH, Chung CY, Cho TJ, Park SS. Correction of genu recurvatum by the Ilizarov method. *J Bone Joint Surg Br*. 1999;81:769–74.
5. Domzalski M, Mackenzie W. Growth arrest of the proximal tibial physis with recurvatum and valgus deformity of the knee. *Knee*. 2009;16(5):412–16.

Nicholas Peterson, Christopher Prior, Selvadurai Nayagam

Case

This adolescent girl with a family history of hypophosphataemic X-linked rickets presented with a deformity of the right knee. The condition was diagnosed early in childhood with bilateral lower limb deformities managed successfully with intermittent use of guided growth through implantation of 8-plates. Just prior to her 13th birthday, recurrence of her lower limb deformities was noted.

Correction was recommended with one side being treated at a time, and treatment of the left side was successfully completed prior to the current presentation.

Clinical inspection showed a mild degree of short stature and varus alignment of the right leg. She walked with a lateral thrust on the right knee during the stance phase. The right knee had no tender areas and had a full range of movement. Stressing into varus with the knee held in slight flexion demonstrated some laxity of the lateral restraints of the knee joint.

Standing x-rays confirmed the varus alignment of the right lower limb with 8-plates from previous surgery remaining in situ (Figure 13.1). Deformity analysis showed that distal femoral and

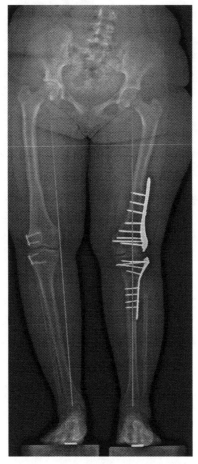

Figure 13.1 Standing full-length views showing a normal mechanical axis on the left lower limb post–corrective surgery and medial axis deviation on the right side.

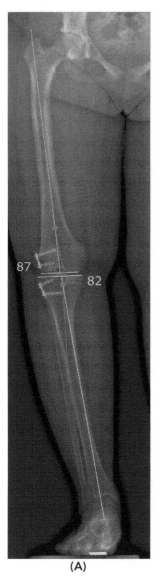
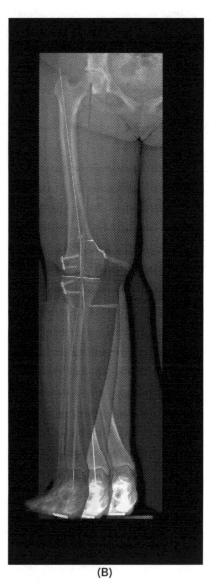

(A)   (B)

Figures 13.2a–13.2b Deformity analysis using population-based normal values indicates deformities in the distal femur and proximal tibia with CORAs located as shown (red dots). Simulation of correction shows a cumulative improvement in the position of the mechanical axis with each level of correction. The intermediate position in the simulation is the contribution from the femoral correction and the final position after the tibial correction is added (A). This final image confirms that normalising the position of the mechanical axis is best achieved by osteotomies of both femur and tibia.

proximal tibial deformities (anatomical LDFA 87°; MPTA 82°) were contributing to the genu varum (Figures 13.2a, 13.2b). The CORA of the deformities was identified using population-based average values as the basis for normal knee alignment (anatomical LDFA 81°; MPTA 87°). A lateral x-ray of the femur showed that there was a procurvatum deformity in the lower half of the femur (Figure 13.3). Assessment of bone age suggested that there was less than two years of growth remaining before skeletal maturity.

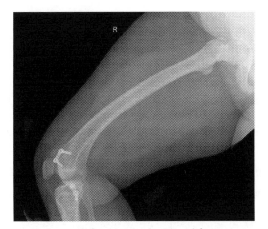

Figure 13.3 There is a procurvatum deformity in the distal femur.

Questions

- What are the problems that need to be addressed in this girl?
- What are the aims of treatment?
- What are the commonly available options for treatment?
- What are the factors that may influence your choice of treatment?
- What treatment would you recommend for this girl?

The Problems That Need to Be Addressed

- Varus deformity of the right knee that has resulted in:
  - An abnormal mechanical axis of the right lower limb
  - Lateral thrust arising from an adduction moment at the knee
  - Risk of gradual stretching of ligamentous and capsular restraints on the lateral side of the knee
- Procurvatum deformity of the right femur

The Aims of Treatment Are to

- Correct the relevant deformities in the femur and tibia such that the mechanical axis is restored to normal.
- Correct the mechanical axis sufficiently to eliminate the knee adduction moment.

Options for Treatment of Genu Varum

- Guided growth[1]
- Osteotomy[2–4]

FACTORS THAT INFLUENCED THE CHOICE OF TREATMENT

- Age of the patient
- Site of deformity
- Associated deformities in other planes
- The patient's preference to avoid external fixation
- Outcome of previous treatment on the contralateral side

The choice of treatment based on these factors is outlined in Table 13.1.

Table 13.1 Factors That Influenced the Choice of Treatment

Factors		Treatment Implications
Age of the patient	13 years—approaching skeletal maturity	Guided growth is not a feasible option as there is too little growth remaining for temporary epiphyseodesis to be effective.
Site of deformity	The distal femur and the proximal tibia are contributing to the deformity	The deformity components in both the femur and the tibia need to be addressed.
Associated deformities in other planes	Procurvatum deformity of the distal femur	Since deformities in two planes are present, correction with the Ilizarov external fixator is a good option.
Patient's preference	The patient will not accept treatment with an external fixator	Osteotomies with acute correction and internal fixation are the only available option in this patient.
Outcome of previous treatment on the contralateral side	The opposite limb was treated with osteotomies and acute correction and external fixator-assisted internal fixation	Since the outcome of treatment of the opposite limb was very satisfactory, the same strategies may justifiably be followed.

How Was the Girl Treated?

The chosen method of treatment was acute correction of deformities by osteotomies and external fixator-assisted internal fixation. This method allows the surgery to be performed in a minimally invasive fashion which, in turn, facilitates recovery. The external fixator is used only intra-operatively to hold and adjust the osteotomy to the desired degree of correction, at which point internal fixation is substituted.

Femur

A rail fixator was used to facilitate compression across the osteotomy prior to internal fixation. The fixator was applied from the medial side (Figure 13.4a). The half-pins were inserted with care to avoid injury to the neurovascular structures (Figure 13.4b). The external fixator was positioned out of the way of the intended internal fixation and substitution carried out whilst the fixator was still holding the corrected deformity under compression.

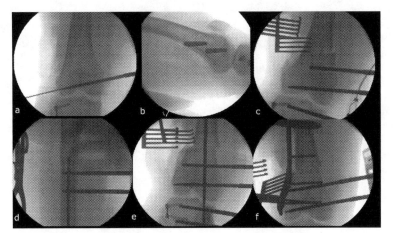

Figures 13.4a–13.4f A sequence of intra-operative x-ray images showing how the rail fixator is applied on the medial side both distal (A) and proximal (D) to the intended osteotomy in the femur. Accurate positioning of the half-pins will allow both coronal and sagittal plane deformities to be corrected acutely after osteotomy (A–D). Lateral translation of the osteotomy (the CORA is proximal to the osteotomy) can be adjusted to optimum (E). The rail fixator can compress the osteotomy in the desired position whilst a plate is applied using the minimally invasive percutaneous plate osteosynthesis (MIPO) technique from the lateral side (F).

The osteotomy was performed through a limited distal femoral incision on the lateral side (Figure 13.4c) The osteotomy was compressed through the fixator and the desired degree of correction confirmed by x-ray (Figures 13.4d, 13.4e). The plate was applied in the extra-periosteal, submuscular plane and fixed without compression (none is needed as this is maintained by the fixator) (Figure 13.4f). The fixator was then removed, and wounds closed.

Tibia

There was a coronal deformity with the CORA at the level of the proximal tibial physis (Figure 13.2a).

The position of the CORA was identified on intra-operative x-ray and a half-pin inserted at this point (Figures 13.5a, 13.5b). With the appropriate sleeve through a Rancho cube placed over this half-pin, a check was then made to see if the holes in the cube were able to trace out a curve centred around the pin (Figures 13.5c, 13.6). Multiple drill holes were made through this hole using drill sleeves (Figures 13.5d, 13.7). The external fixator was applied from the medial side with two half-pins proximal to and two distal to the intended dome osteotomy. An osteotomy of the fibula was made in the proximal third. The half-pins of the rail fixator were inserted in the coronal plane (Figures 13.5e, 13.5f, 13.8).

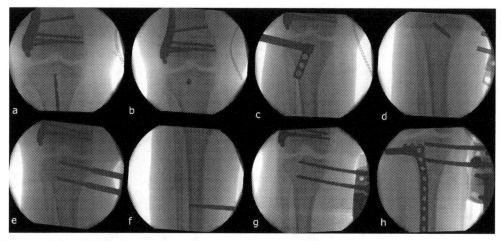

Figures 13.5a–13.5h A sequence of intra-operative x-ray images showing the creation of a dome osteotomy and the application of the rail fixator in the coronal plane from the medial side. The half-pin which mimics the axis of correction of angulation (ACA) placed over the CORA allows a Rancho cube to be rotated about it as a centre (A, B). X-ray screening of this will determine which holes of the Rancho cube are best suited for drilling out the dome osteotomy (C, D). The fixator half-pins are inserted in the coronal plane from the medial side (E, F). After the osteotomy is completed and the desired position obtained, compression can be applied by the fixator before the submuscular plate is fixed from the lateral side (G, H).

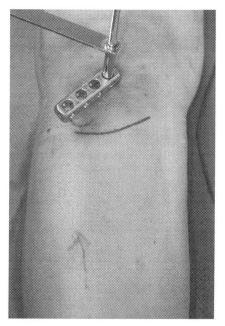

Figure 13.6 Once the decision has been made as to which hole in the Rancho cube is to be used, the curve of prospective drill holes can be marked on the skin and the incision made accordingly.

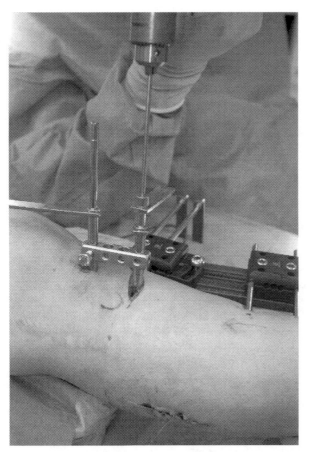

Figure 13.7 Drilling along the curve determined by the Rancho cube rotating around the ACA of the half-pin inserted at the CORA. Care should be taken, and lateral x-ray views carefully observed to avoid over-penetration of the posterior tibial cortex.

The osteotomy was performed by connecting the drill holes and distracted by the fixator to ensure it was complete. Acute correction of angulation was performed, and the osteotomy was compressed (Figure 13.5g). Incisions at the level of proximal and mid-tibia were made, the plane deep to tibialis anterior was developed, and a proximal lateral tibial plate was inserted in this submuscular plane (Figure 13.5h). The plate was fixed in neutral as the compression was maintained by the fixator. The fixator was removed and the wounds closed (Figure 13.9).

Post-Operative Management

Partial weight-bearing was permitted as soon as the patient was comfortable. X-rays at 6 and 12 weeks recorded the progress of healing and restoration of normal alignment of both lower limbs (Figure 13.10).

Comment

Many conditions result in deformities in the coronal and sagittal planes; it is with the former that symptoms arise as both ankle and knee joints compensate well for deformities in the sagittal plane. The minimally invasive method of guided growth is effective in the growing child for

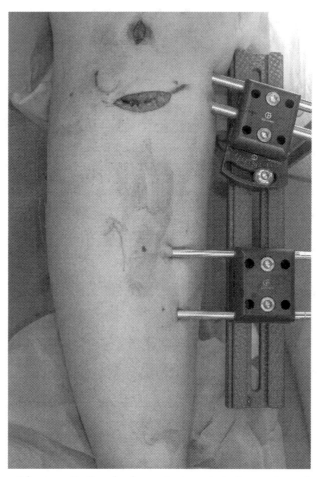

Figure 13.8 The rail fixator will allow for fine adjustments to be made and compression applied across the osteotomy.

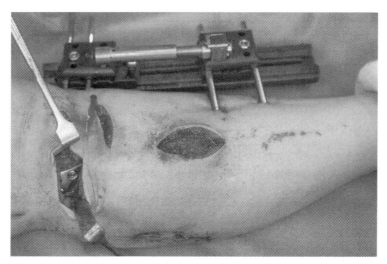

Figure 13.9 Two incisions allow for submuscular plating of the osteotomy. The third anterior incision is that for the dome osteotomy. The sutured incision postero-laterally is that which allowed for the fibular osteotomy.

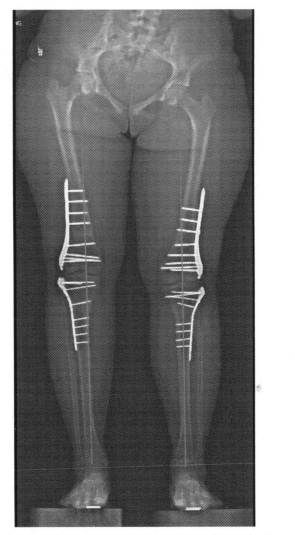

Figure 13.10 Standing full-length view showing a normal mechanical axis on both lower limbs.

coronal plane deformities around the knee. The pre-requisite is that the child has at least two years (and preferably three years) of growth remaining and that the physis is working normally. Correction by osteotomy is applicable at any age. It is a more invasive procedure but is able to address sagittal plane elements of the deformity also. The methods by which this can be achieved include by creating wedges (open or closed) or by use of a dome technique; fixation of the osteotomy can be by means of internal or external fixation.[2-4]

Much concern is raised about the need for bone grafting when performing open-wedge osteotomies; this can be avoided simply by good contact achieved by compression of the osteotomy and the care taken to preserve biological reserve for healing through the minimal access osteotomy and the nature of percutaneous osteosynthesis.

References

1. Stevens PM, Novais EN. Multilevel guided growth for hip and knee varus secondary to chondrodysplasia. *J Pediatr Orthop*. 2012;32(6):626–30.
2. Takahashi T, Wada Y, Tanaka M, Iwagawa M, Ikeuchi M, Hirose D, et al. Dome-shaped proximal tibial osteotomy using percutaneous drilling for osteoarthritis of the knee. *Arch Orthop Trauma Surg*. 2000;120(1–2):32–7.
3. Amer AR, Khanfour AA. Evaluation of treatment of late-onset tibia vara using gradual angulation translation high tibial osteotomy. *Acta Orthop Belg*. 2010;76(3):360–6.
4. Park YE, Song SH, Kwon HN, Refai MA, Park KW, Song HR. Gradual correction of idiopathic genu varum deformity using the Ilizarov technique. *Knee Surg Sports Traumatol Arthrosc*. 2013;21(7):1523–9.

Christopher Prior, Nicholas Peterson, Selvadurai Nayagam

Case

A 12-year-old girl presented with pain on the medial and anterior aspects of both knees related to exertion. There was no significant past medical history and no previous trauma. No symptoms of instability, swelling, giving way or locking were described. The girl had not attained menarche.

Clinical examination showed bilateral symmetrical genu valgum. There was mild femoral anteversion, but otherwise the rotational profile was unremarkable. There was tenderness over the medial aspect of the proximal right tibia without evidence of swelling or erythema. The patella and knee ligaments were stable to stress-testing (Figure 14.1).

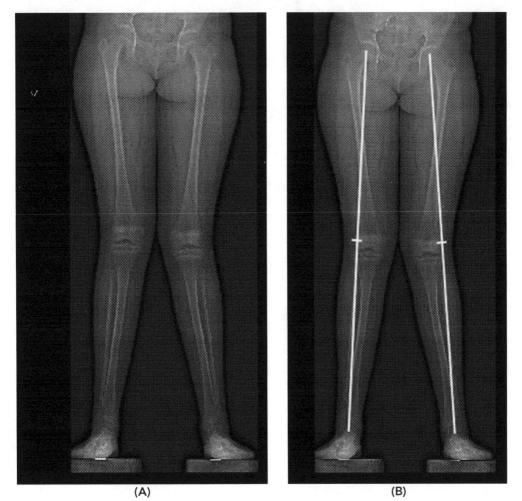

(A)   (B)

Figure 14.1 Weight-bearing AP x-rays demonstrating lateral mechanical axis deviation and the mechanical Lateral Distal Femoral Angle (mLDFA) and Medial Proximal Tibial Angle (MPTA) on both sides.

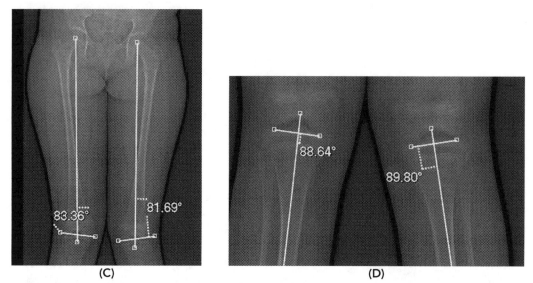

(C) **(D)**

Figure 14.1 (Continued)

A full-length standing AP EOS x-ray revealed bilateral valgus knee alignment with lateral mechanical axis deviation. The mechanical lateral distal femoral angles (mLDFA) were 83° and 82° (normal values 87° ± 3°), and the medial proximal tibial angles (MPTA) were 89° and 90° (normal values 87° ± 3°).[1]

X-rays of the knees were otherwise normal with no suggestion of metabolic bone disease or skeletal dysplasia. MRI of the knees did not reveal any significant pathology within bone or over the pes anserinus on the right side. The cause of pain was attributed to repeated stresses on the medial collateral ligament and medial capsular structures while walking and running.

Questions

- What are the problems related to the right lower limb that need to be addressed in this girl?
- What are the aims of treatment?
- What are the available options for treatment?
- What are the factors that may influence your choice of treatment?
- What treatment would you recommend for this girl?

The Problems That Need to Be Addressed

- Deformity of both knees with mechanical axis deviation
- Bilateral anterior knee pain and pain on the medial aspect of both knees
- Awkward appearance of the limbs
- Abnormal loading of the knees with potential long-term adverse effects

The Aims of Treatment

- Correct the deformities and restore normal mechanical axes of the limbs[2] with the hope of

  o Relieving knee pain
  o Improving the cosmetic appearance
  o Restoring normal loading of the knee

Options for Treatment

- Hemi-epiphyseodesis

  o Medial distal femur
  o Medial proximal tibia
  o Both femur and tibia

- Osteotomy

FACTORS THAT INFLUENCED THE CHOICE OF TREATMENT

- The age of the patient
- Natural history of the deformity
- Site of the deformity
- Status of the growth plates
- Nature of surgery

The factors that influenced the choice of treatment are outlined in Table 14.1.

Table 14.1 Choice of Treatment Based on the Factors Influencing Treatment

Factors		Treatment Implications
Age of the patient	12 years	Spontaneous resolution of physiologic genu valgum may be expected till around the age of 7 years. Thereafter, no resolution occurs. Hence, intervention in this girl is justified.
		Since there is sufficient growth remaining, growth modulation by temporary epiphyseodesis is worth attempting. However, the intervention should not be delayed further as the window of opportunity will close soon.

(Continued)

Table 14.1 (Continued)

Factors		Treatment Implications
Natural history of the deformity	Idiopathic genu valgum	Since there is no underlying metabolic disease or skeletal dysplasia, the deformity is not likely to progress.
Site of the deformity	The deformity is in the distal femur with no contribution from the proximal tibia	Since the deformity is in the distal femur, surgery should be on the femur only.
Status of the growth plates	Healthy growth plates	Guided growth works more predictably if the growth plate is healthy.
Nature of surgery	Guided growth versus osteotomy	Guided growth is far less invasive and far simpler than an osteotomy.

How Was the Child Treated?

Under general anaesthesia with tourniquets, the distal femoral physis was identified and the level marked using fluoroscopy. A small medial longitudinal incision was made centred on the level previously marked. The vastus medialis muscle was identified and retracted anteriorly off the periosteum with care. Attention was paid to avoid injury to the saphenous vein and nerve, medial patellofemoral ligament, the physis and the perichondral ring as inadvertent dissection of the physis could cause permanent growth disturbance.

The 16 mm 8-plate was positioned centrally over the physis on the AP fluoroscopy image and in the centre of the distal femoral physis on the lateral view; it was held in place with a 21-gauge needle inserted through the central hole of the plate directly into the physis. A threaded guidewire was then passed through the centre of the distal hole into the epiphysis, ensuring that the 8-plate was perpendicular to the physis and that the wire was parallel or divergent from the physis. A second threaded guidewire was passed into the metaphysis through the proximal hole of the 8-plate, ensuring that the trajectory would not enter the physis. Two cannulated screws, about one-third the length of the physis, were inserted over the guidewires after some initial pre-drilling. The guidewires were extracted at the end (Figure 14.2).

Final fluoroscopy checks were made to confirm satisfactory location of the plates and the knee flexed and extended to ensure that no soft tissues were trapped or inhibited. A small piece of bone wax was inserted into the cannulated hole at the end of each screw as a plug to prevent intramedullary bleeding into the surrounding tissues. Local anaesthesia was infiltrated around the periosteum before closure.

Post-Operative Management

Post-operative physiotherapy and full weight-bearing with assistance were started on recovery from anaesthesia. At 10 days post-surgery, the wounds were checked and the recovery of knee movements confirmed to be full.

Standing full-length EOS x-ray images were obtained at three months to ensure that the plates were still in the correct position and to monitor for rapid corrections that can occur during growth spurts (Figure 14.3).

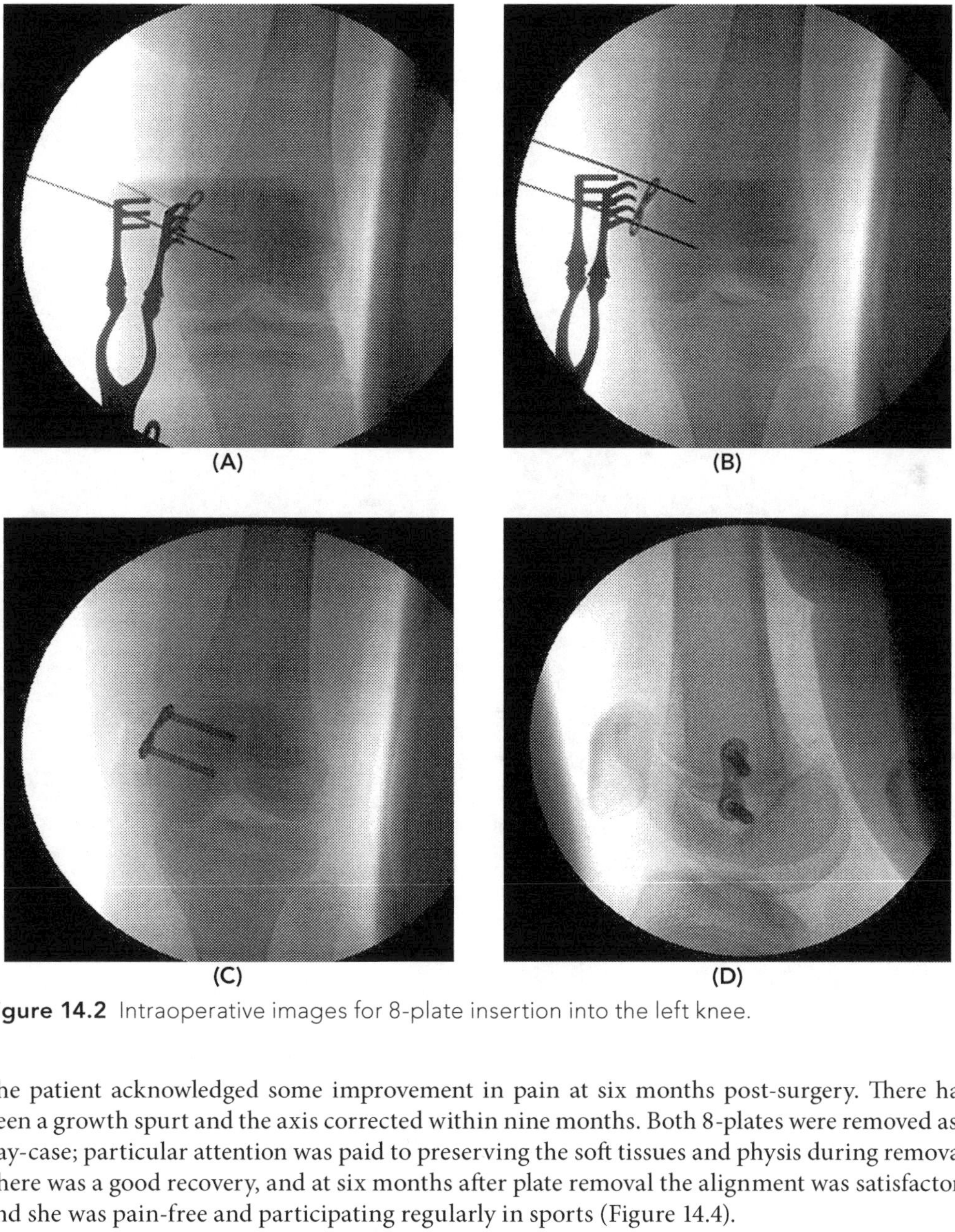

Figure 14.2 Intraoperative images for 8-plate insertion into the left knee.

The patient acknowledged some improvement in pain at six months post-surgery. There had been a growth spurt and the axis corrected within nine months. Both 8-plates were removed as a day-case; particular attention was paid to preserving the soft tissues and physis during removal. There was a good recovery, and at six months after plate removal the alignment was satisfactory and she was pain-free and participating regularly in sports (Figure 14.4).

Comment

Femoral 8-plates correct at an average of 0.7° per month and the tibia corrects at 0.5° per month.[3] Approximately 6° of correction were required on the right knee and 8 on the left. With the patient's age at 12 years and being pre-menarche, there was sufficient time to correct the alignment with femoral 8-plates alone.

The association between lower limb malalignment and future osteoarthritis, in particular the threshold above which intervention is warranted, is controversial.[4] Mild asymptomatic genu valgum in a younger child can be monitored. In this case, there were symptoms, and the mechanical axes were almost outside the lateral compartment of the knee.

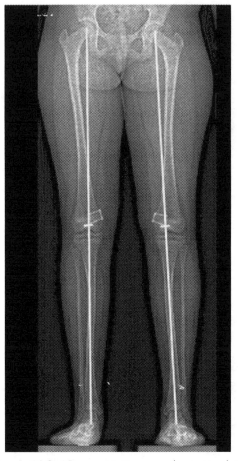 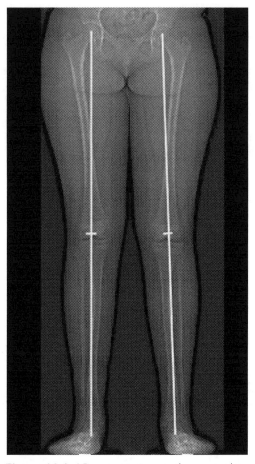

Figure 14.3 AP x-ray at nine months post–plate insertion.

Figure 14.4 AP x-ray at six months post–plate removal.

References

1. Popkov D, Lascombes P, Berte N, Hetzel L, Baptista BR, Popkov A, Journeau P. The normal radiological anteroposterior alignment of the lower limb in children. *Skeletal Radiol.* 2015 Feb;44(2):197–206. doi: 10.1007/s00256-014-1953-z. Epub 2014 Jul 5. PMID: 24997161.
2. Farr S, Kranzl A, Pablik E, Kaipel M, Ganger R. Functional and radiographic consideration of lower limb malalignment in children and adolescents with idiopathic genu valgum. *J Orthop Res.* 2014; 32(10):1362–70.
3. Ballal MS, Bruce CE, Nayagam S. Correcting genu varum and genu valgum in children by guided growth: Temporary hemiepiphysiodesis using tension band plates. *J Bone Joint Surg Br.* 2010 Feb;92(2):273–6.
4. McClure PK, Herzenberg JE. The natural history of lower extremity malalignment. *J Pediatr Orthop.* 2019;39:S14–9. doi: 10.1097/BPO.0000000000001361.

CASE 15: COXA VARA

Leo Donnan

Case

This 4-year-old boy had been attending the facio-maxillary clinic for a minor cleft palate when his parents raised the issue about his short stature and waddling gait. A referral to orthopaedics was made, where he was noted to be below the 1st percentile for height and mild disproportion between his limb and truncal height. He had exaggerated lumbar lordosis and genu valgum. He walked with a waddling gait and complained of tiring easily.

His parents gave no family history of any significant musculoskeletal problems, and his two older siblings were of normal stature and health.

The hip examination was grossly abnormal on both sides with fixed flexion deformities of 15° and further flexion being limited to 100°. Passive hip abduction was only 10° while the hips could be adducted to 60°. Internal and external rotations in extension were within the normal ranges.

The clinical features of proportionate dwarfism were consistent with an underlying bone dysplasia involving both the trunk and extremities. A skeletal survey confirmed the diagnosis of spondyloepiphyseal dysplasia (Figure 15.1). The pelvic radiograph showed complete lack of ossification of the capital femoral epiphysis and suggestion of severe coxa vara with Hilgenreiner epiphyseal (HE) angles >60° on both sides (Figure 15.2).

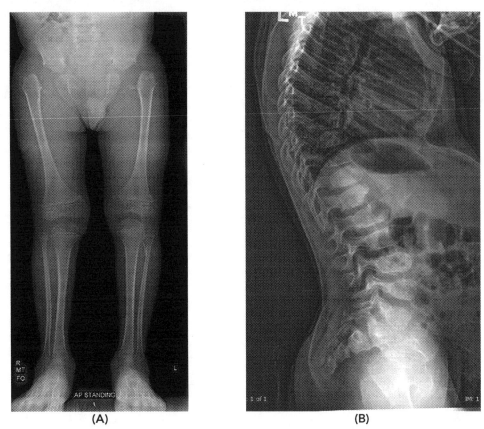

(A)   (B)

Figure 15.1 (A) Generalised epiphyseal changes indicative of a skeletal dysplasia. (B) Platyspondyly, anterior beaking of the vertebral bodies and exaggerated lumbar lordosis.

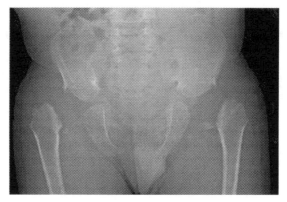

Figure 15.2 Elevated Hilgenreiner epiphyseal angles on both sides.

An arthrogram was performed to assess the shape of the femoral head, its congruency with the acetabulum and how it might respond to a corrective osteotomy (Figure 15.3a, b, c).

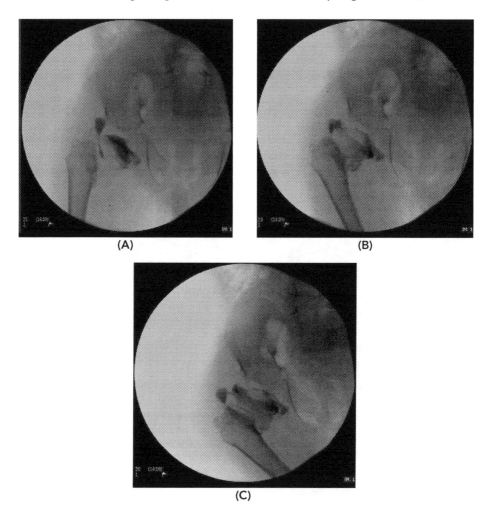

Figure 15.3 Dynamic arthrogram of the hip shows a large un-ossified cartilaginous anlage of the femoral head and neck. The joint is subluxated and incongruous in the neutral position (A). Adduction of the hip considerably improves both the congruency and stability (B, C).

Questions

- What are the problems that need to be addressed in this child?
- What are the aims of treatment?
- What are the available treatment options to fulfil these aims?
- What are the factors that may influence your choice of treatment?
- Based on these points, what treatment would you recommend for this child?
- How long would you follow-up this child after treatment?

The Problems That Need to Be Addressed Are

- Coxa vara (Hilgenreiner epiphyseal angle greater than 60°)

    o   Abductor mechanism dysfunction producing a Trendelenburg gait
    o   Relative trochanteric overgrowth
    o   Hip joint incongruity that can potentially hasten development of degenerative arthrosis
    o   Propensity of progression of coxa vara if untreated and potential risk of recurrence following correction
    o   Propensity to develop genu valgum[1]

- Fixed flexion deformity of the hip

    o   Exaggeration of lumbar lordosis

Aims of Treatment in This Case Are to

- Correct the coxa vara and thereby:

    o   Halt the progression of deformity
    o   Improve the proximal femoral anatomy and mechanics

        ☐   Improve the HE angles
        ☐   Improve the relative trochanteric overgrowth

    o   Reduce the hip joint into a stable position

- Reduce the fixed flexion deformity and thereby:

    o   Reduce the lumbar lordosis

Options for Treatment

- Correct coxa vara

    o   Valgus intertrochanteric femoral osteotomy[2]
    o   Valgus and extension intertrochanteric femoral osteotomy

- Reduce the relative trochanteric overgrowth

    o   Trochanteric epiphyseodesis

        ☐   Drilling of the growth plate
        ☐   Screw epiphyseodesis

FACTORS THAT INFLUENCE THE CHOICE OF TREATMENT

- Age and stature of the child
- Underlying cause of the deformity
- Site of the deformity
- Severity of the deformity
- Range of hip motion
- Presence of degenerative changes
- Other associated medical issues

The choice of treatment based on these factors is outlined in Table 15.1.

Table 15.1 Factors that influenced the choice of treatment

Factors		Treatment Implications
Age and stature	4 year-old with severe short stature	Choice of implant may be limited due to the small size of the bone, and alternative techniques involving fixation with K-wires may be required.[3]
Underlying cause	Spondyloepiphyseal dysplasia	Coxa vara associated with bone dysplasia is likely to progress and may have less reliable treatment outcomes due to abnormal articular collagen.[4]
Site of the deformity	Poor epiphyseal development	Physeal and metaphyseal deformities are more appropriately treated by intertrochanteric rather than sub-trochanteric osteotomies.
Severity of the deformity	HE angle greater that 60°	The high HE angle results in a vertical shearing stress on the physis with the likelihood for progression. When high angles are combined with defective cartilage structure, progression is usually rapid and severe.[5]
Range of hip motion	There is a significant reduction in abduction and a fixed flexion deformity. Importantly, the range of passive adduction is 60° while the passive flexion is only 100°	It is imperative to know that there is enough hip range of motion in the plane of correction being undertaken. A valgus osteotomy requires a good range of adduction which is present. An extension osteotomy requires near normal range of flexion which is only 100°. Excessive reduction of hip flexion by an extension osteotomy could make sitting difficult.
Presence of degenerative changes	The plain radiographs and the arthrogram did not show features of degenerative changes	Degenerative changes of the hip may preclude a proximal femoral osteotomy due to limited range of motion or the risk of worsening the hip loading and accelerating the degenerative process.
Other associated medical issues	Type II collagen disorder due to defects in COL2A1 gene	Spondyloepiphyseal dysplasia affects Type II collagen and is therefore associated with joint laxity. This may lead to cervical spine instability underlining the importance of a thorough screening of the spine prior to any anaesthesia.[6]

How Was This Child Treated?

The arthrogram showed that the hip reduced in adduction with improved congruency in this position. It was planned to perform a valgus osteotomy to reduce the HE angle to 30° and add in 15° of extension using a paediatric blade plate.

With the patient in a supine position, a lateral approach was used to expose the proximal femur. The leg was adducted to 60° and a guide passed high into the trochanter parallel to Hilgenreiner's line up to the level of the physis. The position was checked to be central in the femoral neck by the frog lateral view and the length of blade required determined.

The seating chisel was then passed using the K-wire as a guide and with 15° of extension. A transverse intertrochanteric osteotomy was made, and the definitive blade plate applied to hold the correction without performing any bony resection (Figure 15.4).

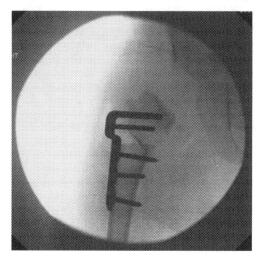

Figure 15.4 Intra-operative correction.

Post-Operative Management

The child spent four weeks in a wheelchair before being mobilised with a walking frame. Once union was solid, a program of abductor muscle strengthening and gait training was implemented.

Follow-Up

Long term follow-up is essential for these types of patients as recurrence of deformity is common[4] and joint degeneration may occur as part of the condition. Twelve months after the surgery (Figure 15.5), the blade plates were removed, and an arthrogram confirmed that the hips were well corrected and stable.

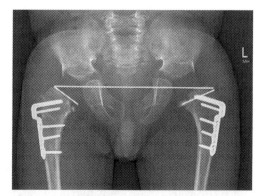

Figure 15.5 Healed osteotomies with improved HE angles just prior to removal of the implants.

At age 9, it was noted that his gait was deteriorating and that the coxa vara was recurring, and a further correction is planned. He was yet to develop a secondary ossification centre in his femoral heads. Following further correction the child must be followed, till skeletal maturity as the risk of recurrence persists and even into adulthood because of the risk of premature degenerative arthritis.

References

1. Shim J, Kim H, Mubarak S, Wenger D. Genu valgum in children with coxa vara resulting from hip disease. *Journal of Pediatric Orthopaedics*. 1997 Mar/Apr;17(2):225–9.
2. Key JA. The classic: Epiphyseal coxa vara or displacement of the capital epiphysis of the femur in adolescence. *Clin Orthop Relat Res*. 2013;471(7):2087–117.
3. Abdelaziz TH, El-Sayed MM. Pauwels' osteotomy for surgical correction of infantile coxa vara. *J Pediatric Orthop B*. 2012;21(4):325–30.
4. Oh C-W, Thacker MM, Mackenzie WG, Riddle EC. Coxa vara. *Clinical Orthopaedics and Related Research*. 2006 Jun;447:125–31.
5. Srisaarn T, Salang K, Klawson B, Vipulakorn K, Chalayon O, Eamsobhana P. Surgical correction of coxa vara: Evaluation of neck shaft angle, Hilgenreiner-epiphyseal angle for indication of recurrence. *J Clin Orthop Trauma*. 2018;10(3):593–8.
6. Fassier F, Sardar Z, Aarabi M, Odent T, Haque T, Hamdy R. Results and complications of a surgical technique for correction of coxa vara in children with osteopenic bones. *J Pediatr Orthop*. 2008;28(8):799–805.

Leo Donnan

Case

At the age of 15, this adolescent girl was experiencing activity-related aching in both groins and intermittent left patellar instability. She was tall for her age and had always been noted to be awkward when walking and running, and she often tripped when she was younger. There was no relevant family history, and her development appeared to have been normal.

When examined, she was noted to walk with in-toeing with a 15° internal foot progression angle and her patellae "squinted" (Figure 16.1a, b). She had mild ligament laxity, a straight spine and no evidence of spinal dysraphism.

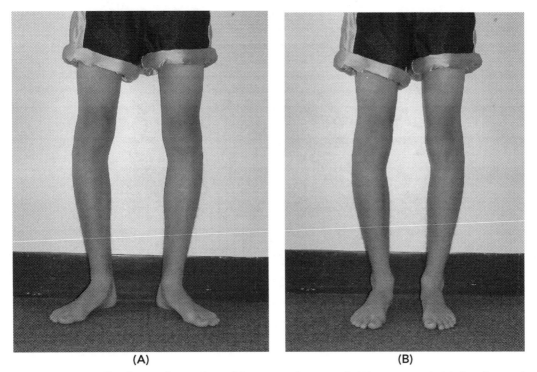

(A)   (B)

Figure 16.1 Patellae facing forwards and feet turned outwards (A) compared with feet forward and patellae turned inward (B).

Measurement of the rotational profile of her lower limbs revealed that with the hips in extension there was 90° of internal rotation and −10° of external rotation, the thigh-foot angles were 10° external on both sides, and the lateral borders of her feet were straight. Examination of her hips, knees and feet was otherwise normal except for mild patellar subluxation in extension with a positive J sign. Neurological examination was normal.

Radiological examination including a standing long leg radiograph and a CT scan to assess the rotational profile of the lower limbs were done (Figures 16.2 and 16.3).[1]

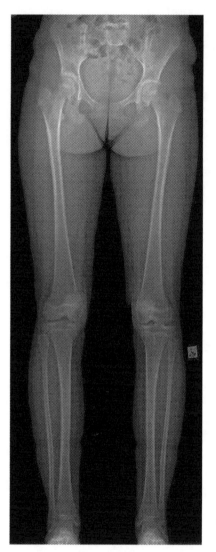

Figure 16.2 Mechanical axis radiograph of her lower limbs showed a normal profile with internally rotated patellae.

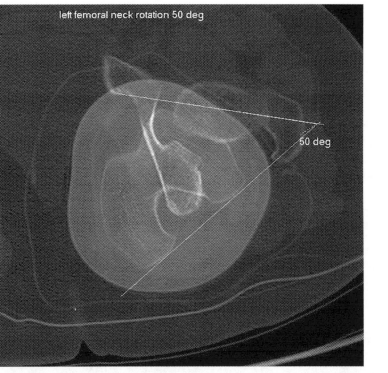

left femoral neck rotation 50 deg

50 deg

Figure 16.3 CT scan for rotational profile showing 50° of femoral anteversion on the gunsight views.[1]

Questions

- What are the problems that need to be addressed?
- What are the aims of treatment?
- What are the available treatment options to fulfil these aims?
- What are the factors that may influence your choice of treatment?
- Based on these points, what treatment would you recommend for this girl?

The Problems That Need to Be Addressed Are

- Excessive femoral anteversion

    - Awkward in-toeing gait
    - Groin pain while walking
    - Patellar instability

Aims of Treatment in This Case Are

- Improve the appearance of gait[2]
- Relieve the groin pain
- Abolish the patellar mal-tracking[3]

Options for Treatment

- Observation
- Gait retraining and pelvic stability exercises
- Femoral de-rotation osteotomy using:

    - Blade plate
    - Intramedullary nail

FACTORS THAT INFLUENCE THE CHOICE OF TREATMENT

- Age of the patient
- Underlying cause of the deformity
- Presence of compensatory external tibial torsion
- Psychological state of the patient

The choice of treatment based on these factors is shown in Table 16.1.

Table 16.1 Outline of the Choice of Treatment Based on Factors Influencing the Decision

Factors		Treatment Implications
Age	15 years—almost reached skeletal maturity (the proximal femoral physis is not completely fused)	When the physis is open, a blade plate device is preferred to minimise the risk of avascular necrosis of the femoral head.[4] Alternatively, if an IM nail is used, the point of entry should be the tip of the trochanter and not the pyriform fossa as the risk of avascular necrosis is less with trochanteric entry.
Underlying cause of the deformity	Idiopathic femoral anteversion (not associated with developmental dysplasia of the hip or neuro-muscular disorders with hip instability)	The correction of femoral anteversion is often needed as an essential part of treatment if it is associated with hip instability of any cause. The indications for correction of isolated idiopathic femoral anteversion are very much more selective.

(Continued)

Table 16.1 (Continued)

Factors		Treatment Implications
Presence of compensatory external tibial torsion ("miserable malalignment syndrome")	"Miserable malalignment"	Some patients with significant femoral anteversion have a relatively normal foot progression angle due to increased external tibial torsion. If this is not identified preoperatively, a femoral de-rotation without concomitant tibial internal rotation osteotomies can result in a severe out-toe gait.[5]
Psychological state of the patient	Acceptance of gait and posture	Many adolescents are unhappy with the way they look, and this can contribute significantly to the symptoms expressed. Surgery may not be justified in minor degrees of anteversion just because the patient is unhappy with the gait pattern. Whilst femoral de-rotation can be a very successful operation, case selection is important.

How Was This Child Treated?

After appropriate evaluation of this girl, it was decided that correction of the rotary mal-alignment would be justified and likely to improve her symptoms. Her anteversion was measured at 50° by CT scan, and she required at least 30° of external rotation to allow a normal foot progression and to allow her to walk with the hips in a neutral position and the patellae facing forward.

With the patient in the lateral position, under image intensifier guidance a 2 mm K-wire was placed transversely just above the femoral condyles. A 2 cm incision was made above the greater trochanter, and a ball-tipped guide wire was introduced from the posterolateral aspect of the greater trochanter (Figure 16.4) and passed down the femoral shaft. The femur was then slowly reamed, watching for any changes in oxygen saturation as a sign of fat embolism.

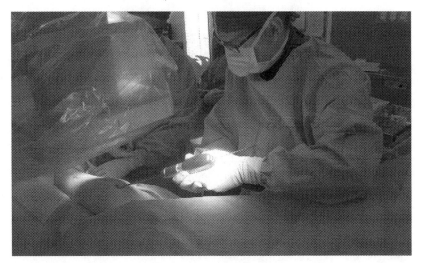

Figure 16.4 Trochanteric entry using a percutaneous approach.

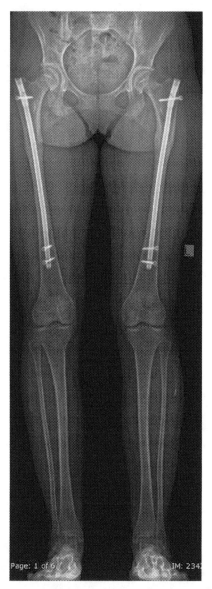

Figure 16.5 Healed de-rotation osteotomies with patellae facing forward.

A subtrochanteric osteotomy was made with an intramedullary saw and final reaming performed to remove any bone spicules at the osteotomy site. The selected nail was passed and locked proximally. The holding jig for the nail was left in place to act as the proximal arm of the goniometer when compared to the distal femoral K-wire. The distal femur was then rotated externally by 30° as measured with a long arm goniometer. This position was held whilst the distal cross bolts were inserted.

Post-Operative Management

Postoperatively, the girl was rested in bed for 24 hours whilst pain and muscle spasm were addressed. Weight-bearing was permitted as tolerated with crutches. Crutches were discarded once callus was visible at the osteotomy sites. After sound union of the osteotomy (Figure 16.5), targeted abductor-strengthening exercises and low-impact activities such as cycling and swimming were encouraged.

Follow-Up

Patients who undergo this procedure should be followed up at four weeks with an X-ray and every month both clinically and radiologically until bridging bone formation at the osteotomy is seen. After that, they should continue with a supervised exercise program and be reviewed at six and 12 months.

This girl returned to playing netball with a more natural running style. Her groin pain completely resolved, but she did have minor irritability from the locking cross bolts, which were removed a year later with good effect. The patellar instability on the left resolved following surgery.

Comment

Some patients will experience irritation from the tip of the nail or the cross bolts which may necessitate nail removal, but in the majority the nail can be retained.

References

1. Schmaranzer F, Lerch TD, Siebenrock KA, Tannast M, Steppacher SD. Differences in femoral torsion among various measurement methods increase in hips with excessive femoral torsion. *Clin Orthop Relat Res.* 2019 May;477(5):1073–83. doi: 10.1097/CORR.0000000000000610. PMID: 30624313; PMCID: PMC6494336.
2. Stambough JB, Davis L, Szymanski DA, Smith JC, Schoenecker PL, Gordon JE. Knee pain and activity outcomes after femoral derotation osteotomy for excessive femoral anteversion. *J Pediatr Orthoped* [Internet]. 2018 Oct 25;38(10):503–9.
3. Imhoff FB, Cotic M, Dyrna FGE, Cote M, Diermeier T, Achtnich A, et al. Dynamic Q-angle is increased in patients with chronic patellofemoral instability and correlates positively with femoral torsion. *Knee Surg Sports Traumatology Arthrosc.* 2020:1–8.
4. Svenningsen S, Apalset K, Terjesen T, Anda S. Osteotomy for femoral anteversion: Complications in 95 children. *Acta Orthop Scand.* 2009;60(4):401–5.
5. Bruce WD, Stevens PM. Surgical correction of miserable malalignment syndrome. *J Pediatr Orthoped.* 2004;24(4):392.

Hitesh Shah and Benjamin Joseph

Case

A 4-year-old girl presented with a severe deformity of the left wrist with shortening of the left forearm (Figure 17.1a–c). She had sustained a fracture of the radius after a fall at 1 year of age, following which she developed progressive deformity of the forearm and wrist. The function of the left hand was compromised, and she had difficulty in fulfilling activities of daily life that required bimanual dexterity. A previous operation attempting to obtain union had failed.

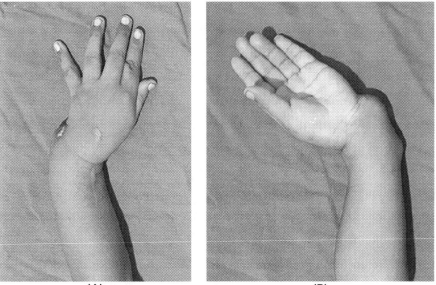

(A)   (B)

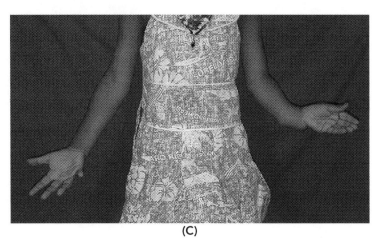

(C)

Figure 17.1 Severe manus valgus deformity (A, B) and shortening of the left forearm. The prominence of the ulnar head at the wrist is evident (C).

On examination, she had a short, bowed left forearm with a radial deviation of the wrist. There were multiple café-au-lait spots on her torso suggestive of Type I neurofibromatosis (Figure 17.2). There was palpable discontinuity of the lower half of the radius with abnormal mobility. Passive movements of the wrist and the forearm were severely restricted. Radiographs of the forearm showed a gap non-union of the shaft of the left radius in the distal half with tapering atrophic ends of the two fragments. The ulna was intact, but it was bowed, and there was dorsal subluxation of the distal ulna with disruption of the inferior radio-ulnar joint (Figure 17.3).

Figure 17.2 Multiple café-au-lait spots on the trunk of the child.

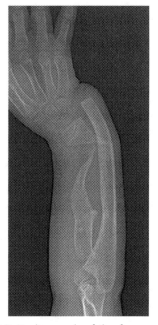

Figure 17.3 Radiograph of the forearm showing the atrophic gap non-union of the radius with bowed ulna and disruption of the inferior radio-ulnar joint.

Questions

- What are the problems that need to be addressed in this child?
- What are the aims of treatment?
- What are the available treatment options to fulfil these aims?
- What are the factors that may influence your choice of treatment?
- Based on these points, what treatment would you recommend for this child?
- How long would you follow-up this child after treatment?

The Problems That Need to Be Addressed Are

- Deformity
  - ○ Bowing of the forearm
  - ○ Valgus deformity of the wrist
- Atrophic gap non-union of the radius
- Joint instability—at inferior radio-ulnar joint
- Limb length inequality
  - ○ Radius much shorter than the ulna
  - ○ Left forearm shorter than the right
- Propensity for recurrence of radial fracture after healing

The Aims of Treatment in This Child

1. Correct the deformities of the forearm and wrist
2. Obtain sound union of the radius
3. Restore integrity of the inferior radio-ulnar joint
4. Restore length relationship between the radius and ulna
5. Reduce the limb length inequality
6. Minimise the risk of re-fracture

Options for Treatment to Fulfil Each Aim

- Correcting deformities of the forearm

  - ○ Osteotomy of bowed ulna

- Correcting deformity at the wrist

  - ○ Restoring length relationship between radius and ulna

- Obtaining union of the radius

  - ○ Excision of pseudarthrosis
  - ○ Bone grafting

    - □ Vascularised bone graft
    - □ Non-vascularised autologous bone graft

  - ○ Internal fixation (intramedullary rod) or external fixation
  - ○ Bone morphogenetic protein (BMP)

- Restoring length relationship between radius and ulna

  - ○ Distraction of radius prior to grafting
  - ○ Obtain union of radius to restore growth of the radius
  - ○ Shorten the ulna

- Reducing limb length inequality

  - ○ Accept shortening
  - ○ Lengthen radius and ulna

- Minimising risk of re-fracture

  - ○ Retain intramedullary rod till skeletal maturity
  - ○ Protective splintage

FACTORS THAT INFLUENCED THE CHOICE OF TREATMENT
• Age of the child • Nature of underlying disease • Complexity of surgery

The choice of treatment based on these factors is outlined in Table 17.1.

Table 17.1 Factors Influencing the Choice of Treatment

Factors		Treatment Implications
Age of the child	4 years	Early surgical intervention is warranted as further delay in treatment will result in further shortening of the limb and aggravation of deformity. This age is adequate to consider vascularised bone grafting. If union of the radius is obtained at this age, there is a good chance of restoration of normal growth of the radius and improvement of the disparity in lengths of the radius and ulna. Once union of the radius is obtained, the bone needs to be protected till skeletal maturity by retaining the intramedullary rod. This is likely to entail rod revision as the bone grows and the initial rod becomes too short to support the site of union.
Nature of underlying disease	Neurofibromatosis Type I	Union is difficult to achieve unless care is taken to excise all the hamartomatous tissue around the non-union site.[1] High union rates have been reported with vascularised bone graft.[2,3] The risk of re-fracture is high till skeletal maturity, and hence the intramedullary rod should be retained till maturity.[4] In addition, using a protective splint is advisable.
Complexity of surgical procedure	Free vascularised fibular graft versus non-vascularised grafting	Free vascularised grafting is a lot more complicated than non-vascularised grafting.

How Was This Child Treated?

Meticulous excision of the pseudoarthrosis of the radius was done; this included excision of the hamartomatous tissue and a 1.5 cm cuff of periosteum from each fragment. A half-centimetre of sclerotic bone was removed from the tips of both fragments of the radius; cortical bleeding was noted from the ends of the radial fragments. The ulna was osteotomised at the apex of the bow. When the radial fragments were held in good apposition, the soft tissues of the forearm were slack. When traction was applied to make the soft tissues taut, gaps were noted between the radial fragments and between the ulnar fragments. Cortical bone graft harvested from the iliac crest was cut into two struts about 3 mm longer than the gaps in the radius and ulna produced by traction. These pieces of iliac bone were prised into the gaps between the fragments of the radius and ulna to function as intercalary grafts under compression. Both the radius and ulna were then fixed with intramedullary Kirschner wires (K-wire), with care taken to confirm that the contact between the fragments and the intercalary grafts was perfect. Additional cortical and cancellous bone graft was harvested from the iliac crest and placed around the site of excised pseudarthrosis of the radius and osteotomy site of the ulna. The wrist deformity improved considerably, but complete correction of the valgus deformity was not achieved. The K-wires were bent and buried under the skin. The wounds were closed, and a long arm cast was applied.

Post-Operative Management

The plaster cast was changed after six weeks, and union of the radius and ulna was monitored with periodic radiographs. The complete union of radius and ulna was achieved after 4.5 months. Active, active-assisted, and passive physiotherapy was started, and normal activities were allowed after 4.5 months. The intramedullary wires were retained. Sequential radiographs (Figure 17.4) showed progress of union. Another important feature evident in these radiographs is that normal growth of the radius has been restored. The position of the articular surface of the radius was proximal to the tip of the ulnar wire at 12 weeks, while it was distal to the tip of the ulnar wire at three years. With resumption of normal radial growth, the normal relationship of the distal ulna to the radius was restored, and the alignment of the wrist was normal three years following surgery (Figure 17.5). The forearm was 3 cm shorter compared to the opposite side. She was able to use the upper limb for all routine activities of daily living.

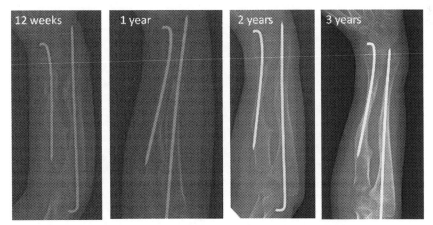

Figure 17.4 Sequential follow-up radiographs of the forearm of the child show progressive healing of the radial pseudarthrosis. Resumption of normal growth of the radius is clearly seen as the relationship between the distal radius and the distal ulna changes; the distal articular margin of the radius moves from being proximal to the tip of the ulna to being distal to it over time.

Follow-Up

Since there is a risk of re-fracture, the child needs to be carefully monitored to revise the intramedullary wires with stouter and longer wires when the current radial wire recedes close to the site of the pseudarthrosis. The child must then be followed up till skeletal maturity.

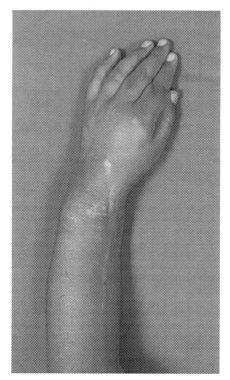

Figure 17.5 The appearance of the limb three years after surgery.

Comment

The case illustrates that restoration of normal growth in a young child can contribute to deformity correction.

References

1. Talab YA. Congenital pseudoarthrosis of the radius: A case report and review of the literature. *Clin Orthop Relat Res.* 1993 Jun;291:246–50. PMID: 8504607.
2. Beris AE, Lykissas MG, Kostas-Agnantis I, Vasilakakos T, Vekris MD, Korompilias AV. Congenital pseudoarthrosis of the radius treated with gradual distraction and free vascularized fibular graft: Case report. *J Hand Surg Am.* 2010 Mar;35(3):406–11. doi: 10.1016/j.jhsa.2009.11.022. Epub 2010 Feb 4. PMID: 20133088.
3. Mathoulin C, Gilbert A, Azze RG. Congenital pseudarthrosis of the forearm: Treatment of six cases with vascularized fibular graft and a review of the literature. *Microsurgery.* 1993;14(4):252–9. doi: 10.1002/micr.1920140408. PMID: 8412635.
4. Narayana Kurup JK, Shah HH. Congenital pseudoarthrosis of the radius in Neurofibromatosis Type 1: An entity not to be missed! *J Orthop.* 2020 Sep 23;22:427–30. doi: 10.1016/j.jor.2020.09.013. PMID: 33029048; PMCID: PMC7527621.

David A Spiegel

Case

A 15-year-and-11-month-old male presented for the evaluation of a curvature in his spine. His medical history was notable for developmental delay, hypotonia, and intermittent lactic acidosis. A formal diagnosis was not established, although a mitochondrial disorder was considered. His cardiac evaluation revealed no abnormalities. He was an independent community ambulator and participated in all activities, including some sports. A standing postero-anterior (PA) radiograph of the thoracolumbar spine demonstrated a right thoracic curve from T5 to L1 of 62° (Figure 18.1a), and he was referred for further medical workup for his undiagnosed lactic acidosis, anticipating that he would require surgical treatment based on the natural history of the curvature. He returned for orthopaedic follow-up seven months later, and the curve had progressed to 85° (Figure 18.1b, c). A bending radiograph over a bolster showed that the curve improved to 53° (Figure 18.1d). Given his rapid progression, an MRI was obtained which revealed no intraspinal anomalies such as a tethered cord or syrinx.

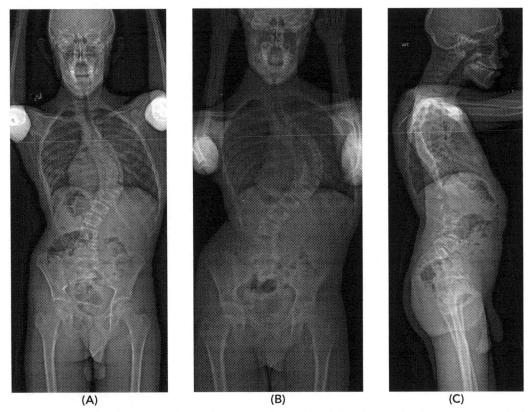

| (A) | (B) | (C) |

Figure 18.1a–18.1d The initial standing PA radiograph of the thoracolumbar spine revealed a Cobb angle of 62° (A) which progressed to 85° (B). The standing lateral radiograph demonstrated mild thoracic hypokyphosis and moderate rotational asymmetry of the rib cage (C). The curve corrected to 53° on a bolster bending radiograph (D).

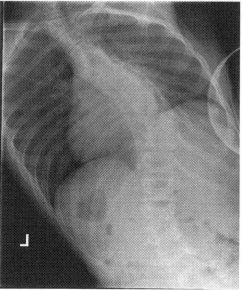

(D)

Figure 18.1 (Continued)

Questions

- What are the problems that need to be addressed?
- What are the aims of treatment?
- What are the commonly available options for treatment?
- What are the factors that may influence your choice of treatment?
- What treatment would you recommend for this boy?
- How long would you follow-up this boy after treatment?

The Problems That Need to Be Addressed Are

- Progressive deformity of the spine
- Chest wall deformity which could impact pulmonary function
- Coronal and sagittal imbalance of trunk relative to pelvis which could potentially result in back pain
- Cosmetic concerns

The Aims of Treatment in This Boy Are to

- Alter the natural history of the spinal deformity by arresting its progression
- Improve spinal alignment and reduce deformity of the rib cage

Options for Treatment

- Bracing
- Posterior spinal fusion with instrumentation with or without spinal osteotomies
- Anterior release followed by an instrumented posterior spinal fusion either during the same operative session or in two stages

---

FACTORS THAT INFLUENCED THE CHOICE OF TREATMENT

- Age of the boy
- Severity of the curve
- Flexibility of the curve
- Rate of curve progression
- Underlying disease and its natural history

The choice of treatment based on these factors is outline in Table 18.1.

Table 18.1 Factors Influencing the Choice of Treatment

Factors		Treatment Implications
Age of the boy	15 years	The risk of progression is very high as he is skeletally immature.
		Growth-sparing surgical strategies such as "growing rods" and Vertical expandable prosthetic titanium rib (VEPTR) may be considered in younger patients but is not appropriate in this 15 year-old boy.
Severity of the curve	85° Cobb angle	Bracing may considered for thoracic curves < 45° in patients who are skeletally immature.
		Since the curve is much more than 45°, bracing is not a justifiable option.
The flexibility of the deformity	The curvature is moderately flexible	Preliminary anterior release and halo traction are not needed, and their risks outweigh the perceived benefits.
		This curve can be managed by a posterior spinal fusion with instrumentation, and Ponte osteotomies could be considered depending on the flexibility under anaesthesia after exposure of the spine.

(Continued)

Table 18.1 (Continued)

Factors		Treatment Implications
Rate of progression of the deformity	The curve progressed from 62° to 85° in seven months	The potential exists for this curve to be life-threatening if progression continues at this rate. Early intervention is mandated in this boy.
The underlying disease and its natural history	The exact diagnosis has not been established	Given the magnitude of the curvature, he would be offered surgical management if the diagnosis was adolescent idiopathic scoliosis, and it is likely that the risk of progression and of future clinical problems such as respiratory impairment are even higher for a non-idiopathic condition (syndromic, neuromuscular).

How Was This Child Treated?

Although a final diagnosis had yet to be established, he was scheduled for surgical treatment given the rapidity of progression and the severity of the deformity. A posterior spinal fusion with instrumentation was planned, with the fusion levels determined by his preoperative standing radiographs and bend films. On the PA radiograph of the thoracolumbar spine, the central sacral line went through the inner wall of the left pedicle at L3, and the neutral vertebra was L4, but L3 had minimal rotation. Based on this information, L3 was selected as the lower instrumented vertebra.[1] When selecting the upper instrumented vertebra, we noted that clinically the left shoulder was lower than the right and T1 was tilted to the left, which led us to select T4. His preoperative right-sided bending radiograph, obtained with a bolster, showed that the curve improved to only 53°.

He underwent a posterior spinal fusion with instrumentation from T4 to L3 without any spinal osteotomies. Facetectomies were performed at each level, and corrective manoeuvres included rod rotation with manual pressure on the thoracic apex, in situ bending, and coupled derotation of the four apical vertebrae. His coronal Cobb angle measured 22° postoperatively, and his thoracic kyphosis measured 25°. Estimated blood loss was 400 cc, and no transfusion was required. His rib hump improved considerably, and there was mild persistent rib asymmetry as seen on the lateral radiograph. The central sacral line is within a centimetre of C7, and his chest is well aligned with his pelvis. While T1 is still tilted a small amount to the left, it appears that the left clavicle is slightly elevated relative to the right, although there were no clinical concerns. He was satisfied with his clinical appearance.

Post-Operative Management

He was admitted to the paediatric intensive care unit for observation and management of his metabolic acidosis, and came to the regular unit on postoperative day two. He sat up on the first day, and was discharged home on post-operative day six without any complications. At three years of follow-up, he is doing well clinically, although he did report some right peri-scapular pain at one of the visits which responded well to physical therapy. On examination, his spine remained well balanced with no loss of correction. His radiographs revealed good deformity correction and balance of his shoulders and chest wall relative to his pelvis (Figure 18.2a, b). The young man needs to be followed up for late complications.

Comment

There are no studies that we are aware of concerning scoliosis in patients with metabolic diseases such as chronic lactic acidosis or mitochondrial disease, so the decision making was based on

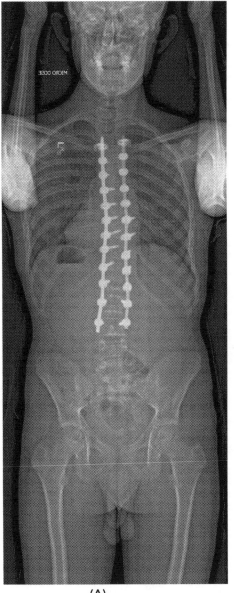 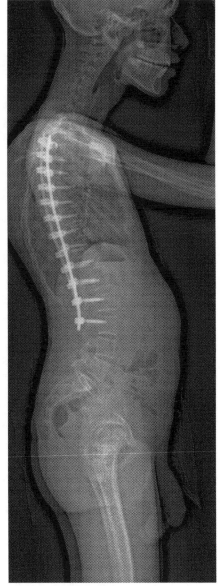

(A)   (B)

Figure 18.2a–18.2b A standing PA radiograph three years following instrumented spinal fusion demonstrated adequate curve correction and coronal balance with level shoulders (A), while the lateral demonstrated normal sagittal contours and balance with mild residual rotational deformity of the ribs (B).

accumulated experience with the natural history for adolescent idiopathic scoliosis (AIS) of the thoracic spine, where curvatures beyond 50° usually progress slowly into adulthood at between 0.5–1° per year.[2–6] The vast majority of idiopathic curves do not impact life expectancy and the quality of life, but patients who develop large thoracic curves commonly have chronic back pain, pulmonary impairment, and significant cosmetic concerns.[2–6]

While life expectancy is rarely impacted by adolescent idiopathic scoliosis, early-onset idiopathic or non-idiopathic curves can lead to premature death. They are more likely to become severe, and curves beyond 100° can be associated with pulmonary hypertension, right ventricular hypertrophy, cor pulmonale, and death.[2-4] In our case, the boy had an undiagnosed metabolic disease, was skeletally immature, and had a curve that progressed rapidly to 85°. We would anticipate progression of the curve could have impaired pulmonary function and potentially altered life expectancy.

The surgical strategy was not influenced by the diagnosis in this boy, and the preoperative planning was based on principles for AIS.[7,8] With regard to the selection of levels, while saving motion segments is very important, clinical experience suggests that there is an increased risk of imbalance and progression of curves below the instrumented segments in patients with connective tissue diseases or syndromes when "fusing short", so it is better to be conservative with the selection of levels in these circumstances. There are also likely differences in the rate of complications between idiopathic scoliosis and non-idiopathic curvatures. Chung et al found that relative to patients treated surgically for AIS, patients with syndromic scoliosis had almost a three times higher risk of complications including neurologic injuries, procedural and device-related complications, and durotomy.[8] Major inpatient complications were 10 times higher for the syndromic cohort.[8]

References

1. Trobisch PD, Ducoffe AR, Lonner BS, Errico TJ. Choosing fusion levels in adolescent idiopathic scoliosis. *J Am Acad Orthop Surg*. 2013;21:519–28.
2. Weinstein SL, Dolan LA, Spratt KF, Peterson KK, Spoonamore MJ, Ponseti IV. Health and function of patients with untreated idiopathic scoliosis: A 50-year natural history study. *JAMA*. 2003;289:559–67.
3. Weinstein SL, Dolan LA, Cheng JC, Danielsson A, Morcuende JA. Adolescent idiopathic scoliosis. *Lancet*. 2008;371:1527–37.
4. Weinstein SL. The natural history of adolescent idiopathic scoliosis. *J Pediatr Orthop*. 2019;39:S44–6.
5. Ascani E, Bartolozzi P, Logroscino CA, et al. Natural history of untreated idiopathic scoliosis after skeletal maturity. *Spine (Phila Pa 1976)*. 1986;11:784–9.
6. Agabegi SS, Kazemi N, Sturm PF, Mehlman CT. Natural history of adolescent idiopathic scoliosis in skeletally mature patients: A critical review. *J Am Acad Orthop Surg*. 2015;23:714–23.
7. Tambe AD, Panikkar SJ, Millner PA, Tsirikos AI. Current concepts in the surgical management of adolescent idiopathic scoliosis. *Bone Joint J*. 2018;100-B:415–24.
8. Chung AS, Renfree S, Lockwood DB, Karlen J, Belthur M. Syndromic scoliosis: National trends in surgical management and inpatient hospital outcomes: A 12-year analysis. *Spine (Phila Pa 1976)*. 2019;44:1564–70.

David A Spiegel

Case

A 17-year old-male presented for evaluation of a progressive spinal deformity in the upper thoracic spine (Figure 19.1a–e). Diagnoses of cutis marmorata telangiectatica congenita syndrome, congenital hydrocephalus, macrocephaly, growth hormone deficiency, hypothyroidism, and Chiari malformation with basilar invagination had been made previously. He also had a history of a vertebro-basilar ischemic stroke at 1 year of age. At the age of 1 year, he underwent C1–2 laminectomy with Chiari decompression and partial resection of his cerebellar tonsils. At 12 years of age, a repeat intradural decompression was abandoned due to adhesions. The following year, he was diagnosed with a syrinx and underwent a T4 laminectomy and placement of a syringo-pleural shunt. A follow-up MRI revealed that the syrinx was still present but was slightly smaller (Figure 19.2a, b).

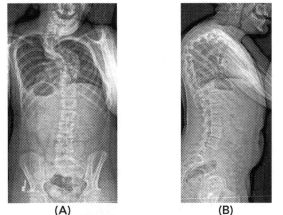

(A)　　　　　　　　　　　(B)

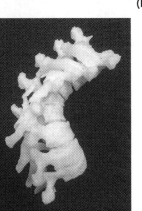
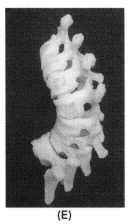

(C)　　　　　　　　(D)　　　　　　　　(E)

Figure 19.1a–e Standing PA and lateral radiographs of the thoracolumbar spine demonstrated a high thoracic kyphoscoliosis which was sharp and angular (A, B). A PA radiograph of the thoracolumbar spine (A) demonstrated a left-sided curve of 68° curve from T1 to T6, and a right-sided curve of 48° from T6 to T11. The lateral view of the thoracolumbar spine (B) revealed a sharp angular kyphosis measuring 88° and centred at T4–T6, and the deformity had progressed 27° over seven months. The CT scan and the reconstructed images were used to generate a 3-D model (c = front, d = right side, e = left side).

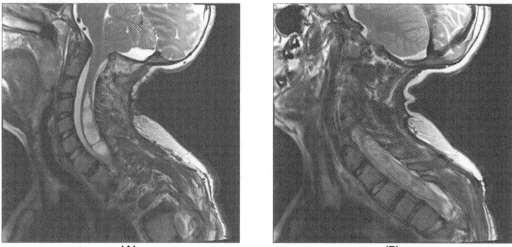

(A)   (B)

Figure 19.2a, b Sagittal images from his latest MRI demonstrate a persistent syrinx.

He did not have headaches, neurologic symptoms, or back pain, and on examination there were no abnormal neurologic findings. The spine was well balanced with level shoulders in the coronal plane. In the sagittal plane, he had a sharp upper thoracic gibbus with anterior translation of his head and shoulders relative to his lower spine.

Questions

- What are the problems that need to be addressed?
- What are the aims of treatment?
- What are the commonly available options for treatment?
- What are the factors that may influence your choice of treatment?
- What treatment would you recommend for this boy?
- How long would you follow-up this boy after treatment?

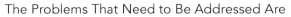

The Problems That Need to Be Addressed Are

- Progressive deformity of the spine
- High risk of neurologic impairment with further curve progression
- High risk of surgical complications
- Cosmetic deformity (gibbus)

The Aims of Treatment in This Boy Are to

- Alter the natural history of the spinal deformity and avoid neurologic complications by arresting its progression
- Achieve some correction of the deformity
- Avoid surgical complications

Options for Treatment

- Arresting progression of the deformity by achieving spinal fusion

  - Posterior spinal fusion
  - Anterior spinal fusion

- Deformity correction

  - Halo traction
  - Spinal osteotomies
  - Vertebral column resection

FACTORS THAT INFLUENCED THE CHOICE OF TREATMENT

- Age of the boy
- Rate of progression of deformity
- Severity and morphology of the curve
- Flexibility of the curve
- Location of the curve
- Status of the neural axis
- Effect of previous spinal operations
- Anticipated risk-benefit ratio

The choice of treatment based on these factors is outlined in Table 19.1.

Table 19.1 Choice of Treatment Based on the Factors Influencing Treatment

Factors		Treatment Implications
Age of the boy	17 years	Although likelihood of progression is less in patients who are skeletally mature, in this case the magnitude of deformity is sufficient to anticipate continued progression after skeletal maturity.
Rate of progression of the deformity	Rapid progression (the curve progressed from 62° to 90° in seven months)	Urgent intervention is required as the deformity is likely to continue to progress, resulting in spinal cord injury or paralysis.

(Continued)

Table 19.1 (Continued)

Factors		Treatment Implications
Severity and morphology of the curve	88° Cobb angle Sharp and angular curve	High risk of neurological complications of surgery.
The flexibility of the deformity	Rigid curve	Preliminary halo traction may only yield partial correction of the deformity; spinal osteotomies or vertebral column resection may be required if further correction is planned.
Location of the curve	Upper thoracic	Anterior exposure of the upper thoracic spine in the presence of severe kyphotic deformity is fraught with major risks to vital structures.
Status of neural axis	Shunted hydrocephalus Persistent syringomyelia following syringo-pleural shunting	Increased risk of neurologic injury with deformity correction.
Effect of previous spinal operations	Previous laminectomy	Higher risk of pseudarthrosis of posterior spinal fusion.
	Previous syringo-pleural shunt	Risk of damage to the shunt while undertaking spinal deformity correction.
	Previous laminectomy and shunt	Adhesions may increase the risk of neural damage during surgery.
Risk-benefit ratio	Risk-benefit ratio of spinal fusion	Benefit of preventing progression and risk of neurologic compromise outweighs risks of surgery.
	Risk-benefit ratio of achieving complete correction of spinal deformity	Risk of intra-operative neurologic injury while attempting complete correction outweighs benefits. Partial correction of the spinal deformity is a more realistic goal.
	Risk-benefit ratio of anterior spinal surgery versus posterior instrumentation and fusion	Risks of intra-operative complications are very high with anterior spinal surgery for kyphosis in the upper thoracic spine and they outweigh the potential benefits.

How Was This Boy Treated?

We discussed with the parents and explained in detail:

- The natural history of the deformity and the extremely high risk of neurologic deterioration with further curve progression if left untreated
- Our goals of treatment:

  o to fuse the spine to prevent curve progression
  o to obtain only modest correction of the deformity as full correction was likely to be associated with an extremely high risk of intra-operative neurologic injury

given the location of the deformity (upper thoracic spine), the nature of the curve (rigid, sharp, angular), and the abnormal neural axis (hydrocephalus, persistent syringomyelia).

- The options of treatment and the attendant risks:
  - o Instrumented spinal fusion
  - o A period in halo traction followed by an instrumented spinal fusion
  - o More aggressive, high-risk strategy of two- or three-column osteotomy or vertebral column resection

After this discussion, we elected to place him in halo traction for three weeks and then perform an instrumented posterior spinal fusion. We elected not to proceed with more complex osteotomies after discussion with family and with surgical colleagues.

We also counselled the family that there was an increased risk of pseudarthrosis due to the previous laminectomy and the kyphosis.

The first procedure involved placement of a halo with two pins anteriorly and four pins posteriorly, each tensioned to 6 inch/pound as a previous head CT scan suggested that his skull was quite thin. He tolerated this procedure well, and neurophysiologic monitoring suggested that his signals were consistent with those obtained at his previous neurosurgical procedures, and there was no change with our starting weight of 15 pounds. We then gradually increased the traction weight to a maximum of 40 pounds over two weeks, and obtained a lateral radiograph of the cervical spine in traction every few days to make sure the cervical spine was not over-distracted (Figure 19.3a). He worked with physical therapy to maintain strength, and ambulated regularly while in traction, and was able to travel around the hospital in a wheelchair while in traction. Images obtained with maximum traction demonstrated significant improvement in the coronal alignment, with only a modest improvement in the sharp angular kyphosis from 90 to approximately 75 degrees (Figure 19.3b, c).

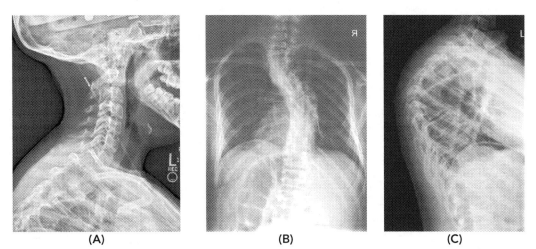

(A) (B) (C)

Figure 19.3a–c Periodic lateral radiographs of the cervical spine were obtained to ensure that the spine did not become over-distracted (A). Both the PA and lateral images revealed improvements in alignment while in 40 pounds of traction (B, C).

After three weeks, he was taken to the operating room for the instrumented posterior spinal fusion from T2 down to T12. He was placed in 15 pounds of traction after positioning. Interestingly, our neurophysiologic monitoring team noted an improvement in his motor signals relative to the data obtained at the time of his previous neurosurgical procedures and when traction was applied. The spine was exposed with care taken to isolate and protect the syringo-pleural shunt. While the facet joints had been preserved with the previous laminectomy, they had become elongated across the apex of the deformity. Pedicle screws were placed where technically possible, as the CT scan demonstrated markedly abnormal anatomy and several of the pedicles could not accommodate screws. We preserved the supraspinous and interspinous ligaments between T1 and T2. He tolerated the procedure well, did not receive a blood transfusion, and had stable monitoring signals throughout. His postoperative radiographs (Figure 19.4a, b) show that the kyphosis had improved to 65°. His sagittal balance (as evaluated by C7 relative to the postero-superior corner of the sacrum) had improved but was still not normal.

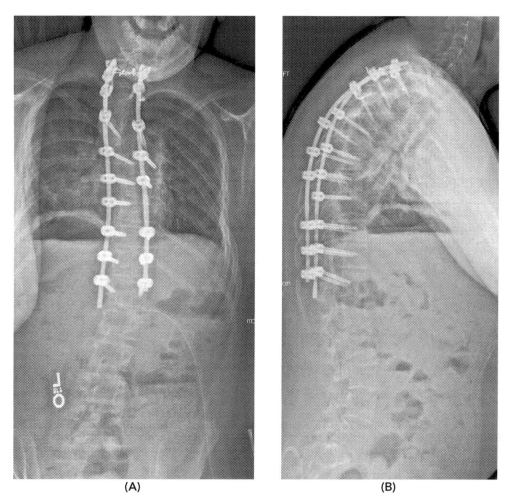

(A)   (B)

Figure 19.4a, b Standing PA (A) and lateral (B) images show improvement in scoliosis and the kyphosis, with a kyphotic angle of 65°.

Postoperative Management

He was admitted to the paediatric intensive care unit for overnight observation, and he remained hemodynamically stable with a normal neurologic examination. He was mobilised to a chair on the first postoperative day, and was beginning to ambulate on the second postoperative day. He was discharged home on the fourth postoperative day. He was placed in a cervico-thoracic orthosis for the first six weeks postoperatively, and was started on physical therapy for strengthening the neck and spinal musculature after the bracing was discontinued. His family was satisfied with his clinical appearance and alignment as the gibbus was no longer seen.

Given the risks of pseudarthrosis and of progressive deformity above or below the instrumented segments, he will require close follow-up over many years.

Comment

There is limited information in the literature concerning post-laminectomy kyphosis of the thoracic spine in children and adolescents.[1-5] Reports suggest that around 46% of children under 15 years of age who undergo multilevel laminectomy may develop spinal deformity. The propensity for developing a deformity is highest in the cervical region and less in the thoracic and thoracolumbar regions.[3,5] The frequency of spinal deformity following multi-level laminoplasty is not less than that observed after laminectomy.[6]

While several early studies suggested that an anterior spinal fusion be used to treat progressive kyphotic deformities,[1,3] the vast majority of kyphotic deformities are currently managed by a posterior-only approach with procedures of varying complexity. The general principles are well outlined in a review of Scheuermann's kyphosis.[7] While an isolated posterior spinal fusion with instrumentation is considered for flexible deformities, the addition of multiple posterior osteotomies (Ponte osteotomies) affords greater correction while shortening the spine, which lowers the risk of neurologic injury (Figure 19.5a-e). In the most severe and rigid deformities, either a two-column (pedicle subtraction osteotomy) or three-column osteotomy (vertebral column resection) can be considered, but these procedures have the highest risk of complications.[7]

The risks of neurologic injury are greater in patients with kyphosis (3.7%) than in those with scoliosis (1%).[8] Li et al presented a classification system for stratifying risk of neurologic injury with vertebral column resections to treat severe and stiff cases of kyphoscoliosis based on severity of the curve and pre-existing neurologic impairment, and found that there was a 29% risk of a monitoring alert and 14% risk of neurologic injury when there was an asymptomatic pre-existing neurologic abnormality such as a syrinx and a sharp angular curve with a sagittal Deformity Angular Ratio (DAR, degree of curve divided by the number of vertebrae in the curve) of <20.[9] There was a 100% risk of an alert and 25% risk of injury if the DAR was 20–31.[9] In this case, the DAR was 16.2.

Another complication of posterior surgery for kyphosis is proximal or distal junctional kyphosis[7,10] which may be prevented by fusing to the vertebra beyond the first lordotic disc[7,10] and to the sagittal stable vertebra, namely the most proximal vertebra that is touched by a vertical line extending upwards from the posterior corner of the sacrum. It is also helpful to avoid damage to the supporting soft tissues above the instrumented segments (supraspinous and infraspinous ligaments, ligamentum flavum, facet joints), to use hooks at the top of the construct, include the proximal end vertebra of the curve, and to avoid overcorrection of the deformity by having the final degree of kyphosis at the upper range of normal values, between 40 and 50°.[7,10]

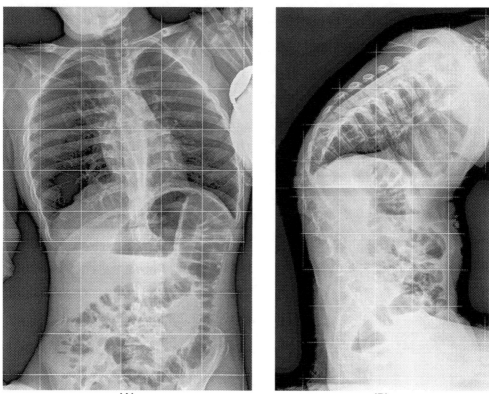

(A)

(B)

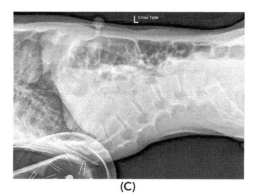

(C)

Figure 19.5a–e This second case illustrates a progressive thoracolumbar kyphosis in a neuro-muscular patient who lost the ability to look straight (A, B). His curve was rigid on supine hyper-extension bolster bending radiograph (C), and he was treated with an instrumented posterior spinal fusion, including multiple Ponte osteotomies to restore alignment (D, E).

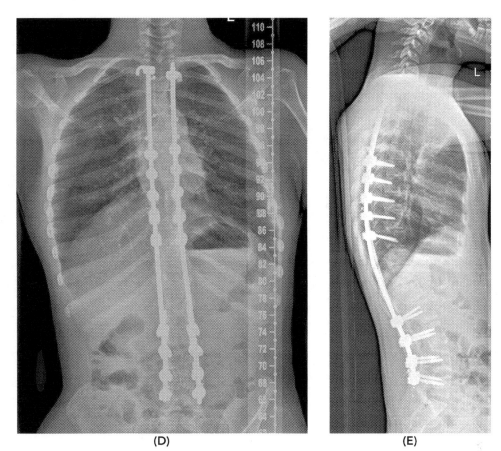

(D)   **(E)**

Figure 19.5 (Continued)

References

1. Lonstein JE. Post-laminectomy kyphosis. *Clin Orthop Rel Res.* 1977;128:93–100.
2. Yasuoka S, Peterson HA, MacCarty CS, et al. Incidence of spinal column deformity after multilevel laminectomy in children and adults. *J Neurosurg.* 1982;57:441–5.
3. Yasuoka S, Peterson HA, Laws ER Jr., et al. Pathogenesis and prophylaxis of postlaminectomy deformity of the spine after multilevel laminectomy: Difference between children and adults. *Neurosurgery.* 1981;9:145–52.
4. Otsuka N, Hey L, Hall JE. Postlaminectomy and postirradiation kyphosis in children and adolescents. *Clin Orthop Rel Res.* 1998;354:189–94.
5. Papagelopoulos PJ, Peterson HA, Ebersold MJ, et al. Spinal column deformity and instability after lumbar or thoracolumbar laminectomy for intraspinal tumors in children and young adults. *Spine.* 1997;22:442–51.
6. McGirt MJ, Garces-Ambrossi GL, Parker SL, et al. Short-term progressive spinal deformity following laminoplasty versus laminectomy for resection of intradural spinal tumors: Analysis of 238 patients. *Neurosurgery.* 2010;66:1005–12.
7. Sardar ZM, Ames RJ, Lenke L. Scheuermann's kyphosis: Diagnosis, management, and selecting fusion levels. *J Am Acad Orthop Surg.* 2019;27:e462–72.
8. Fu KMG, Smith JS, Polly DW Jr., et al. Morbidity and mortality associated with spinal surgery in children: A review of the Scoliosis Research Society morbidity and mortality database. *J Neurosurg Pediatrics.* 2011;7:37–41.

9. Li XS, Fan HW, Huang ZF, et al. Predictive value of spinal cord function classification and sagittal Deformity Angular Ratio for neurologic risk stratification in patients with severe and stiff kyphoscoliosis. *World Neurosurg.* 2019;123:e787–96.
10. Mika AP, Mesfin A, Rubery PT, Molinari R, Kebaish KM, Menga EN. Proximal Junctional kyphosis: A pediatric and adult spinal deformity surgery dilemma. *JBJS Rev.* 2019;7:e4.

Hitesh Shah

Case

An 8-year-old girl presented with a deformity of the neck first noted by her parents in infancy. She had been treated with physiotherapy for a few months without any appreciable improvement. On examination, the child had a right-sided torticollis with the head tilted to the right and the face and chin rotated to the left. The right sternocleidomastoid muscle was contracted. Lateral bending of the neck to the left side and rotation of the neck to the right were restricted; other movements of the neck were normal (Figure 20.1a, b, c). There was no obvious facial asymmetry. Her vision was normal as was her neurologic examination. Radiographs of her cervical spine were normal.

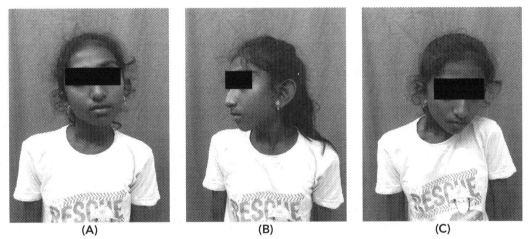

| (A) | (B) | (C) |

Figure 20.1 Right-sided torticollis in a girl. Her head is tilted to the right, and her face and chin are rotated to the left (A). Rotation of her neck to the right is reduced (B), and on attempting left lateral bending the right sternomastoid stands out very prominently (C).

Questions

- What are the problems that need to be addressed?
- What are the aims of treatment?
- What are the available treatment options to fulfil these aims?
- What are the factors that may influence your choice of treatment?
- Based on these points, what treatment would you recommend for this child?
- How long would you follow-up this child after treatment?

The Problems That Need to Be Addressed in This Girl Are

- Deformity of the neck due to contracture of the right sternocleidomastoid muscle
- Restriction of neck movements

The Aims of Treatment in This Girl Are

- Correct the deformity and restore the range of motion of the neck
- Avoid recurrence of the deformity
- Avoid an unsightly surgical scar
- Avoid diplopia

Options for Treatment to Fulfil Each Aim

- To correct the deformity and to restore the range of motion of the cervical spine

  - Manual stretching and proper positioning
  - Botulinum toxin injection
  - Release of the sternomastoid

    - Percutaneous release of sternocleidomastoid
    - Endoscopic lengthening
    - Open lengthening of sternocleidomastoid

- To avoid recurrence of the deformity

  - Manual stretching and proper positioning
  - Adequate lengthening of sternocleidomastoid

- To avoid unsightly scar

  - Use an incision along Langer's lines if scar is in a visible area
  - Use a scar hidden by the hair line

FACTORS THAT INFLUENCED THE CHOICE OF TREATMENT

The factors that influenced the choice of treatment of torticollis were:

- The age of the child
- Aetiology of torticollis
- The severity of deformity with facial asymmetry

The choice of treatment based on these factors is shown in Table 20.1.

Table 20.1 Factors Influencing the Choice of Treatment

Factors		Treatment Implications
The age of the child	8 years	Children less than 1 year of age may be effectively treated with muscle stretching and appropriate positioning.[1,2] Surgical intervention is usually required in older children.[3]
Aetiology of torticollis	Congenital muscular torticollis	Stretching or surgical release of the sternocleidomastoid is the treatment for congenital muscular torticollis.[2,3,4] The treatment of non-muscular torticollis is quite different.[5]

Table 20.1 (Continued)

Factors		Treatment Implications
The severity of deformity and presence of facial asymmetry	Moderate deformity with no gross facial asymmetry	The results are better with mild to moderate deformity with less than 30-degree restriction of range of motion and without facial asymmetry. A unipolar release may suffice for less severe deformity, while a bipolar release may be required for a severe deformity.[6]

How Was This Girl Treated?

The girl was treated with open unipolar lengthening of the sternocleidomastoid with a transverse incision just above the clavicle. Both the sternal and clavicular insertions of the sternocleidomastoid muscle were released.

Post-Operative Management

The girl was treated in halter traction after the surgery. Five days later, a Minerva cast in a mildly over-corrected position was applied. The cast was removed after six weeks, and the range of motion exercises were started. The passive stretching of the sternocleidomastoid was done for six months.

Follow-Up

The girl was followed up regularly for two years. Her vision was perfect. She and her parents were satisfied with the cosmetic outcome of the surgery. The range of motion of the neck improved significantly (Figure 20.2). No further follow-up is warranted as recurrences usually occur within two years.

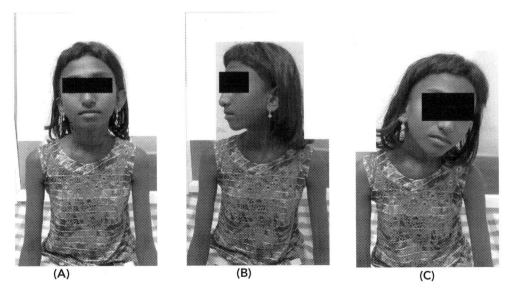

(A) (B) (C)

Figure 20.2a, b, c Two years following surgery, the deformity is well corrected; the head is not tilted (A) and the range of neck movements has improved (B, C).

Comment

Eight years is a late age to perform a torticollis correction as facial asymmetry may develop by that time. If significant facial asymmetry has developed, the cosmetic outcome is poor even if the deformity per se is corrected.

References

1. Cheng JC, Tang SP, Chen TM, Wong MW, Wong EM. The clinical presentation and outcome of treatment of congenital muscular torticollis in infants: A study of 1,086 cases. *J Pediatr Surg.* 2000;35:1091–6.
2. Cheng JCY, Wong MWN, Tang SP, et al. Clinical determinants of the outcome of manual stretching in the treatment of congenital muscular torticollis in infants. *J Bone Joint Surg Am.* 2001;83:679–87.
3. Cheng JC, Tang SP. Outcome of surgical treatment of congenital muscular torticollis. *Clin Orthop Relat Res.* 1999;362:190–200.
4. Joyce MB, de Chalain TM. Treatment of recalcitrant idiopathic muscular torticollis in infants with botulinum toxin type a. *J Craniofac Surg.* 2005;16:321–7.
5. Do TT. Congenital muscular torticollis: Current concepts and review of treatment. *Curr Opin Pediatr.* 2006;18(1):26–9. doi: 10.1097/01.mop.0000192520.48411.fa.
6. Shim JS, Noh KC, Park SJ. Treatment of congenital muscular torticollis in patients older than 8 years. *J Pediatr Orthop.* 2004;24(6):683–8. doi: 10.1097/00004694-200411000-00016.

DISLOCATIONS

Randall T Loder

Case

A 27-month-old girl had a waddling gait from when she started walking at 13 months of age. The parents had also noted some popping of the right hip. She was breech presentation, born by vaginal delivery. Physical examination demonstrated a bilateral painless, Trendelenburg gait; hip abduction was 40 degrees on the right and 50 degrees on the left, and both trochanters were proximally located. An AP radiograph of the pelvis confirmed bilateral developmental disloca-tion of the hips (Figure 21.1). The femoral heads were high, and they had begun to form false acetabulae. The true acetabulae were dysplastic.

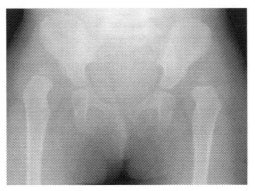

Figure 21.1 An AP radiograph of the pelvis demonstrating bilateral developmental hip disloca-tions with pseudo acetabulae and dysplasia of the true acetabulae.

Questions

- What are the problems that need to be addressed in this girl?
- What are the aims of treatment?
- What are the available treatment options to fulfil these aims?
- What are the factors that may influence your choice of treatment?
- Based on these points, what treatment would you recommend for this child?
- How long would you follow-up this child after treatment?

The Problems That Need to Be Addressed Are

- Bilateral hip dysplasia
  - Hip dislocation
  - Acetabular dysplasia
  - Femoral anteversion
- Risk of re-dislocation following reduction
- Risk of developing late complications following treatment
  - Late acetabular dysplasia
  - Avascular necrosis and proximal femoral growth disturbance
  - Leg length inequality

The Aims of Treatment in This Girl Are to

- Obtain and maintain stable, concentric reduction of the hips
- Monitor acetabular growth and correct progressive acetabular dysplasia
- Monitor proximal femoral growth and signs of avascular necrosis
- Obtain equal leg lengths by skeletal maturity

Options for Treatment to Fulfil Each Aim

Obtaining and maintaining stable, concentric reduction of the hip dislocations

- Closed reduction of the hips following skeletal traction
- Open reduction with femoral shortening/rotational osteotomy and pelvic osteotomy

If late acetabular dysplasia occurs, repeat pelvic osteotomy

- Salter innominate, Steel or Tonnis triple osteotomy if the triradiate cartilage is open
- Periacetabular osteotomy (Ganz) if the triradiate cartilage is fused

If limb length inequality develops

- Timed epiphyseodesis of the longer limb

FACTORS THAT INFLUENCED THE CHOICE OF TREATMENT

• Age of the child
• Unilateral versus bilateral dislocations
• Associated bony deformity
 	
  o Acetabular dysplasia
  o Femoral anteversion

The choice of treatment based on these factors is shown in Table 21.1.

Table 21.1 Factors Influencing the Choice of Treatment

Factors		Treatment Implications
Age of the child	27 months	The results of closed reduction are poor in this age group, and hence open reduction is preferred.[1]

Table 21.1 (Continued)

Factors		Treatment Implications
		Acetabular dysplasia and femoral anteversion can be corrected at the same time as the open reduction.[2,3]
Unilateral versus bilateral dislocations	Bilateral dislocation	Bilateral simultaneous open reductions are fraught with poor outcomes and are more difficult to treat with a higher complication rate than unilateral dislocations.[3] Staged open reduction is often selected though the treatment time is more protracted.
Position of the femoral head in relation to the acetabulum	High dislocation (Tonnis 4 or International Hip Dysplasia Institute [IHDI] class 4)[3–5]	Femoral shortening should be considered as it will facilitate reduction, reduce the risk of avascular necrosis, increase stability and reduce the risk of re-dislocation.[2,3]
Presence of acetabular dysplasia	True acetabular dysplasia is present	Stability after reduction is greatly improved by correcting the acetabular dysplasia at time of reduction.[2,3]
Presence of femoral anteversion	Femoral anteversion present	Stability of reduction can be improved by performing a femoral de-rotation osteotomy.[2,3]

How Was This Girl Treated?

Bilateral, staged open reductions of the hips with proximal femoral shortening and rotational osteotomy and Pemberton pelvic osteotomy were performed. The right hip was operated first at 29 months of age and the left hip at 34 months of age. Satisfactory concentric reductions of both hips were obtained as seen in the radiograph at age 4 years 11 months (Figure 21.2a).

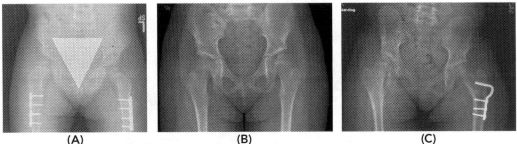

(A)   **(B)**   **(C)**

Figure 21.2 (A) An anteroposterior radiograph at 4 years 11 months of age after bilateral open reductions, femoral shortening/rotational osteotomies, and Pemberton pelvic osteotomies. (B) An anteroposterior radiograph at age 10 years 10 months demonstrating left coxa valga and a very horizontal proximal femoral physis, likely due to a proximal femoral growth disturbance. The lateral centre-edge angles are 25 degrees on the right and 11 degrees on the left. (C) An anteroposterior radiograph at the age of 11 years 4 months after a left proximal femoral varus osteotomy. The left lateral centre-edge angle is now 23 degrees.

However, the centre-edge angles progressively decreased over time. At age 10 years 10 months (Figure 21.2b), there was progressive left proximal femoral valgus likely due to a mild proximal femoral growth disturbance.[6] A proximal femoral varus osteotomy was performed on the left to correct the valgus deformity (Figure 21.2c).

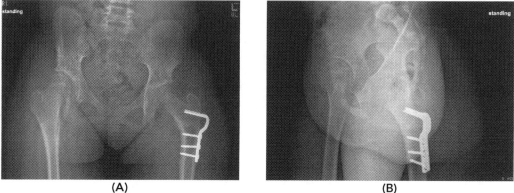

(A)   (B)

Figure 21.3 (A) An anteroposterior radiograph demonstrating a lateral centre-edge angle of 15 degrees. (B) A false-profile radiograph demonstrating reduced anterior femoral head coverage with an anterior centre-edge angle of 17 degrees and a horizontal sourcil.

Discomfort in the right groin began at the age of 12 years. Radiographs demonstrated mild acetabular dysplasia with a decreased lateral centre-edge angle (Figure 21.3a) and anterior centre-edge angle (Figure 21.3b). As the triradiate cartilage had closed, a Ganz periacetabular osteotomy was performed (Figure 21.3c) on the right. Eventually, a Ganz periacetabular osteotomy was performed on the left hip, which had become symptomatic. The final result is shown in Figure 21.4; the lateral centre-edge angles are 33 degrees on the right and 35 degrees on the left.

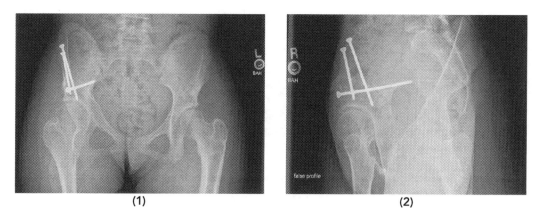

(1)   (2)

Figure 21.3c An anteroposterior radiograph (1) and a false profile radiograph (2) after a Ganz periacetabular osteotomy had been performed. Note that the sourcil on the false profile radiograph is now sloping downward. The anterior centre-edge angle is now 27 degrees.

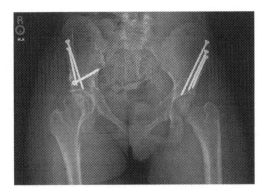

Figure 21.4 The latest follow-up radiograph at 15 years 1 month of age demonstrates excellent bilateral femoral head coverage.

Post-Operative Management

Spica cast immobilization was used for six weeks after each of the initial open reductions and femoral or pelvic osteotomies. An arthrogram was performed at the six-week mark to assess stability and determine if further spica casting was necessary.

For the later femoral varus and peri-acetabular osteotomies, bed-to-wheelchair transfers and non–weight bearing for four weeks was used, followed by progressive weight bearing and muscle strengthening physiotherapy, especially the hip abductors.

Follow-Up

The girl was followed until complete maturity of the hip and triradiate physeal closure.

The final correction was excellent (Figure 21.4). We hope that since the final peri-acetabular osteotomies were done before the age of 25 years, the need for total hip arthroplasty will be delayed significantly.[7]

Comment

- Diagnosis of bilateral hip dislocations can be delayed due to symmetric findings.[1]
- In general, the outcome of bilateral DDH surgery is less favourable than that for unilateral DDH.[3]
- The outcomes of the modern periacetabular osteotomy for residual dysplasia are promising, but the long-term outcomes are still not completely known.[7–9]

References

1. Vitale MG, Skaggs DL. Developmental dysplasia of the hip from six months to four years of age. *J Am Acad Orthop Surg.* 2001;9(6):401–11.
2. Galpin RD, Roach JW, Wenger DR, Herring JA, Birch JG. One-stage treatment of congenital dislocation of the hip in older children, including femoral shortening. *J Bone Joint Surg [Am].* 1989;71-A(5):734–41.
3. Tennant SJ, Hashemi-Nejad A, Calder P, Eastwood DM. Bilateral developmental dysplasia of the hip: Does closed reduction have a role in management? Outcome of closed and open reduction in 92 hips. *J Pediatr Orthop.* 2019;39(4):e264–71.
4. Narayanan U, Mulpuri K, Sankar WN, Clarke NMP, Hosalkar H, Price CT, et al. Reliability of a new radiographic classification for developmental dysplasia of the hip. *J Pediatr Orthop.* 2015;35(5):478–84.

5. Ramo BA, Rocha ADL, Sucato DJ, Jo C-H. A new radiographic classification system for developmental hip dysplasia is reliable and predictive of successful closed reduction and late pelvic osteotomy. *J Pediatr Orthop.* 2018;38(1):16–21.
6. Campbell P, Tarlow SD. Lateral tethering of the proximal femoral physis complicating the treatment of congenital hip dysplasia. *J Pediatr Orthop.* 1990;10(1):6–8.
7. Wells J, Millis M, Kim Y-J, Bulat E, Miller P, Matheney T. Survivorship of the Bernese periacetabular osteotomy: What factors are associated with long-term failure? *Clin Orthop.* 2017;475(2):396–405.
8. Clohisy JC, Barrett SE, Gordon JE, Delgado ED, Schoenecker PL. Periacetabular osteotomy for the treatment of severe acetabular dysplasia. *J Bone Joint Surg [Am].* 2005;87-A(2):254–9.
9. Ziran N, Varcadipane J, Kadri O, Ussef N, Kanim L, Foster A, et al. Ten- and 20-year survivorship of the hip after periacetabular osteotomy for acetabular dysplasia. *J Am Acad Orthop Surg.* 2019;27(7):247–55.

David A Spiegel

Case

A 6-year-old boy with spastic quadriplegia cerebral palsy (GMFCS 5) presented for the evaluation of an abnormal radiograph of the pelvis noted by his physical medicine and rehabilitation specialist, taken as part of an institutional hip-screening protocol. He did not have any hip pain, although he had some restrictions in hip motion which did not impair his seating, or the ability to dress him and provide perineal hygiene. His medical history was notable for cerebral cortical dysgenesis, hypopituitarism, adrenal insufficiency, seizures, and profound developmental delay. On physical examination, there were bilateral hip flexion contractures of approximately 25°, and his passive abduction was approximately 20° bilaterally. There was no hip pain while the range of motion was being tested. The radiograph of the pelvis demonstrated bilateral hip dysplasia with coxa valga, severe subluxation, and acetabular dysplasia (Figure 22.1).

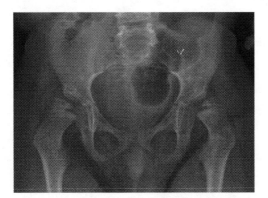

Figure 22.1 The AP radiograph of the pelvis demonstrates bilateral hip subluxation with a break in Shenton's line and bilateral coxa valga, a migration percentage of 64% on the right and 88% on the left. The acetabular indices are elevated at 30° bilaterally. There is mild flattening of the epiphysis on the right side.

Questions

- What are the problems that need to be addressed?
- What are the aims of treatment?
- What are the commonly available options for treatment?
- What are the factors that may influence your choice of treatment?
- What treatment would you recommend for this boy?
- How long would you follow-up this boy after treatment?

The Problems That Need to Be Addressed Are

- Displacement of both hips with associated soft tissue contractures and dysplasia of the proximal femur and acetabulum.
- Risk of progressive subluxation proceeding to dislocation over time, which may then result in altered posture, challenges with perineal care, chronic pain, and a decrease in health-related quality of life (HRQOL).[1,2,3]

The Aims of Treatment in This Boy Are to

- Restore concentric reduction of the hips.
- Minimize the risk of progressing to painfully dislocated hips and poor HRQOL.

Options for Fulfilling the Aims of Treatment

- Reconstructive surgery
  - Soft tissue release (adductors, gracilis, iliopsoas)
  - Proximal femoral osteotomy (varus derotation and shortening)
  - Acetabuloplasty (volume-reducing procedure such as Dega or San Diego)
- Salvage surgery
  - Proximal femoral valgus osteotomy with or without resection of the femoral head and neck
  - Sub-trochanteric resection of the proximal femur
  - Total hip replacement (ambulators)
  - Prosthetic replacement with a total shoulder prosthesis

FACTORS THAT INFLUENCED THE CHOICE OF TREATMENT

- The age of the child
- The extent of migration
- Presence of contractures
- Presence of adaptive bony changes
  - Femur
    - Coxa valga
    - Anteversion
  - Acetabulum
- Shape of the femoral head and presence of arthritic changes
- Location of acetabular deficiency

The choice of treatment based on these factors is outlined in Table 22.1.

Table 22.1 Factors That Influenced the Choice of Treatment

Factors		Treatment Implications
Age of the child	6 years	Younger patients have a greater risk of remodelling, and while no cutoff has been

(Continued)

Table 22.1 (Continued)

Factors		Treatment Implications
		established for age the author prefers to wait until 5–6 years of age to perform reconstructive surgery if at all possible.
The extent of migration	Migration percentages of 64% and 88%	Hips with a migration percentage beyond approximately 60% will all go on to dislocate, and a significant number of chronically dislocated hips will become painful.[1] This implies that early intervention is mandated in this boy.
Presence of contractures	Flexion and adduction contractures are present	The adductors and the iliopsoas need to be released.
Presence of adaptive bony changes in the proximal femur	Coxa valga and femoral anteversion are present	A varus de-rotational osteotomy (VDRO) is indicated in this boy.
Presence of acetabular dysplasia and the location of acetabular deficiency	Acetabular dysplasia is present, and the deficiency is likely to be posterior or global in cerebral palsy (unlike in developmental dysplasia where the acetabular deficiency is anterolateral)	In order to improve the coverage of the femoral head posteriorly, a technique that permits that should be chosen. The Dega acetabuloplasty or the San Diego procedure can improve posterior cover.
The shape of the femoral head and arthritic changes	The femoral head has retained adequate sphericity with minimal deformation, and there are no arthritic changes in the hip	This justifies reconstructive surgery aimed at reducing the femoral head into the acetabulum. There is no role for any form of salvage surgery in this boy.

How Was This Child Treated?

After discussion with the family, at the age of 7-years-and-8-months he underwent reconstructive surgery on both hips. An epidural catheter was placed, and under general anaesthesia, the adductor longus, gracilis, and some fibres of the adductor brevis were released till 45° of abduction was achieved. A varus derotation osteotomy was then performed at the inter-trochanteric level. The femur was shortened by 1.5 cm by excising a trapezoidal segment of bone from the distal fragment of the femur. The excised bone segments were preserved for use during the acetabuloplasty. The iliopsoas was released from the lesser trochanter. The femur was fixed such that the neck-shaft angle was about 100° (Figure 22.2a). Since the hips reduced at this point, an open reduction was not required. A San Diego acetabuloplasty was performed, with care taken to enhance posterior and lateral coverage by placing of the first wedge of bone graft posteriorly.

Post-Operative Management

A spica cast was not utilised owing to adequate fixation at the time of surgery, given an increased risk of insufficiency fractures, especially the distal femur post-operatively (our practice has been

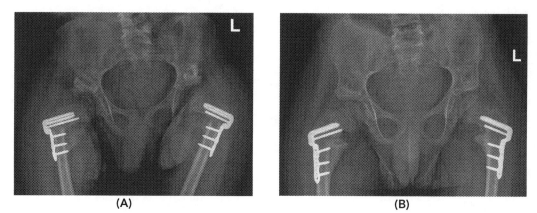

Figure 22.2a, b Radiographs immediately postoperatively (A) and at nine months follow-up (B) demonstrate that both hips are well reduced.

to only use a spica cast when an open reduction and capsulorrhaphy were required). The child was managed overnight in the surgical intensive care unit owing to medical comorbidities. He was placed in a soft abduction pillow which was maintained for six weeks. He was then graduated to night-time use of the device for six months. Weight-bearing was restricted for six weeks, after which he was gradually placed back into a stander. Nine months following surgery, the hips are well reduced, and the acetabular development is satisfactory (Figure 22.2b). The child needs to be followed up with annual radiographs till he is skeletally mature to ensure that the hip displacement does not recur.

Comment

Hip dysplasia is extremely common in children with cerebral palsy with profound neurologic impairment, and up to 90% of children with GMFCS 5 will have progressive dysplasia at some point of time.

Studies on the natural history of hip displacement in cerebral palsy suggest that maintaining the hips in a well-reduced position will lead to better long-term outcomes as compared to hips that are subluxated or dislocated.[2,3] This has led to the establishing of screening protocols which identify progressive displacement early on when the hips are still amenable to reconstructive surgery. Though isolated soft tissue releases are ineffective in arresting displacement, especially in GMFCS 4–5 patients, they may be justified in young children to delay the need for bony reconstruction until a time where the risks of revision surgery are less. Current evidence supports the use of a combined femoral osteotomy and a volume-reducing pelvic osteotomy such as the Dega or the San Diego acetabuloplasty.[4–10]

One area of controversy has been whether or not to surgically treat the contralateral side when it is essentially normal radiographically. A contralateral VDRO balances limb lengths and symmetry around the pelvis, but it remains controversial whether the contralateral "normal" hip is more likely to displace without surgery. In cases in which the range of motion is normal and there are no radiographic changes of displacement or dysplasia, the author will discuss the pros and cons of contralateral VDRO and typically offers bilateral surgery, especially in patients with considerable growth remaining. If the family is not interested in contralateral VDRO, then it is still important to perform an adductor release if range of motion is not normal. While no conclusive data has been presented in the literature, the current trend has been to perform a contralateral soft tissue release and a VDRO.

One of the challenging decisions is whether to reconstruct a hip with an obviously deformed femoral head with or without cartilage erosion. The decision must be individualised based on the age of the patient and the magnitude and chronicity of the pathology, as there is some evidence that the femoral head can partially remodel,[10] and non-ambulatory children may be less likely to experience pain due to decreased loading, although this has not been proven.

Recently there has been some interest in using guided growth with a screw to prevent migration, and while this strategy may be appropriate and relevant in earlier stages of disease, further study will be required to define the indications.

References

1. Miller F, Bagg MR. Age and migration percentage as risk factors for progression in spastic hip disease. *Dev Med Child Neuro.* 1995;37:449–55.
2. Lins LAB, Watkins CJ, Shore BJ. Natural history of spastic hip disease. *J Pediatr Orthop.* 2019;39(6, Suppl 1):S33–7.
3. Ramstad K, Jahnsen RB, Terjesen T. Severe hip displacement reduces health-related quality of life in children with cerebral palsy. *Acta Orthop.* 2017;88:205–10.
4. McNerney NP, Mubarak SJ, Wenger DR. One-stage correction of the dysplastic hip in cerebral palsy with the San Diego acetabuloplasty: Results and complications in 104 hips. *J Pediatr Orthop.* 2000;20:93–103.
5. Miller F, Girardi H, Lipton G, Ponzio R, Klaumann M, Dabney KW. Reconstruction of the dysplastic spastic hip with peri-ilial pelvic and femoral osteotomy followed by immediate mobilization. *J Pediatr Orthop.* 1997;17:592–602.
6. Mallet C, Ilharreborde B, Presedo A, Khairouni A, Mazda K, Penneçot GF. One-stage hip reconstruction in children with cerebral palsy: Long-term results at skeletal maturity. *J Child Orthop.* 2014;8:221–8.
7. Terjesen T. Femoral and pelvic osteotomies for severe hip displacement in nonambulatory children with cerebral palsy: A prospective population-based study of 31 patients with 7 years' follow-up. *Acta Orthop.* 2019;90:614–21.
8. El-Sobky TA, Fayyad TA, Kotb AM, Kaldas B. Bony reconstruction of hip in cerebral palsy children Gross Motor Function Classification System levels III to V: A systematic review. *J Pediatr Orthop B.* 2018;27:221–30.
9. Shore BJ, Graham HK. Management of moderate to severe hip displacement in nonambulatory children with cerebral palsy. *JBJS Rev.* 2017;5:e4.
10. Rutz E, Vavken P, Camathias C, Haase C, Jünemann S, Brunner R. Long-term results and outcome predictors in one-stage hip reconstruction in children with cerebral palsy. *J Bone Joint Surg Am.* 2015;97:500–6.

Hitesh Shah and Benjamin Joseph

Case

A 10-year-old girl presented with a painless limp which was noticed ever since she recovered partially from a febrile episode associated with acute flaccid paralysis involving both lower limbs at 1.5 years of age. At no point was there sensory impairment or loss of bowel and bladder control. The muscle weakness of both lower limbs improved over the next two years, but some residual weakness remained.

On examination, fixed pelvic obliquity was present and the right hip was flexed, abducted, and externally rotated, while the left hip was adducted and flexed. Passive internal and external rotations of the left hip were exaggerated. The left hip abductor power was Grade 3 (MRC grade), and the hip flexor power was Grade 4. The quadriceps power was Grade 2 on the right side and Grade 4 on the left. There was a 15-degree fixed flexion deformity of the right knee. Both feet were totally flail, but there were no fixed deformities of the feet. There was an apparent limb-length inequality with apparent shortening of the left lower limb. The lumbar spine was mobile, and there was no fixed lumbar scoliosis. She walked with a knee-ankle-foot orthosis on the right lower limb and an ankle-foot orthosis on the left. Without her braces, she walked with high stepping during the swing phase of both limbs and with a hand-on-thigh gait during the stance phase on the right side. The radiograph of the pelvis showed subluxation of the left hip with acetabular dysplasia and marked pelvic obliquity (Figure 23.1).

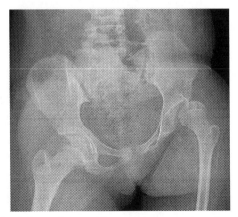

Figure 23.1 Radiograph of the pelvis and lower lumbar spine showing marked pelvic obliquity. The left hip is subluxated with over 50% of the femoral head outside the acetabular margin. The acetabulum is dysplastic, and there is no coxa valga.

Questions
- What are the problems that need to be addressed?
- What are the aims of treatment?
- What are the available treatment options to fulfil these aims?
- What are the factors that may influence your choice of treatment?
- Based on these points, what treatment would you recommend for this child?
- How long would you follow-up this child after treatment?

The Problems That Need to Be Addressed Are

- Pelvic obliquity secondary to:
  - ○ Fixed abduction deformity of the right hip
  - ○ Fixed adduction deformity of the left hip
- Subluxation of the left hip secondary to:
  - ○ Pelvic obliquity (Figure 23.2)[1,2]

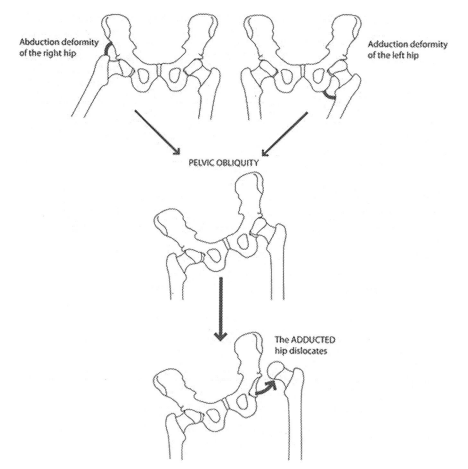

Figure 23.2 Diagrammatic representation of the pathogenesis of paralytic hip dislocation. (Modified from Figure 26.1 Paediatric Orthopaedics—A System of Decision-making 2nd Edition.)

  - ○ Muscle imbalance around the hip[1,2]
  - ○ Acetabular dysplasia[1,2]
- Abnormal gait pattern secondary to:
  - ○ Apparent shortening of the left lower limb due to pelvic obliquity
  - ○ Muscle weakness around left hip, right knee and both feet
  - ○ Subluxation of the left hip

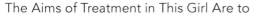

The Aims of Treatment in This Girl Are to

- Correct pelvic obliquity
- Obtain a stable concentric reduction of the left hip
- Improve the gait pattern by achieving the previous two aims

Options for Treatment to Fulfil Each Aim

- Correcting pelvic obliquity
    - Correction of adduction deformity of the left hip
    - Correction of abduction deformity of the right hip
        - Soft tissue release
        - Proximal femoral osteotomy
- Obtaining a stable concentric reduction of the left hip
    - Correct pelvic obliquity
    - Improve muscle balance
        - Tendon transfer (iliopsoas transfer to the greater trochanter[3])
        - Augmenting the power of hip abductors (e.g., increasing the resting length of the muscle fibres by trans-iliac lengthening[4])
        - Weakening the hip adductors and flexors
    - Correct acetabular dysplasia
        - Innominate osteotomy[4,5]
        - Acetabular shelf procedure

FACTORS THAT INFLUENCED THE CHOICE OF TREATMENT

- The severity of adduction and abduction deformities
- Power of muscles around the subluxating hip
- Quality of hip reduction obtained during surgery

The choice of treatment based on these factors is shown in Table 23.1.

Table 23.1 Factors Influencing the Choice of Treatment

Factors		Treatment Implications
Severity of adduction and abduction deformities of the hip	To be decided during surgery	If the adduction and abduction deformities of the hips can be corrected and pelvic obliquity resolved by soft tissue release, there is no need for femoral osteotomies. Proximal femoral osteotomies are only needed if significant residual deformities are present following soft tissue release.
Power of muscles around the subluxating hip	Grade 3 hip abductors Grade 4 hip flexor	A muscle should ideally have Grade 5 power to be transferred. In this instance, the hip's flexor power is only Grade 4. For this reason, restoring muscle balance should be by weakening the deforming muscle (e.g., by lengthening or releasing it).

(Continued)

Table 23.1 (Continued)

Factors		Treatment Implications
Quality of hip reduction obtained during surgery	Concentric reduction	If a concentric reduction of the left hip is obtained by correcting deformities of both hips, a pelvic osteotomy that reorients the dysplastic acetabulum should be considered. If the reduction is sub-optimal, a shelf procedure may be done.

How Was This Girl Treated?

The girl was treated with release of contracted structures around the respective hips; on the right side, the sartorius, tensor fascia lata, rectus femoris, anterior fibres of gluteus medius, and the iliopsoas were released, and on the left side the adductor longus and brevis and the iliopsoas were released. The hip could then be reduced. In order to address the acetabular dysplasia, a pelvic osteotomy akin to a Salter osteotomy was done. A large wedge of autologous iliac graft was driven into the gap in an attempt distract the pelvic fragments, and the osteotomy was fixed with two Kirschner wires (Figure 23.3).

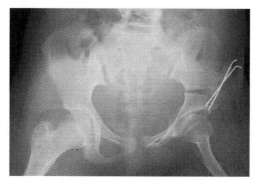

Figure 23.3 Radiograph showing pelvic osteotomy with reorientation of the acetabulum and a small amount of intra-pelvic lengthening of the limb.

Post-Operative Management

The child was kept in bed on bilateral above-knee skin traction for three weeks, following which she was discharged. Weight-bearing was deferred till the pelvic osteotomy had united.

Follow-Up

Six years after surgery, the hip remains stable (Figure 23.4), and when seen last, 11 years following the hip stabilisation, there is no pelvic obliquity, the limb lengths are equal, and the left hip is well reduced with very satisfactory acetabular coverage of the femoral head. Further follow-up is needed only if any symptoms develop.

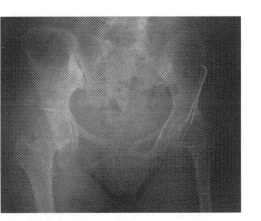

Figure 23.4 Radiograph of the pelvis six years following the surgery, showing that the left hip is well centred in the acetabulum.

Comment

- We attempted to minimise the muscle imbalance around the left hip by releasing the adductors and the iliopsoas. In addition, the pelvic osteotomy with a wide-open wedge could have increased the resting length of the gluteus medius muscle and augmented its power to some degree.
- In order to reduce the extent of bracing, a supracondylar femoral extension osteotomy of the right knee was performed close to skeletal maturity. This stabilised her knee, and she discarded the knee-ankle-foot orthosis on her right limb and began ambulating with bilateral ankle-foot-orthoses.

References

1. Joseph B, Watts H. Polio revisited: Reviving knowledge and skills to meet the challenge of resurgence. *J Child Orthop.* 2015;9(5):325–38. doi: 10.1007/s11832-015-0678-4.
2. Lau JH, Parker JC, Hsu LC, Leong JC. Paralytic hip instability in poliomyelitis. *J Bone Joint Surg Br.* 1986;68:528–33.
3. Mustard WT. A follow-up study of iliopsoas transfers for hip instability. *J Bone Joint Surg Br.* 1959;41:289–98.
4. Lee DY, Choi IH, Chung CY, Ahn JH, Steel HH. Triple innominate osteotomy for hip stabilisation and transiliac leg lengthening after poliomyelitis. *J Bone Joint Surg Br.* 1993;75(6):858–64.
5. Sierra RJ, Schoeniger SR, Millis M, Ganz R. Periacetabular osteotomy for containment of the non-arthritic dysplastic hip secondary to poliomyelitis. *J Bone Joint Surg Am.* 2010;92(18):2917–23. doi: 10.2106/JBJS.I.00753.

CASE 24: TERATOLOGIC DISLOCATION OF THE HIP – MULTIPLE CONGENITAL CONTRACTURES

Hitesh Shah

Case

A 1-year-old girl presented with dislocation of the left hip, hyper-extension of both knees, rocker-bottom deformities of both feet and flexion deformities of both wrists. She was the second child in the family and was born by a normal delivery. She had typical features of multiple congenital contractures. All the deformities and dislocations were rigid and could not be corrected passively. Radiographs of the pelvis and knee joints confirmed dislocations of both knee joints and left hip (Figure 24.1a, b, c). The child could not crawl or stand, and hand function was severely compromised.

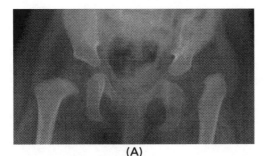

(A)

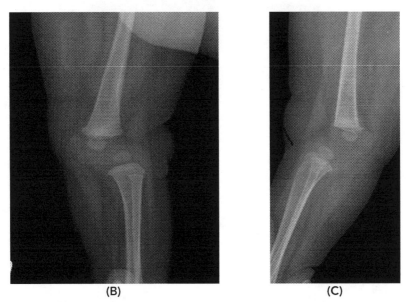

(B)   **(C)**

Figure 24.1 Radiographs of the pelvis (A) and both knee joints (B, C) show dislocations of the left hip and both knee joints.

Questions

- What are the problems that need to be addressed in this child?
- What are the aims of treatment?
- What are the available treatment options to fulfil these aims?
- What are the factors that may influence your choice of treatment?
- Based on these points, what treatment would you recommend for this child?
- How long would you follow-up this child after treatment?

The Problems That Need to Be Addressed in This Young Child Are

- Multiple rigid joint deformities and dislocations of the upper and lower extremities
- Severely compromised upper and lower limb function

The Aims of Treatment in This Child Are to

- Correct deformities and dislocations that are contributing to functional limitations to facilitate independence in the activities of daily living

The overall management of this child entails treatment of each deformed or dislocated joint in a planned sequence. Once the sequence of treatment is decided, the problems related to each individual joint need to be defined and addressed.

Problems Related to the Left Hip Joint

- Rigid unilateral dislocation

  o   Risk of not achieving a concentric reduction

- Stiffness of the joint due to contractures of soft tissue

  o   Risk of residual stiffness even if reduction is satisfactory

Aims of Treatment of the Left Hip

- Achieve a stable concentric reduction
- Retain as much motion of the hip as possible

Options for Treatment to Fulfil Each Aim

- Achieving a stable concentric reduction

  o   Open reduction of the hip joint by medial approach[1]
  o   Open reduction of the hip joint by anterolateral approach[2]

- Retaining motion of the hip

  o   No attempt to reduce the hip (accept the dislocation)

FACTORS THAT INFLUENCED THE CHOICE OF TREATMENT

- Age of the child
- Unilateral versus bilateral hip dislocations
- Associated knee dislocation
- The extent of muscle weakness and severity of upper limb involvement
- Likelihood of walking

The choice of treatment of the dislocated hip based on these factors is shown in Table 24.1.

Table 24.1 Factors Influencing the Choice of Treatment of Hip Dislocation

Factors		Treatment Implications
The age of the child	1 year old	Children younger than 1 year may be treated by medial open reduction of the hip. Children between 1 and 2 years of age may be treated by anterolateral open reduction of the hip.[3,4] In children over the age of 2 years, unreduced bilateral hip dislocations may be ignored and not be reduced.
Unilateral or bilateral hip dislocation	Unilateral dislocation (left)	An attempt at reduction of unilateral hip dislocation must be made to prevent limb length inequality and asymmetry of the pelvis.[3,4,5]
The extent of muscle weakness and severity of upper limb involvement	Mild/moderate muscle weakness Wrist deformities present Involvement of elbows and shoulders not severe	Children with profound weakness and severe upper limb involvement may have a poor prognosis for independent walking. Hip dislocation should be left alone in such a situation.[6,7] Hip dislocation in a child with good ambulatory potential should be treated more aggressively.[3,4,5]
Presence of other musculoskeletal anomalies	Bilateral knee dislocation, bilateral congenital vertical talus, bilateral wrist flexion deformities	The sequence of treatment needs to be planned. Reduction of knee dislocation takes precedence as it will enable knee flexion and relaxation of the hamstrings, both of which may facilitate successful reduction of the hip.[8] The flexed knee is also essential for dealing with contracture of the gastroc-soleus while correcting the vertical talus. The hip dislocation may then be addressed either in a separate sitting or be treated simultaneously with reduction of the knee dislocation.[9]

How Was This Girl Treated?

The girl was treated with staged surgical procedures. First, bilateral quadricepsplasty was done to reduce the knee joints. Ninety-degree knee flexion was achieved after the surgery. Both feet were then corrected with soft tissue release after three months. The left hip dislocation was treated last of all with open reduction through the anterolateral approach six months later.

A concentric stable reduction of the hip was achieved without having to shorten the femur.

Post-Operative Management

A hip spica was applied immediately following surgery; this was changed, and a fresh spica was applied at six weeks. The second hip spica was retained for another six weeks, and mobilisation was started thereafter with bilateral ankle-foot orthoses to support the feet.

Follow-Up

The girl was followed up regularly. At the five-year follow-up, both knees and the operated hip joint had excellent function. Radiographs of the hip taken at 5, 12 and 16 years of age showed good development of the left hip that is well centred and concentric (Figure 24.2a, b, c).

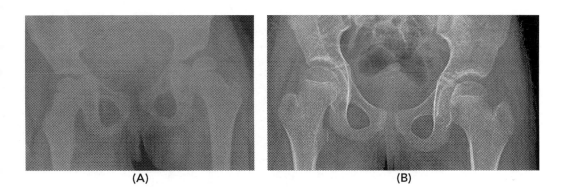

(A)

(B)

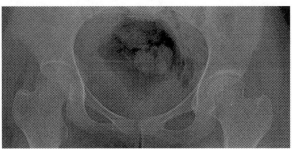

(C)

Figure 24.2 Radiographs of the pelvis at the ages of 5 years (A), 12 years (B) and 16 years (C) show a well reduced hip and good development of the hip joint.

Comment

Dorsal carpal wedge osteotomies were also performed to improve hand function at 12 years of age. Further follow-up is needed only if fresh symptoms develop.

References

1. Wada A, Yamaguchi T, Nakamura T, Yanagida H, Takamura K, Oketani Y, et al. Surgical treatment of hip dislocation in amyoplasia-type arthrogryposis. *J Pediatr Orthop B*. 2012;21:381–5.
2. Szoke G, Staheli LT, Jaffe K, Hall JG. Medialapproach open reduction of hip dislocation in amyoplasia-type arthrogryposis. *J Pediatr Orthop*. 1996;16:127–30.
3. Bradish C. The hip in arthrogryposis. *J Child Orthop*. 2005;9(6):459–63. https://doi.org/10.1007/s11832-015-0693-5.
4. Fassier A, Wicart P, Dubousset J, Seringe R. Arthrogryposis multiplex congenita: Long-term follow-up from birth until skeletal maturity. *J Child Orthop*. 2009;3(5):383–90. https://doi.org/10.1007/s11832-009-0187-4.

5. B K AR, Singh KA, Shah H. Surgical management of the congenital dislocation of the knee and hip in children presented after six months of age. *Int Orthop.* 2020 Dec;44(12):2635–44. doi: 10.1007/s00264-020-04759-8.

6. Gruel CR, Birch JG, Roach JW, Herring JA. Teratological dislocation of the hip. *J Pediatr Orthop.* 1986;6:693–702.

7. Lloyd-Roberts GC, Lettin AWF. Arthrogryposis multiplex congenita. *J Bone Joint Surg Br.* 1970;52(3):494–508.

8. Tercier S, Shah H, Joseph B. Quadricepsplasty for congenital dislocation of the knee and congenital quadriceps contracture. *J Child Orthop.* 2012;6(5):397–410. doi: 10.1007/s11832-012-0437-8.

9. Johnston CE. Simultaneous open reduction of ipsilateral congenital dislocation of the hip and knee assisted by femoral diaphyseal shortening. *J Pediatr Orthop.* 2011;31(7):732–40. https://doi.org/10.1097/BPO.0b013e31822f1b24.

Hitesh Shah

Case

A 2-year-old girl presented with a painless limp first noted some months earlier. She was a pre-term child with a history of neonatal sepsis at around 10 days of age, for which she was treated with parenteral antibiotics. She apparently recovered from this, and her developmental milestones were normal.

On examination, the left lower limb was a centimetre shorter than the right. Passive movements of the hip were not painful. The ranges of motion of the left hip were normal except for internal rotation which was exaggerated. She walked with a painless, short-limb, Trendelenburg limp on the left. Radiographs of the pelvis displayed a subluxated left hip with a broken Shenton line, mild acetabular dysplasia, a markedly increased medial joint space and the femoral neck pointing to the lateral margin of the acetabulum. The ossific nucleus of the capital femoral epiphysis was much smaller than that of the normal hip and was situated eccentrically in relation to the lateral half of the femoral metaphysis (Figure 25.1).

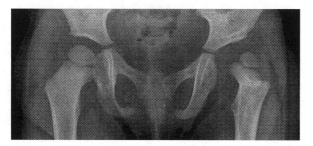

Figure 25.1 Subluxation of the left hip with acetabular dysplasia and a small femoral ossific nucleus that is eccentrically located.

A radiograph of the pelvis taken in 15 degrees of abduction and full internal rotation of the hips revealed improved coverage of the left femoral head with the femoral neck pointing to the triradiate cartilage (Figure 25.2). The neck shaft angle was only marginally increased; this suggested that excessive femoral anteversion was the major cause of subluxation.

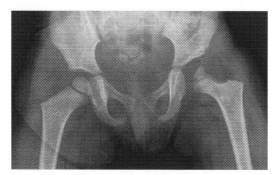

Figure 25.2 Subluxation reduced with modest abduction and full internal rotation of the hip.

Since the ossific nucleus of the femoral epiphysis was so small and eccentrically located, there was a possibility that the medial part of the epiphysis may have been destroyed, and in order to exclude this, an arthrogram was performed. The arthrogram showed a well-formed cartilaginous epiphysis that was congruous with the acetabulum (Figure 25.3).

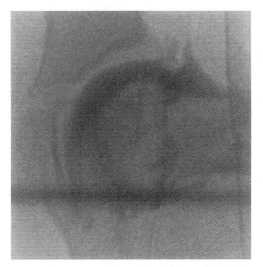

Figure 25.3 Arthrogram of the hip showing a near normal cartilaginous contour of the femoral head that is congruent with the acetabulum.

Questions

- What are the problems that need to be addressed in this child?
- What are the aims of treatment?
- What are the available treatment options to fulfil these aims?
- What are the factors that may influence your choice of treatment?
- Based on these points, what treatment would you recommend for this child?
- How long would you follow-up this child after treatment?

The Problems That Need to Be Addressed in This Child Are

- Instability of the left hip due to:
  - Excessive femoral anteversion
  - Mild coxa valga
  - Mild acetabular dysplasia
- Shortening of the left lower limb of 1 cm

The Aims of Treatment in This Girl Are to

- Restore stability of the hip
- Correct the shortening of the limb by skeletal maturity

Options for Treatment to Fulfil Each Aim

- Instability of the hip
  - Correction of femoral anteversion and coxa valga by a proximal femoral osteotomy
  - Open reduction of the hip if the previous measure fails to achieve a concentric reduction

- Limb length inequality
  - Observation
  - Timed contralateral epiphyseodesis, if needed, in due course
  - Timed limb lengthening, if needed, in due course

FACTORS THAT INFLUENCED THE CHOICE OF TREATMENT

- Age of the child
- Status of the femoral head
- Status of the femoral neck
- Status of acetabulum
- Type of instability
- Severity of shortening

The choice of treatment based on these factors is shown in Table 25.1.

Table 25.1 Factors Influencing the Choice of Treatment

Factors		Treatment Implications
Age of the child	2 years	The child is too young to consider any intervention for limb length inequality. At this point, observation is all that is justified.

(Continued)

Table 25.1 (Continued)

Factors		Treatment Implications
Status of the femoral head	Entire femoral head is present and congruent with the acetabulum in abduction and internal rotation of the hip (though the ossification is delayed, partial and eccentric)	If the femoral head was destroyed, there would be little value in correcting the femoral anteversion. Similarly reducing a distorted, irregular or incongruent femoral head may be associated with poor outcomes.[1,2,3] In this child as the femoral head is rounded, reducing it into the acetabulum to restore a congruent joint is justified.
Status of the femoral neck	Intact and anteverted with mild coxa valga	Correction of the anteversion and coxa valga by a proximal femoral osteotomy is indicated as the hip reduces well on internal rotation and abduction.
Status of acetabulum	Mild acetabular dysplasia	The acetabular dysplasia (confirmed on the arthrogram) is mild, and if the subluxation can be corrected by addressing the femoral anteversion, the acetabular dysplasia may improve over time.
Type of instability (subluxation versus dislocation)	Subluxation	Subluxation can be managed without having to open the joint capsule; dislocation may require a formal open reduction.[2,3,4]
Shortening	1 cm	Such mild shortening at this age can be left alone and closely monitored to see if shortening increases to an extent that it warrants intervention.

How Was This Girl Treated?

The girl was examined under anaesthesia, and an arthrogram was done. As the subluxation was well corrected by internally rotating and abducting the hip, a sub-trochanteric open-wedge varus derotation osteotomy was performed. The distal fragment was rotated laterally by 45 degrees and adducted by 20 degrees and fixed with a contoured dynamic compression plate (DCP) and screws. Concentric reduction of the hip was confirmed with an arthrogram (Figure 25.4).

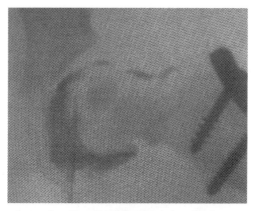

Figure 25.4 Arthrogram done after proximal femoral de-rotation, varus osteotomy shows that with the hip in the neutral position the femoral head is well centred in the acetabulum.

Post-Operative Management

In view of the fact that the osteotomy was an open-wedge osteotomy (Figure 25.5a), she was kept non–weight bearing for six weeks, and after union of the osteotomy was confirmed, weight bearing was permitted (Figure 25.5b). The implants were removed after a year. A year later, the acetabular development had improved, and the femoral head remained well reduced (Figure 25.5c).

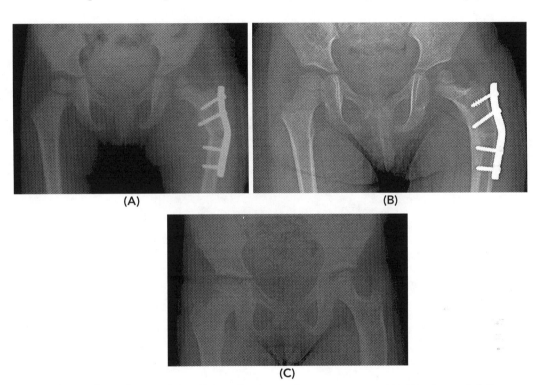

(A) (B)

(C)

Figure 25.5a, b, c Sequential radiographs: immediate post-operative (A), six-week follow-up (B), two-year follow-up (C).

Follow-Up

The girl was followed up annually, and at the eight-year follow-up, she was normally active and had no symptoms related to the hip. The hip examination was normal. Shortening of the limb of 1 cm was still present. A radiograph of the pelvis showed a well-centred femoral head, very satisfactory acetabular development and excellent remodelling of the osteotomy site (Figure 25.6).

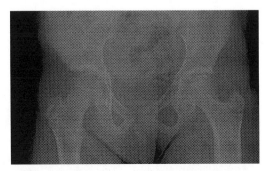

Figure 25.6 Radiograph of the pelvis eight years following surgery.

Comment

The child needs to be followed up until skeletal maturity to keep a check on hip development and shortening.

References

1. Choi IH, Pizzutillo PD, Bowen JR, Dragann R, Malhis T. Sequelae and reconstruction after septic arthritis of the hip in infants. *J Bone Joint Surg Am*. 1990;72:1150–65.
2. Johari AN, Dhawale AA, Johari RA. Management of post septic hip dislocations when the capital femoral epiphysis is present. *J Pediatr Orthop B*. 2011;20:413–21.
3. Rastogi P, Agarwal A. Management of post septic sequelae of hips with dislocation in children [published online ahead of print, 2020 Jul 24]. *Int Orthop*. 2020. doi: 10.1007/s00264-020-04743-2.
4. Forlin E, Milani C. Sequelae of septic arthritis of the hip in children: A new classification and a review of 41 hips. *J Pediatr Orthop*. 2008;28(5):524–8. doi: 10.1097/BPO.0b013e31817bb079.

Hitesh Shah and Benjamin Joseph

Cases

a. A 2-week-old neonate presented with hyperextension of both knees since birth. He was the first child of the family; he was born at full term by a normal delivery. There were no features of generalised ligament laxity or facial dysmorphism. Both the hips, feet and upper limbs were normal. The hyperextended knees could not be passively flexed beyond 5 degrees. Ultrasound of both knees showed anterior dislocation of the knee joint (Figure 26.1).

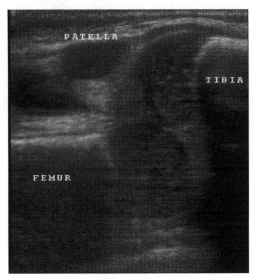

Figure 26.1 Ultrasound of the knee showing anterior dislocation of the joint.

b. A 7-month-old girl presented with hyperextension of the right knee and dislocation of right hip since birth. She was the first child of the family, born at full term by a normal delivery. Features of generalised ligament laxity were present. Both feet, the opposite lower limb and both upper limbs were normal. There was recurvatum deformity of the right knee, and passive flexion was not possible beyond 5 degrees. Radiographs of hip and knee joints showed dislocation of both the right knee and the right hip (Figure 26.2).

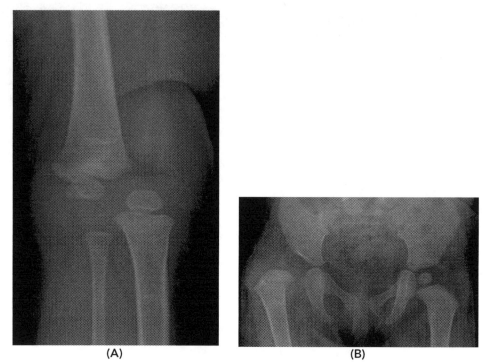

(A)   **(B)**

Figure 26.2 Lateral radiograph of the right knee of the infant showing dislocation (A) and antero-posterior radiograph of the infant's pelvis showing dislocation of the right hip (B).

Questions
- What are the problems that need to be addressed in these infants?
- What are the aims of treatment?
- What are the available treatment options to fulfil these aims?
- What are the factors that may influence your choice of treatment?
- Based on these points, what treatment would you recommend for these infants?
- How long would you follow-up these children after treatment?

The Problems Related to the Knee That Need to Be Addressed in Both These Infants Are

- Dislocation of the knee
- Contracture of the quadriceps muscle which may not yield to stretching, necessitating quadricepsplasty

The Aims of Treatment in These Infants Are to

- Obtain reduction of the knee dislocation
- Obtain knee flexion of 90 degrees to perform activities of daily living
- Avoid excessive weakening of the quadriceps muscle
- Avoid complications of treatment

   o Fracture of the femur or tibia
   o Instability of the knee

Options for Treatment to Fulfil Each Aim

- Obtaining reduction of the knee dislocation and obtaining knee flexion of 90 degrees

   o Serial manipulation and cast application
   o Pavlik harness
   o Percutaneous quadriceps tenotomy
   o Quadricepsplasty and open reduction

- Maintaining the strength of the quadriceps muscle

   o Reduction of the dislocation by non-operative means
   o If quadricepsplasty is required, avoiding excessive lengthening of the muscle

- Avoiding complications of treatment

   o Prevent iatrogenic fractures by

      □ Avoiding forceful manipulation
      □ Resorting to early quadricepsplasty if response to stretching is poor

   o Prevent knee instability

      □ Avoiding release of collateral ligaments during surgery

FACTORS THAT INFLUENCED THE CHOICE OF TREATMENT
• The age of the child
• The underlying disease and its natural history
• The severity of knee deformity
• Presence of other anomalies of the lower limb

The choice of treatment based on these factors is shown in Table 26.1.

Table 26.1 Factors Influencing the Choice of Treatment

Factors		Treatment Implications
The age of the child	a. Fourteen days b. Seven months	Children under 6 months of age can be treated with a trial of serial manipulation and cast application.[1,2]
The underlying disease and its natural history	a & b. Idiopathic congenital dislocation of the knee	Children with a syndromic association or multiple congenital contractures often require surgical intervention.[3]
The severity of knee deformity	Complete dislocation of the knee	The results of serial manipulation are good in children with hyperextension of the knee joint without proximal migration of the tibia. Surgical intervention is often required with complete dislocation and proximal migration of the tibia.[4,5]
Presence of other musculoskeletal anomalies	a. No associated anomalies b. Associated developmental dysplasia (DDH) of the ipsilateral hip	When associated DDH is present, the reduction of the knee should precede reduction of the hip as relaxation of the hamstrings (once flexion of the knee has been achieved) will facilitate reduction of the hip.[1,2]

How Were These Infants Treated?

a. The boy was treated with gentle longitudinal traction on the tibia with gradual flexion of the knee joint. The correction obtained was maintained with an above-knee anterior plaster slab. Sequential weekly manipulation and plaster slab application was commenced. Both knee joints were reduced, and flexion to 90 degrees was achieved after three manipulations. The reduction of the knee joints was confirmed with ultrasound scans. The infant was then fitted with a Pavlik harness which was worn for 23 hours a day for six weeks.

b. The girl was treated with a quadricepsplasty through a lateral incision.[2] The collateral ligaments were untouched. Knee flexion to 90 degrees was obtained at surgery. The knee joint was immobilised with an above-knee plaster slab for three weeks, after which the knee was mobilised. The hip was then treated with closed reduction and spica application. A concentric stable reduction was obtained (Figure 26.3). The spica was retained for three months.

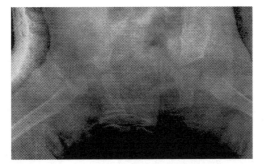

Figure 26.3 Radiograph of the pelvis showing satisfactory reduction of the right hip.

Follow-Up

a. The boy was followed up to the age of 6 years. On the last follow-up, there were no deformities; both knee joints had excellent function with full knee flexion (Figures 26.4a, b, c, d) and normal quadriceps power. A final follow-up at skeletal maturity is planned.

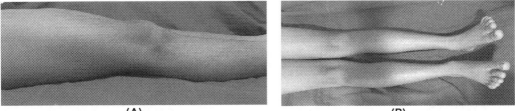

(A) (B)

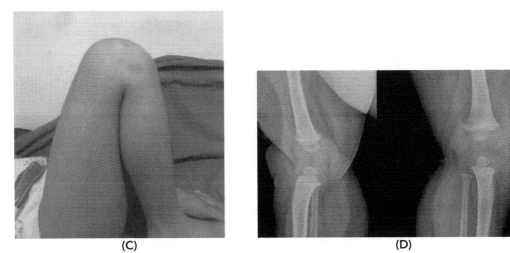

(C) (D)

Figure 26.4 Clinical photographs (A–C) and radiographs (D) after six years following closed reduction of bilateral congenital dislocation of the knees.

b. The girl was followed up till the age of 7 years, at which time both the knee and hip were well reduced and functioning normally (Figure 26.5a, b, c). She needs to be followed till skeletal maturity.

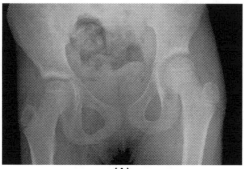

(A)

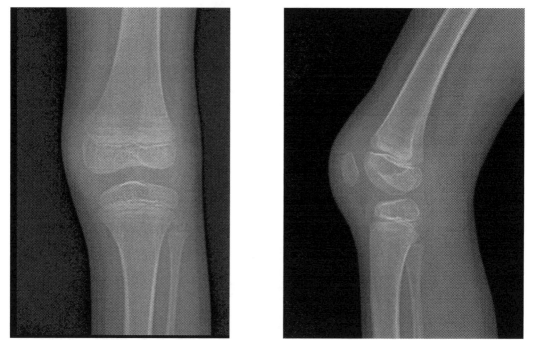

(B)   (C)

Figure 26.5 Radiographs of hips and right knee at 7 years of age show a well-centred right hip (A) and normal alignment of the tibia and femur of the right knee joint (B, C).

References

1. B K AR, Singh KA, Shah H. Surgical management of the congenital dislocation of the knee and hip in children presented after six months of age. *Int Orthop.* 2020 Dec;44(12):2635–44. doi: 10.1007/s00264-020-04759-8.
2. Tercier S, Shah H, Joseph B. Quadricepsplasty for congenital dislocation of the knee and congenital quadriceps contracture. *J Child Orthop.* 2012;6(5):397–410. doi: 10.1007/s11832-012-0437-8.

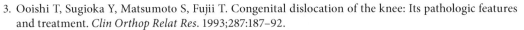

3. Ooishi T, Sugioka Y, Matsumoto S, Fujii T. Congenital dislocation of the knee: Its pathologic features and treatment. *Clin Orthop Relat Res*. 1993;287:187–92.

4. Ahmadi B, Shahriaree H, Silver CM. Severe congenital genu recurvatum. *J Bone Joint Surg Am*. 1979;61:622–4.

5. Curtis BH, Fisher RL. Congenital hyperextension with anterior subluxation of the knee. *J Bone Joint Surg Am*. 1969;51:255–69.

CASE 27: CONGENITAL DISLOCATION OF THE PATELLA

Hitesh Shah and Benjamin Joseph

Case

A 3-month-old male infant presented with a deformity and a puckered area of skin on the outer aspect of the left knee which were noted at birth (Figure 27.1a). He was born at term by a normal vaginal delivery. He was thriving well and was otherwise quite healthy. Examination revealed that there was a fixed flexion deformity of 70 degrees with normal further flexion. The leg was externally rotated (Figure 27.1b). The patella was not palpable in the front of the knee but was palpated on the lateral aspect of the knee. The area of puckered skin was not adherent to the underlying structures.

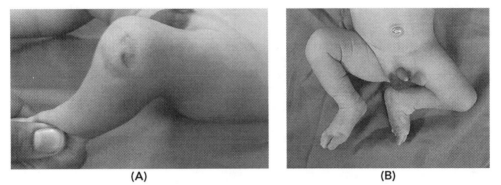

(A)   (B)

Figure 27.1 Appearance of the left knee. Puckering of the skin on the antero-lateral aspect of the knee is seen (A). The knee is flexed, and the leg is externally rotated (B).

Ultrasound scans of the knee confirmed that the patella was not in its normal position (Figure 27.2a) and that it was located on the lateral aspect of the knee (Figure 27.2b).[1] The patella was of a reasonable size.

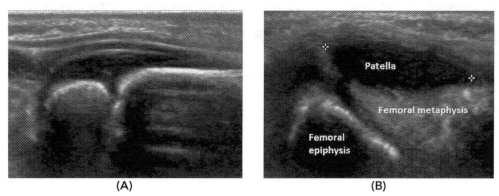

(A)   **(B)**

Figure 27.2 Longitudinal ultrasound scan of the front of the knee shows that the patella is not in its normal position (A). Longitudinal scan on the lateral aspect of the knee shows the patella in relation to the distal femur (B).

Questions

- What are the problems that need to be addressed?
- What are the aims of treatment?
- What are the available treatment options to fulfil these aims?
- What are the factors that may influence your choice of treatment?
- Based on these points, what treatment would you recommend for this infant?
- How long would you follow-up this child after treatment?

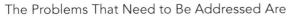

The Problems That Need to Be Addressed Are

- Flexion deformity of the left knee and external rotation deformity of the leg
- Dislocated patella

The Aims of Treatment in This Infant Are to

- Correct the deformities
- Obtain a stable reduction of the patellar dislocation

Options for Treatment to Fulfil Each Aim

- Correcting flexion deformity of the knee and external rotation of the leg

  - Passive stretching
  - Soft tissue release[2–4]

    - Ilio-tibial band and lateral intermuscular septum
    - Vastus lateralis
    - Hamstrings
    - Posterior capsule of the knee

- Obtaining a stable reduction of the dislocated patella[2–4]

  - Soft tissue release (as earlier) and advancement of the vastus medialis
  - Medial shift of the patellar tendon insertion
  - Semitendinosus tenodesis

FACTORS THAT INFLUENCED THE CHOICE OF TREATMENT

- Age at surgery
- Response to sequential release of contracted lateral structures and augmentation of medial structures in terms of:
  - Correction of the flexion deformity of the knee
  - Achieving stable reduction of the patella

The choice of treatment based on these factors is outlined in Table 27.1.

Table 27.1 Factors That Influenced Treatment

Factors		Treatment Implications
Age	Infant	Delay in treatment makes reduction of the dislocation more difficult necessitating more extensive release at the expense of weakening the quadriceps.

(Continued)

Table 27.1 (Continued)

Factors		Treatment Implications
Response to sequential release of lateral structures and augmentation of medial structures	Correcting the deformity	If the knee can be extended to <10 degrees short of full extension after releasing the ilio-tibial band, the lateral intermuscular septum and the vastus lateralis, no further release is required. If more than 10 degrees of flexion deformity persists, hamstring lengthening may be considered. Release of the posterior capsule of the knee is seldom required.
	Achieving stable reduction of the patella	If the patella remains reduced after release of the ilio-tibial band, lateral intermuscular septum and the vastus lateralis and advancement of the vastus medialis, nothing further needs to be done. If the patella is still unstable, lateral half of the patellar tendon insertion may be transferred medially (Roux-Goldthwaite). If the patella is still unstable after all these measures, semitendinosus tenodesis should be done.

How Was This Infant Treated?

Serial casting was done at weekly intervals; the flexion deformity decreased to 30 degrees, and no further correction could be achieved. At the age of 10 months, surgery was performed. Under general anaesthesia, through a lateral parapatellar incision, the ilio-tibial band was divided and a segment of the lateral intermuscular segment was excised. The vastus lateralis was released from the lateral border of the patella and erased from its origin on the distal femur and allowed to retract proximally. The lateral capsule of the knee was opened close to the lateral border of the patella from a point 2 cm proximal to the superior pole of the patella to a point 2 cm distal to the lower pole of the patella. Care was taken to ensure that there were no adhesions between the patella and the lateral surface of the femur. The patella was reduced into the shallow patellar groove on the femur. The vastus medialis was stretched and thin; it was advanced laterally onto the front of the patella and anchored with non-absorbable sutures.

The knee was gently flexed to 90 degrees and extended fully; the patella dislocated when the knee was flexed. The patellar tendon was split into two slips, and the lateral slip was carefully divided close to its insertion, taking care to avoid damaging the growth plate. The lateral half of the patellar tendon was passed posterior to the intact medial half of the tendon and advanced as far medially as possible and anchored to the periosteum with non-absorbable sutures. The stability of reduction was checked again, and at this point the patella remained in the normal position on flexing the knee. The wound was closed, and a plaster-of-Paris cast was applied with the knee in extension.

Post-Operative Management

The cast was removed after six weeks, and physiotherapy to encourage knee bending and quadriceps strengthening was started. The child was not co-operative but over the course of the next year started walking and sitting with his knee flexed.

Follow-Up

He was followed up annually. At the age of 9, he was functioning normally. The quadriceps power was Grade 4+ on the MRC scale. He had a 5-degree extension lag, but he did not complain of tripping or falling. There were no deformities at the knee, and x-rays showed normal alignment of the knee and a slightly smaller patella on the left which was well reduced (Figure 27.3). A final review at skeletal maturity is planned.

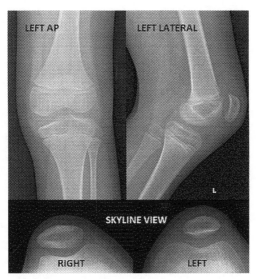

Figure 27.3 X-rays of the knee of the child at 9 years of age. The left patella is smaller than the right but is well formed and well reduced.

References

1. Koplewitz BZ, Babyn PS, Cole WG. Congenital dislocation of the patella. *Am J Roentgenol*. 2005 May; 184(5):1640–6. doi: 10.2214/ajr.184.5.01841640. PMID: 15855131.
2. Ghanem I, Wattincourt L, Seringe R. Congenital dislocation of the patella. Part I: Pathologic anatomy. *J Pediatr Orthop*. 2000 Nov–Dec;20(6):812–16. doi: 10.1097/00004694-200011000-00023. PMID: 11097261.
3. Wada A, Fujii T, Takamura K, Yanagida H, Surijamorn P. Congenital dislocation of the patella. *J Child Orthop*. 2008 Mar;2(2):119–23. doi: 10.1007/s11832-008-0090-4. Epub 2008 Mar 4. PMID: 19308591; PMCID: PMC2656798.
4. Paton RW, Bonshahi AY, Kim WY. Congenital and irreducible non-traumatic dislocation of the patella: A modified soft tissue procedure. *Knee*. 2004 Apr;11(2):117–20. doi: 10.1016/S0968-0160(03)00074-7. PMID: 15066622.

CASE 28: RADIAL HEAD DISLOCATION

Nick Green and James A Fernandes

Case

A 12-year-old girl with multiple hereditary osteochondromatosis (MHO) was referred with an increasingly painful, short and bowed left forearm (Figure 28.1). The deformity was first noticed at age 5. Later pain and decreased motion interfered with gymnastics. Certain movements such as placing her hand behind her head were not possible and appearance of the limb was a cause of embarrassment.

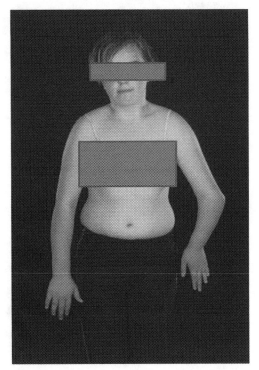

Figure 28.1 Demonstrates cubitus varus, a short forearm segment and a visible dislocated radial head with lateral prominence.

She had cubitus varus, a prominent postero-laterally dislocated radial head, a bowed ulna and a short forearm. Supination was markedly restricted and painful. She had a fixed flexion deformity of 40 degrees of the elbow (Figure 28.2) and varus/valgus instability at her elbow.

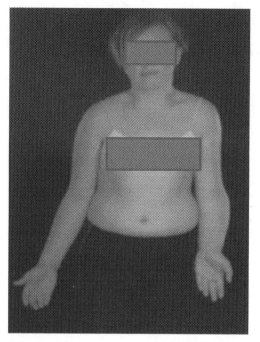

Figure 28.2 Demonstrates her manoeuvre to compensate for her reduced supination by extending, adducting and externally rotating her shoulder.

Radiographs confirmed the radial head dislocation, a short and angulated distal ulna with distal radial and ulnar osteochondromas but no evidence of carpal shift (Figure 28.3).

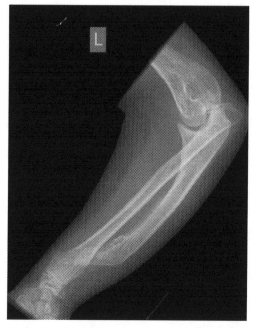

Figure 28.3 Lateral radiograph showing the posterior component of the dislocation, apex posterior distal ulnar angulation (oblique plane in reality) and an anterior distal radial and ulnar osteochondroma. Also note the lack of distal carpal support from the ulna.

Questions

- What are the problems that need to be addressed?
- What are the aims of treatment?
- What are the treatment options to fulfil each aim?
- What are the factors that influenced the choice of treatment?
- Based on these points, what treatment would you recommend for this child?

The Problems That Need to Be Addressed Are
- Radial head dislocation and elbow instability
- Ulnar shortening and distal angular deformity
- Distal radial and ulnar osteochondromata inciting abnormal growth

The Aims of Treatment in This Girl Are to
- Reduce the radial head dislocation and restore elbow stability
- Relieve pain
- Improve the range of supination of the forearm
- Improve the appearance of the limb
- Prevent recurrence of the dislocation and deformity

Options for Treatment to Fulfil Each Aim[1–7]
- Reducing the radial head
  - Restoring length of the ulna
    - Acute lengthening
    - Gradual lengthening
- Relieving pain and improving forearm supination
  - Reduce the radial dislocation
- Improving the appearance of the limb
  - Restore length of the ulna and correct deformity
  - Reduce the prominence of the dislocated radial head
    - Reduce radial head dislocation
    - Resect the radial head
- Prevent recurrence
  - Remove osteochondromata from the ulna and radius

FACTORS THAT INFLUENCED THE CHOICE OF TREATMENT
- Age of the child
- Severity of symptoms
- Cause of ulnar growth retardation
- Cause of radial head dislocation

The factors that influence treatment are shown in Table 28.1.

Table 28.1 Choice of Treatment Based on the Factors That Influenced the Decision

Factors		Treatment Implications
Age of the child	12 years	Whilst reconstructive surgery can be performed at most ages using external fixation, earlier treatment is preferable[4] as it should equate to better outcome. Radial head resection may be considered after skeletal maturity but is unacceptable at this age.
Severity of symptoms	Severe pain and significant loss of motion	The source of pain is probably from the dislocated radial head. Reduction of the radial head is justified.
Cause of ulnar growth retardation	Presence of osteochondroma on the distal ulna	An osteochondroma in the distal ulna compromises normal growth of the ulna. Excision of the distal osteochondroma should be part of the strategy to prevent recurrence following treatment.
Cause of radial head dislocation	Disparity in lengths of the radius and ulna	Restoration of normal relative lengths of the radius and ulna is essential to enable reduction of the radial head. Maintenance of this relationship is necessary to prevent re-dislocation.

How Was This Girl Treated?

Stage 1
A 130 mm by 5/8ths Ilizarov ring and a 130 mm full ring were attached to the proximal ulna. This ring block was connected to a full 130 mm ring distally by two parallel hinges placed in the coronal plane in the convex side of the planned osteotomy, with the motor on the concave radial side. The frame construct was secured to the ulna with one critical radio-ulnar wire and a combination of wires and half pins. A percutaneous proximal ulnar osteotomy was performed and lengthening performed at ¼ mm 3 times per day. This distracted the distal ulnar segment coupled with the radius allowing the radial head to move distally (Figure 28.4). When there was adequate clearance of the radial head beyond the capitellum, the hinges were unlocked and differential distraction continued to allow further lengthening and apex ulnar angulation of the ulna facilitating indirect reduction of the radial head.

Stage 2
Mild lateral and posterior subluxation were visible on intra-op fluoroscopy. Further apex ulnar angulation and re-orientation of the hinges allowed apex anterior angulation to move the radial head anteriorly. Two DRS 3 mm screws were inserted into the distal ulna beyond its distal angulation deformity and secured to a two-hole rancho cube. A percutaneous osteotomy was performed at the apex of the ulnar deformity and acute correction obtained.

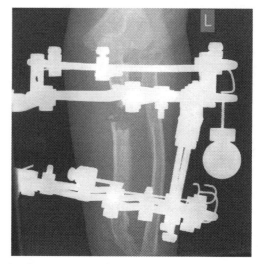

Figure 28.4 AP radiograph after stage 1 of only axial distraction. The regenerate is slow to form, the hinges are still locked, and the radial head is not yet clear of the capitellum and laterally translated. Apex ulnar angulation (oblique plane) of the distal ulnar deformity is visible.

Post-Op

Distraction continued at 3 × 1 mm at the motor and ½ mm at the hinges. This medialised the radial head, but residual posterior translation persisted (Figure 28.5). The hinges and motor were then altered in clinic to achieve satisfactory radio-capitellar alignment. The final correction was to compress and dock the radial head gently onto the capitellum.

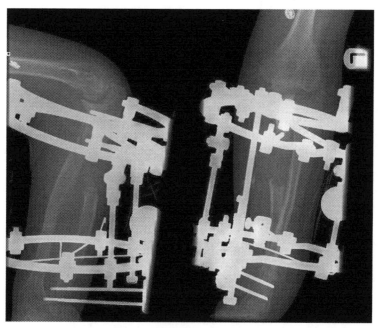

Figure 28.5 Lateral and AP radiographs eight weeks after stage 2 demonstrating the improved alignment of the distal ulna after the second osteotomy. The proximal regenerate is still slow to form. The radial head is well aligned on the AP film but still posteriorly translated on the lateral.

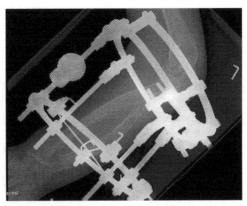

Figure 28.6 Lateral radiograph after the motors and hinges have been changed to create an apex anterior angulation to anteriorise the radial head. Also note the carpal support now present from the ulnar lengthening. The distal osteotomy has healed, and the proximal regenerate is consolidating after autologous bone grafting.

The proximal osteotomy was slow to consolidate, and she underwent bone grafting and DRS pin removal (Figure 28.6). After consolidation at the proximal site, the frame was removed, and a hinged cast-brace was applied for four weeks. After rehabilitation, function improved, and pain reduced (Figures 28.7 and 28.8).

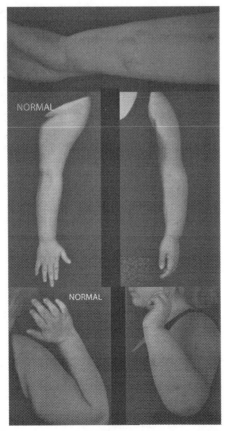

Figure 28.7 At the final follow-up at skeletal maturity, function of the elbow is excellent. Elbow extension and flexion compares well with the normal side.

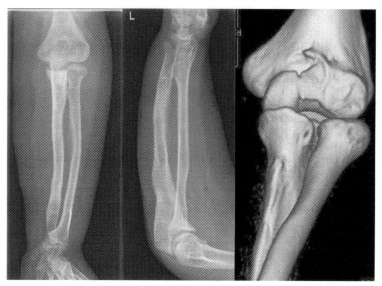

Figure 28.8 Radiographic appearance at skeletal maturity. The radial head is well reduced.

Comments

The senior author recommends a correction program that concentrates on one degree of freedom at a time.

- First, axial lengthening to provide adequate clearance of not only the bony radius and capitellum but also their articular cartilage.
- Second, the lateral translation of the radial head is corrected.
- Third, the posterior translation of the radial head is corrected.
- Fourth, excess axial distraction at the radio-capitellar joint is reversed.

As demonstrated in this case, this can be done with the Ilizarov technique, but can be achieved with less outpatient hardware adjustment using the Taylor spatial frame.

References

1. D'Ambrosi R, Barbato A, Caldarini C, Biancardi E, Facchini RM. Gradual ulnar lengthening in children with multiple exostoses and radial head dislocation: Results at skeletal maturity. *J Child Orthop.* 2016 Apr;10(2):127–33.
2. Masada K, Tsuyuguchi Y, Kawai H, Kawabata H, Noguchi K, Ono K. Operations for forearm deformity caused by multiple osteochondromas. *J Bone Joint Surg Br.* 1989;71(1):24–9.
3. Lluch A. The Sauvé-Kapandji procedure: Indications and tips for surgical success. *Hand Clin.* 2010 Nov;26(4):559–72.
4. Ip D, Li YH, Chow W, Leong JC. Reconstruction of forearm deformities in multiple cartilaginous exostoses. *J Pediatr Orthop B.* 2003 Jan;12(1):17–21.
5. Stanton RP, Hansen MO. Function of the upper extremities in hereditary multiple exostoses. *J Bone Joint Surg Am.* 1996 Apr;78(4):568–73.
6. Ferguson DO, Fernandes JA. Frame assisted radial head reduction in children: In proceedings of British Limb Reconstruction Society: 2017 March leeds. *The Bone and Joint Journal.* Published online in Orthopaedic Proceedings. 2018; 99-B(Supp 13).
7. Cho YJ, Jung ST. Gradual lengthening of the ulna in patients with multiple hereditary exostoses with a dislocated radial head. *Yonsei Med J.* 2014 Jan;55(1):178–84.

DIAPHYSEAL BONE LOSS

CASE 29: DIAPHYSEAL BONE LOSS OF THE RADIUS

Hitesh Shah and Benjamin Joseph

Case

A boy aged 8 presented with deformity of the right wrist and compromised function of the right upper limb. At the age of 4, he had developed osteomyelitis of the radius, for which he underwent an operation to drain pus. Over the course of the intervening four years, a deformity of the wrist developed and progressed.

The right forearm was shorter than the left; the lower end of the ulna was very prominent, and there was a severe manus valgus deformity. The ulna was normally palpable throughout its length, but there was palpable discontinuity of the radius in the middle third of the forearm. Pronation and supination of the forearm were markedly diminished. The shoulder, elbow and hand appeared normal, but the grip strength was weak. Radiographs of the forearm showed that there was loss of bone in the middle third of the diaphysis and the proximal end of the radius, dislocation of the inferior radio-ulnar joint and a severe manus valgus deformity (Figure 29.1).

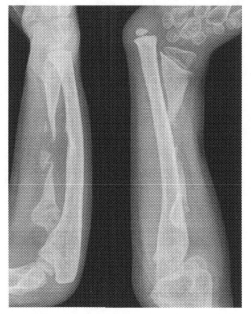

Figure 29.1 There is a loss of the diaphysis in the middle third of the radius. The distal one-fourth of the radius is intact, but the inferior radio-ulnar joint is dislocated. There is a severe manus valgus deformity. Fragments of the radius are present in the proximal half of the forearm, but the radial head is missing.

Questions

- What are the problems that need to be addressed?
- What are the aims of treatment?
- What are the available treatment options to fulfil these aims?
- What are the factors that may influence your choice of treatment?
- Based on these points, what treatment would you recommend for this child?
- How long would you follow-up this child after treatment?

The Problems That Need to Be Addressed Are

- Discontinuity of the radius with bone loss involving the proximal and mid-diaphysis
- Manus valgus deformity

The Aims of Treatment Are

- Restoring bony continuity between normal bone articulating with the humerus at the elbow and normal bone articulating with the carpus at the wrist
- Correcting manus valgus deformity

Treatment Options for Restoring Continuity of the Bones

- Restore continuity of the radius by bone grafting[1,2]
- Restore continuity of the radius by bone transport
- Fix proximal two thirds of the ulna to the distal third of the radius and create a single bone forearm[3,4]

FACTORS TO TAKE INTO CONSIDERATION WHILE PLANNING TREATMENT

- Integrity of the radio-humeral joint
- Length of the distal segment of the radius

The factors that influenced treatment are shown in Table 29.1.

Table 29.1 Factors That Influenced the Choice of Treatment

Factors		Treatment Implications
Integrity of the radio-humeral joint	The radial head is missing	If the radial head is not articulating normally with the humerus, it is futile to graft the gap in the radius. For this reason, the first two treatment options entailing procedures to restore continuity of the radius are not appropriate.
Length of the distal segment of the radius	The distal segment of the radius is of sufficient length to permit adequate fixation to the proximal fragment of the ulna.	Reconstruction with fixation of the distal radial segment to the ulna is a feasible option.

How Was the Boy Treated?

The ulna was divided at the junction of the middle and distal thirds, and the proximal segment of the ulna was fixed to the distal radius fragment with a plate and screws (Figure 29.2).

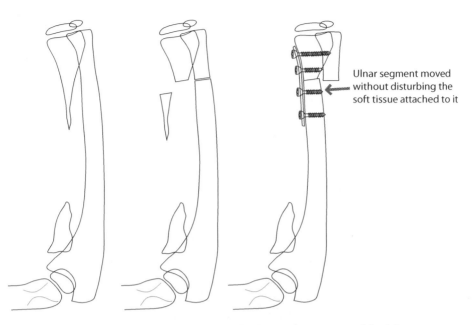

Ulnar segment moved
without disturbing the
soft tissue attached to it

Figure 29.2 Diagram showing the technique of reconstruction. (Modified from Figure 73.3, *Paediatric Orthopaedics—A System of Decision-making* 2nd Ed.)

The distal end of the ulna was fixed to the radius with a Kirschner wire across the radio-ulnar joint (Figure 29.3).

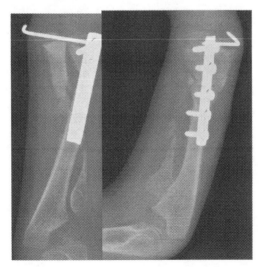

Figure 29.3 The ulna was divided at the junction of the middle and distal third. The proximal fragment of the ulna was fixed to the distal fragment of the radius with plate and screws. The inferior radio-ulnar joint was transfixed with a Kirschner wire.

Sound union occurred and two years later, the plate and screws were removed. At that time, screw epiphyseodesis of the distal ulna was performed.

Follow-Up

At the final follow-up at the age of 18 years, the right forearm is shorter than the left. The manus valgus deformity has been well corrected (Figure 29.4); the hand function is good with a good grasp and release (Figure 29.5a, 29.5b), and there is sound union between the radius and ulna (Figure 29.6a, 29.6b).

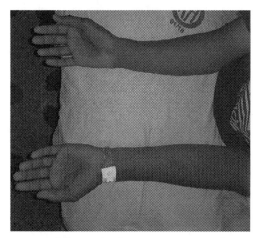

Figure 29.4 Some shortening of the right forearm persists; the manus valgus deformity is corrected.

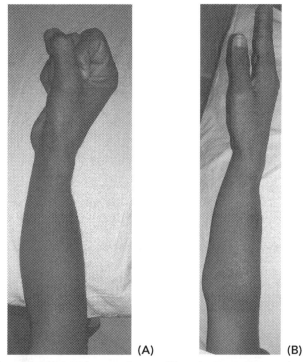

(A)   (B)

Figure 29.5 Good hand function with normal grasp (A) and release (B) was observed at the age of 18.

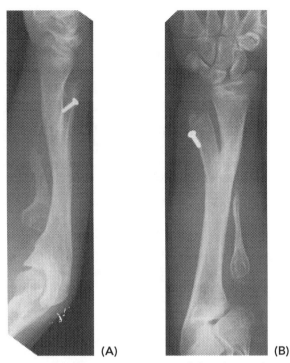

(A)   **(B)**

Figure 29.6a, b The radiographs show sound union of the ulna to the radius; the radio-carpal and the ulno-humeral joints appear well aligned.

Comment

In this boy, creating a single-bone forearm was the only viable option since the radial head was missing. This is a simple option in such situations, but there is a paucity of reports of this operation.

References

1. Lawal YZ, Garba ES, Ogirima MO, et al. Use of non-vascularized autologous fibula strut graft in the treatment of segmental bone loss. *Ann Afr Med*. 2011;10(1):25–8. doi: 10.4103/1596-3519.76571.
2. Swamy MK, Rathi A, Gupta V. Results of non-vascularised fibular grafting in gap non-union of long bones in paediatric age group. *J Clin Orthop Trauma*. 2013;4(4):180–4. doi: 10.1016/j.jcot.2013.09.001.
3. Peterson HA. The ulnius: A one-bone forearm in children. *J Pediatr Orthop B*. 2008;17(2):95–101. doi: 10.1097/bpb.0b013e3282f54849.
4. Wang H, Jiang W, Wei X, Rui Y, Sun Z. Ulnius formation for forearm fracture with segmental radial defect. *Int J Clin Exp Med*. 2015;8(10):17835–8. Published 2015 Oct 15.

DEFICIENCIES

CASE 30: FIBULAR HEMIMELIA

Caroline M Blakey and James A Fernandes

A 4-year-old boy presented with an 8 cm leg length discrepancy, predominantly arising from the tibial segment on the right. He was born at term following an uncomplicated pregnancy and had no other dysmorphic features. He had complete absence of the fibula, antero-medial bowing of the tibia, well-covered hips, retroversion of the femur and distal femoral valgus with a hypoplastic lateral femoral condyle (Figure 30.1a–c). There was minimal difference in femoral lengths. He had deficiency of the anterior cruciate ligament with some anterior subluxation of the tibia. He had a four-ray foot which was in 25° equinus and the hindfoot was in 15° valgus. The hindfoot was stiff with evidence of tarsal coalition and a mid-foot break. Spine examination was normal. MRI imaging of the limb was done, and it ruled out the presence of a fibrocartilaginous fibular anlage.

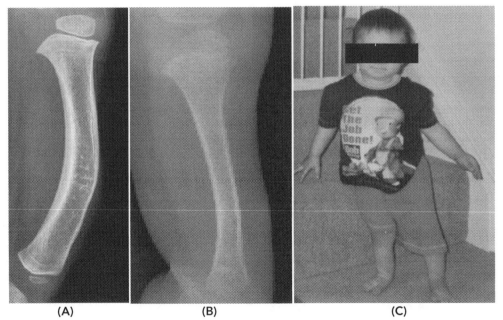

| (A) | (B) | (C) |

Figure 30.1a, b, c Radiographs in infancy show that the fibula is absent and there is anterior (A) and medial bowing of the tibia (B). The clinical photograph at presentation (C).

The predicted leg length discrepancy at skeletal maturity was calculated to be 14 cm.

Questions
- What are the problems that need to be addressed in this boy?
- What are the aims of treatment?
- What are the commonly available options for treatment?
- What are the factors that may influence your choice of treatment?
- What treatment would you recommend for this boy?
- How long would you follow-up this boy after treatment?

The Problems That Need to Be Addressed Are

- Significant limb-length inequality
- Deformities of the
  - knee
  - tibia
  - ankle and foot
- Instability of the knee and ankle

The Aims of Treatment in This Boy Are to

- Equalise leg length by skeletal maturity
- Correct deformities of the knee, tibia, ankle and foot
- Improve the stability of the knee and ankle

Options for Treatment

- Options for equalising limb lengths
  - Contralateral epiphyseodesis and orthosis
  - Multiple lengthening procedures +/− epiphyseodesis of the contralateral limb (biological reconstruction)
  - Ablate the foot and prosthetic fitting
- Options for correcting deformities
  - Knee (genu valgum)
    - □ Hemi-epiphyseodesis of the distal femur
    - □ Distal femoral osteotomy
  - Tibia (antero-medial bow)
    - □ Osteotomy and acute correction (if lengthening not planned)
    - □ Osteotomy and gradual correction during lengthening
- Options for stabilising joints
  - Knee
    - □ Anterior cruciate ligament reconstruction
  - Ankle
    - □ Reconstruction of a "lateral malleolus"
    - □ Ankle fusion

FACTORS THAT INFLUENCED THE CHOICE OF TREATMENT

- Age of the child
- Severity of fibular deficiency
- Status of the foot (number of toes, severity of deformity, function)
- Ankle and hindfoot deformity
- Status of the knee
- Extent of limb length inequality
- Complexity and duration of treatment

The choice of treatment based on these factors is outlined in Table 30.1.

Table 30.1 Factors That Influenced Decision-Making

Factors		Treatment Implications
Age of the child	4 years	A Syme's or Boyd disarticulation can be offered when multiple limb-lengthening procedures are considered unacceptable.[1,2] Amputation is a good option if performed around the age of 9 to 14 months. The child will get accustomed to the use of the prosthesis around the walking age. This child is older than the optimal age for amputation of the foot.
Severity of fibular deficiency	Complete agenesis of the fibula	Mild forms of congenital fibular deficiency, with minimal length inequality, may be treated with orthotics and timed epiphyseodesis of the contralateral limb.[3] In this child, the deficiency and shortening are more severe and consequently more elaborate treatment is warranted.
Status of the foot	Four rays present. Ankle function good	In children with salvageable feet, deformity and limb-lengthening procedures have been shown to have good outcomes.[4] A minimum of three rays, and a plantigrade ankle, are considered as prerequisites to preserve the foot.[5] As four rays are present amputation can be avoided.
Ankle and hindfoot deformity	Equinovalgus	Equinovalgus deformity of the ankle can complicate lengthening. While various procedures to stabilise the ankle have been described, ankle fusion may become necessary.[6,7]
Status of the knee	Anterior cruciate ligament deficiency. Genu valgum due to lateral condylar hypoplasia	Limb lengthening requires adjacent joint stability. The instability is not severe at present but should be carefully monitored during lengthening.[8] Genu valgum will require additional surgery over the course of treatment with guided growth.[9]
Extent of limb length inequality	8 cm shortening at age 4. Predicted discrepancy of a minimum of 14 cm	Since complications increase during lengthening of more than 20% length discrepancy, arresting growth or shortening of the contralateral limb in conjunction may be required in this child. Shortening osteotomy of the contralateral limb can also be considered for residual length discrepancy but is less commonly accepted by parents especially if the final height of the child is likely to be below average.
Complexity and duration of treatment	Foot ablation and prosthetic fitting versus biological reconstruction	Foot ablation and prosthetic fitting involves one simple operation in a single hospital admission. Biological reconstruction requires multiple admissions to hospital, and this should be considered when discussing options for limb-lengthening procedures with the family. Treatment will have an impact on family life including other siblings and will interrupt schooling on multiple occasions. Long-term sequelae in terms of secondary complications including pain, restricted function and risk of hip, knee and ankle OA in early adulthood need to be considered.

The parents were seen in the multidisciplinary limb deficiency clinic as part of the preparation and obtaining informed consent. Extensive discussions took place with the family, regarding the treatment options and implications of each option. The parents were able to meet with other children and families who had been through both treatment options. The parents were then given the choice of ablative reconstruction and biological reconstruction.

How Was This Child Treated?

The boy was treated by biological reconstruction with multiple lengthening procedures, correction of angular deformity and contralateral limb epiphyseodesis as outlined next in Table 30.2. (Figure 30.2a–d).

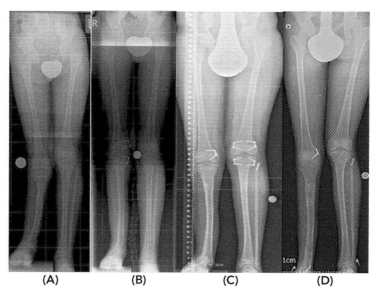

| (A) | (B) | (C) | (D) |

Figure 30.2 Sequential x-rays at (A) age 7 following first lengthening, bifocal genu valgum, (B) age 11 post–guided growth, (C) age 14 post–contralateral epiphyseodesis, (D) final follow-up.

Table 30.2 Sequence of procedures to reconstruct the limb

Age	Problems to Be Addressed	Procedure Undertaken
5 years	8 cm of shortening Oblique deformity of the tibia 22° in the frontal plane 27° in the sagittal plane	Two-stage procedure using all-wire Ilizarov construct with foot protection. Initial correction of apex antero-medial tibial bow through distal corticotomy and tendoachilles tenotomy, followed by second stage lengthening through a proximal corticotomy. Three-centimetre length achieved in total.
8 years	7 cm of shortening Bifocal valgus deformities and distal procurvatum (common rebound phenomenon seen in this pathology) with a functional and well-balanced foot	Further staged tibial lengthening with three-ring tibial frame spanning the ankle. Hindfoot osteotomy with acute medial translation to correct hindfoot valgus, further closed TA lengthening. Second-stage proximal tibial osteotomy with 5 cm target length. Botox to medial and lateral heads of gastrocnemius to reduce pain and improve rehabilitation compliance. Monitoring of the knee joint for any aggravation of instability with focussed physiotherapy input.

(Continued)

Table 30.2 (Continued)

Age	Problems to Be Addressed	Procedure Undertaken
10 years	Genu valgum	Guided growth right medial distal femur and proximal tibia.
13 years	3 cm shortening Genu valgum-rebound phenomenon Laterally translated foot Stiff ankle	Right medial distal femoral guided growth to correct genu valgum. Left pan genu temporary epiphyseodesis to reduce leg length discrepancy.
16 years	6 cm LLD Valgus mal-alignment right knee Valgus hindfoot	Two-stage surgery; corrective osteotomy and realignment with right ankle fusion and 5 cm total lengthening.

Post-Operative Management

At each stage of lengthening, knee protection with bracing was included and the knee was carefully monitored for subluxation. On removal of each frame, a cast brace was applied to manage anterior translation of the tibia. A fixed flexion deformity developed but was corrected with reduction of any anterior subluxation.

The tibia was osteopenic after correction, and was protected with an ankle foot orthosis, raised to account for any leg length discrepancy. In 2018, ring sequestrum was noted at a distal wire site, and he returned to theatre for curettage but has since done well.

Follow-Up

He was followed up until age 19; he had >95° knee flexion (Figure 30.3a–c), there was some residual genu valgum, but no further surgery has been undertaken. He was discharged with no requirement of adult transition or follow-up. He went on to complete university and currently works in the civil service.

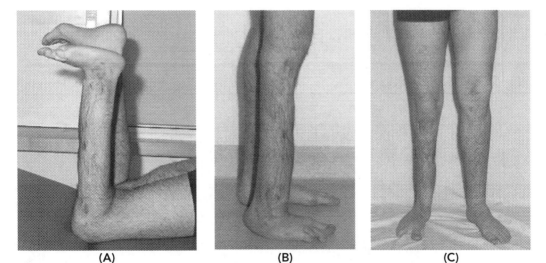

(A)   (B)   (C)

Figure 30.3 a–c Clinical photographs at final follow-up.

References

1. Weston GW, Sakai D, Wood W. Congenital longitudinal deficiency of the fibula: Follow-up of treatment by Syme amputation. *J Bone Jt Surg Am*. 1976;58(4):492–6.
2. Fulp T, Davids J, Meyer L, Blackhurst D. Longitudinal deficiency of the fibula: Operative treatment. *J Bone Jt Surg Am*. 1996;78(5):674–82.
3. Hamdy RC, Makhdom AM, Saran N, Birch J. Congenital fibular deficiency. *Journal of the American Academy of Orthopaedic Surgeons*. 2014:22(4):246–55.
4. Birch JG, Paley D, Herzenberg JE, Morton A, Ward S, Riddle R, et al. Amputation Versus staged reconstruction for severe fibular hemimelia. *JBJS Open Access*. 2019;4(2):e0053.
5. Birch JG, Lincoln T, Mack P, Birch C. Congenital fibular deficiency: A review of thirty years' experience at one institution and a proposed classification system based on clinical deformity. *J Bone Jt Surg Am*. 2011;93(12):1144–51.
6. Paley D. Surgical reconstruction for fibular hemimelia. *Journal of Children's Orthopaedics*. 2016;10(6):557–83.
7. Exner GU. Bending osteotomy through the distal tibial physis in fibular hemimelia for stable reduction of the hindfoot. *J Pediatr Orthop B*. 2003;12(1):27–32.
8. Cooper A, Fernandes J. Lower limb deficiency syndromes. *Orthop Trauma*. 2016;30(6):547–52.
9. Saldanha K, Blakey C, Broadley P, Fernandes J. Defining patho-anatomy of the knee in congenital longitudinal lower limb deficiencies. *J Limb Lengthening Reconstr*. 2016;2(1):48–54.

Nick Green and James A Fernandes

Case

A 3-month-old boy was referred for multiple congenital deficiencies involving all four limbs. He had bilateral tibial hemimelia with the right more severely affected, right single bone forearm with a single digit and left proximal radio-ulnar synostosis with an index-middle finger syndactyly and mild ectrodactyly of the palm. His gestational history had been significant for one episode of heavy bleeding at six weeks. There was no family history of congenital deficiency, and a genetics referral eventually confirmed a normal chromosome count. He had normal facies and spine.

Examination of the Lower Extremities

Right lower limb: There was no palpable patella or tibial anlage; a dimple was present anteriorly over the knee. There was a marked flexion contracture and gross instability of the knee. The foot was fixed in severe equinovarus.

Left lower limb: The knee was near normal except for a prominent fibular head which suggested tibio-fibular diastasis. He had a five-ray foot in equinovarus which had been unsuccessfully treated by the Ponseti method elsewhere. He had internal tibial torsion of 40 degrees and hindfoot equinus. The knee was stable, and the tibial segment appeared short. When he began walking at 13 months, he walked with 70-degree internal foot progression angle.

Pull-down mechanical axis radiograph (Figure 31.1) and MRI scan under general anaesthesia demonstrated right Jones 1a tibial hemimelia and left Jones 4 tibial hemimelia with the talus wedged between the tibio-fibular diastasis.[1,2]

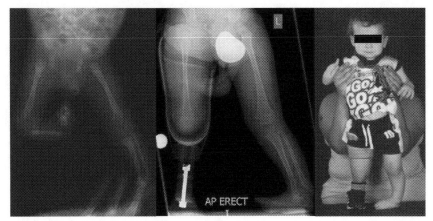

Figure 31.1 Pull down mechanical axis radiograph aged 6 months.

Questions
- What are the problems that need to be addressed?
- What are the aims of treatment?
- What are the options to treat each aim?
- What are the factors that influence choice of treatment?
- Based on these points, what treatment would you recommend for this child?

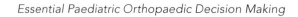

The Problems That Need to Be Addressed Are

- Gross leg length discrepancy (right-sided mesomelic shortening)
- Deficiencies

    o Bilateral tibial hemimelia
    o Right single bone forearm with single ray hand
    o Left radio-ulnar synostosis with syndactyly and mild ectrodactyly

- Deformities

    o Flexion deformity right knee
    o Bilateral equinocavovarus

- Joint instability

    o Right knee

        □ Absent extensor mechanism
        □ Gross multi-directional instability[3]

    o Left ankle

        □ Tibiofibular diastasis

The Aims of Treatment in This Boy Are to[1]

Achieve maximal independent mobility with the least number of interventions by:

- Equalising or compensating for short right limb
- Enabling walking with a stable right knee and plantigrade feet
- Optimising upper limb function

Options for Treatment to Fulfil Each Aim[4,5]

- Equalising or compensating for right-sided short limb

    o Extension prosthesis
    o Right knee disarticulation and above-knee prosthesis
    o Brown's procedure (fibular centralisation) and staged lengthening[6,7]
    o Weber-type patellar arthroplasty using fibula[8,9] and staged lengthening

- Enabling walking with a stable right knee

    o Managing right knee instability and extensor mechanism deficiency

        □ Ablation (knee disarticulation) and prosthetics
        □ Knee fusion (femur to fibula)
        □ Weber-type patellar arthroplasty using centralised fibula[8,9]

- Providing plantigrade feet

    o Right-sided ablation and prosthetics
    o Left foot amputation
    o Left-sided foot and ankle reconstruction

- Optimising upper limb function

    o Release of syndactyly
    o Orthotics/Prosthetics

FACTORS THAT INFLUENCED THE CHOICE OF TREATMENT

- Age of the child
- Severity of limb length inequality
- Quadriceps function
- Single or multiple limb deficiencies
- Parents' acceptance or rejection of protracted multi-stage surgery with attendant risks of complications
- Parents' acceptance or rejection of through knee amputation of right leg.

The choice of treatment option based on these factors is shown in Table 31.1.

Table 31.1 Factors influencing the choice of treatment

Factors		Treatment Implications
Age of the child	Infant	If an amputation is performed in the infant, it is easy for the child to accept the prosthesis.
Severity of limb length inequality	Severe shortening with grossly unstable "knee" and "ankle"	Though staged lengthening of the right fibula is feasible, one can anticipate multiple complications in view of grossly abnormal knee and ankle joints even following any form of reconstruction.
Quadriceps function	No quadriceps function on the right side	Reconstruction may have a poor outcome in the absence of quadriceps function. Knee-disarticulation is a relatively simple and definitive operation with a low complication profile.
Single or multiple limb deficiencies	Deficiencies in all four extremities	Amputation of the left foot is not a good option since he has multiple limb deficiencies—a salvaged lower limb will be easier for him in the long term versus bilateral lower limb amputations.
Parents' acceptance of treatment options	The parents accepted disarticulation of the right knee and reconstruction of the left ankle and foot.	

Summary of Treatment Planned for the Lower Limbs

- **Right leg:** Disarticulation of the knee and prosthesis
- **Left Leg:** Two-stage reconstruction: First a supra-talar bi-osseous osteotomy to create a plantigrade foot position and later a "U" osteotomy to increase Spherion (Foot) height to improve shoe-wear.

How Was This Boy Treated?

The disarticulation of the right knee was performed at 17 months of age. Skin from the first webspace of the amputated foot was used as a full thickness graft to aid syndactyly release by the plastic surgeons under the same anaesthetic. He adapted well to the prosthesis provided after the wound had healed (Figure 31.2).

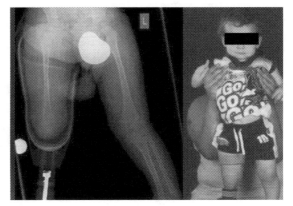

Figures 31.2 and **31.3** Radiograph and clinical photograph post–through-knee disarticulation, aged 2.

Stage 1: Left Leg

At age 2, in-toeing of the left leg was addressed (Figure 31.3). A supra-malleolar, supra-talar tibio-fibular osteotomy was performed and gradual correction with lengthening effected using a hybrid TSF and Ilizarov frame construct capturing the hindfoot (Figure 31.4). There was a delay in union of the tibial regenerate that was resolved with autologous bone grafting as a separate procedure.

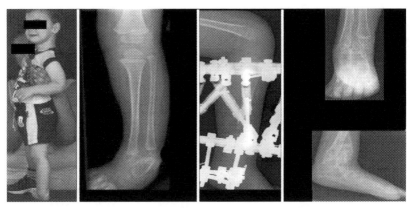

Figure 31.4 Clinical photo and radiographs prior to surgery and following bi-osseous supratalar supramalleolar osteotomy at age of 2 years.

A plantigrade foot and neutral foot progression angle greatly improved his walking, but his sub-malleolar height remained small with limited choice of footwear. He developed a 15-degree recurrence of his equinus, with slight varus and supination and so stage 2 was planned at the age of 5 to both increase his sub-malleolar height for optimising shoe wear and restore his plantigrade foot position.

Stage 2: Hindfoot U Osteotomy and Foot Frame Using TSF

A 2 cm curvilinear incision was made similar to Ollier's approach. White needles were placed in the subtalar joint and neck of talus (Figure 31.5a). Curved and U osteotomes were used to create a U osteotomy, and mobility was confirmed with a triple test of using a McDonald to palpate the completeness of the osteotomy, manual feel for crepitus and radiographic evidence of translation at the osteotomy sites (Figure 31.5b & 31.5c). A TSF foot frame was constructed with a proximal tibial 130 mm full ring with two crossing olive wires. A saddle wire passed through the proximal talar fragment was also secured to the proximal ring. A Butt ring parallel with the sole of the foot was secured with two crossing olive wires in the calcaneus and additional wires in the forefoot and midfoot. Hexapod struts connected the tibial and Butt ring. Mild acute distraction was performed.

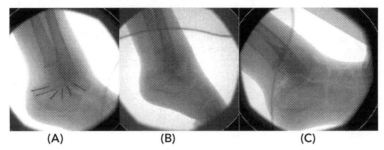

(A) (B) (C)

Figure 31.5 Intra-operative fluoroscopy showing technique of U osteotomy with white needles marking out osteotomy level and stress views showing mobility at osteotomy.

Post-Operative Care

Calibrated TSF protocol radiographs were taken based on the proximal reference ring, and TraumaCad was used to plan the correction. Distraction commenced day 1 post-op 1 mm per day for 10 days to prevent premature consolidation and create adequate clearance at osteotomy to permit subsequent deformity correction. After removal of the frame, a below-knee weight-bearing cast was applied for four weeks until an ankle foot orthosis was ready.

Follow-Up

A femoral discrepancy in length became apparent, and the right side was 3 cm shorter at age 11. In order to accommodate a knee mechanism in his prosthesis, which requires perhaps 8–10 cm of femoral discrepancy to have knee joints at the same height, an epiphyseodesis of the shorter right femur stump was planned and performed aged 11. His increasing leg length discrepancy is easily managed by altering his prosthesis.

At latest follow-up aged 13, he walks independently with his prosthesis (Figures 31.6 and 31.7). He is a keen horse rider but is troubled by some discomfort at the medial aspect of his left ankle where there is the bony prominence of his abnormally inclined distal tibial epiphysis that is still growing. At skeletal maturity, this will be sculpted to alleviate his symptoms.

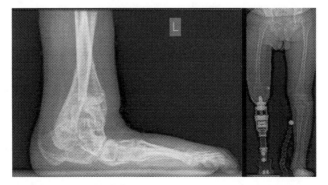

Figure 31.6 Recent radiographs of left foot showing reconstruction results and mechanical axis views with prosthesis.

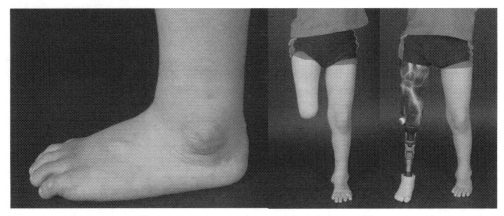

Figure 31.7 Recent clinical photos showing plantigrade left foot with increased sub-malleolar height, right through knee amputation both with and without prosthesis.

Comment

The traditional reconstructive method for Jones Type 1 tibial hemimelia is Brown's fibular centralisation.[7] His reported success has not been replicated by subsequent authors due to progressive knee flexion contracture, instability and poor range of motion. More complex and multistage techniques have been described by Weber and Paley with varied success and no long-term outcomes and a definite requirement for ongoing orthotic and/or prosthetic use.[9,10]

References

1. Jones D, Barnes J, Lloyd-Roberts GC. Congenital aplasia and dysplasia of the tibia with intact fibula: Classification and management. *J Bone Joint Surg Br.* 1978;60(1):31–9.
2. Tokmakova K, Riddle EC, Kumar SJ. Type IV congenital deficiency of the tibia. *J Pediatr Orthop.* 2003;23(5):649–53.
3. Saldanha KA, Blakey CM, Broadley P, Fernandes JA. Defining patho-anatomy of the knee in congenital longitudinal lower limb deficiencies. *J Limb Lengthen Reconstr.* 2016;2:48–54.
4. Herring JA, Birch JG. *The child with a limb deficiency.* IL: American Academy of Orthopaedic Surgeons; 1998. ISBN13:9780892031757.
5. Cooper A, Fernandes J. Lower limb deficiency syndromes. *Orthopaedics and Trauma.* 2016;30–36: 547–52.
6. Simmons E, Ginsburg G, Hall J. Brown's procedure for congenital absence of the tibia revisited. *Journal of Pediatric Orthopedics.* 1996;16:85–9, 10.
7. Brown FW, Pohnert WH. Construction of a knee joint in meromelia tibia: A fifteen-year follow-up study: Abstract. *J Bone Joint Surg Am.* 1972;54:1333.
8. Weber M. New classification and score for tibial hemimelia. *J Child Orthop.* 2008;2(3):169–75.
9. Weber M. A new knee arthroplasty versus Brown procedure in congenital total absence of the tibia: A preliminary report. *J Pediatr Orthop B.* 2002;11(1):53–9.
10. Paley D. Tibial hemimelia: New classification and reconstructive options. *J Child Orthop.* 2016 Dec; 10(6):529–55. doi: 10.1007/s11832-016-0785-x. Epub 2016 Dec 1. PMID: 27909860; PMCID: PMC5145835.

Nick Green and James A Fernandes

Case

A 2-year-old boy presented with severe shortening of his left lower limb predominantly in the thigh segment. His left foot was at the mid-tibial level of his sound right leg. Passive hip abduction was reduced, and excessive hip adduction was present. His limb lay in an externally rotated attitude. Mild genu valgum was present and the anterior and posterior cruciate ligaments were lax. He had a five-ray foot with free ankle and subtalar movements, but his ankle was in slight valgus on standing. Plain radiographs of the pelvis showed typical coxa vara deformity with no ossified connection between the femoral head and shaft (Figure 32.1). CT, MRI and a hip arthrogram done under general anaesthesia confirmed a mobile hip joint with a pseudarthrosis in continuity of the proximal femur associated with coxa vara, femoral retroversion and acetabular dysplasia. The leg length discrepancy was entirely in the femur.

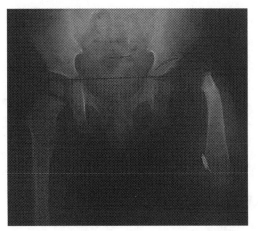

Figure 32.1 Radiograph showing the short femur with coxa vara and acetabular dysplasia. The non-ossified segment of the femoral neck is outlined.

The predicted shortening at skeletal maturity was estimated to be approximately 27 cm.

Questions

- What are the problems that need to be considered in this boy?
- What are the aims of treatment?
- What are the available treatment options to fulfil these aims?
- What are the factors that may influence the family's choice of treatment?
- Based on these points, what treatment would you recommend for this boy?
- How long would you follow-up this boy after treatment?

The Problems That Need to Be Addressed Are

- Severe degree of shortening
- Deformities

    o Acetabular dysplasia
    o Coxa vara
    o Retroversion of the femur
    o Genu valgum
    o Ankle valgus

- Soft tissue anomalies

    o Partially or completely absent knee cruciate ligaments predisposing to instability especially with lengthening[1]

- Joint instability

    o Acetabular dysplasia predisposing to hip instability especially with lengthening[2]
    o Knee instability due to absence or laxity of the cruciate ligaments of the knee

- Pseudarthrosis of the femoral neck

The Aims of Treatment in This Boy Are to

Achieve a functional and painless left leg which allows efficient gait by:

- Equalising limb lengths or compensating for shortening
- Correcting deformities
- Correcting joint instability at the knee and preventing hip instability
- Facilitating union of the pseudarthrosis of the femoral neck

Options for Treatment to Fulfil Each Aim

- Equalising limb lengths or compensating for shortening

    o Extension prosthesis
    o Above-knee prosthesis (following ablation of the foot)
    o Staged limb lengthening
    o Staged limb lengthening combined with contralateral epiphyseodesis
    o Staged limb lengthening and contralateral femoral shortening

- Correction of deformities

    o Acetabular dysplasia—acetabuloplasty
    o Coxa vara and femoral retroversion—proximal femoral valgus de-rotation osteotomy
    o Genu valgum—guided growth

- Correcting joint instability at the knee

    o Knee ligament reconstruction
    o Knee fusion

- Preventing hip instability

    o Correct acetabular dysplasia by Dega-type osteotomy

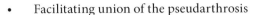

- Facilitating union of the pseudarthrosis

  - Improving neck-shaft angle, internal fixation with or without bone grafting or bone morphogenetic protein (BMP)

Summary of Options for Treatment

- **Non-surgical prosthetic management**:

  - Hip not treated and extension prosthesis provided +/− guided growth for lesser deformities.
  - Non-surgical prosthetic management is generally not recommended. Although surgical risks are near-avoided, abnormal hip biomechanics, knee joints at different levels and worsening hip and knee flexion contractures all compromise efficient gait. The aesthetic result is also poor. However, this may be the only option in some areas of the world.

- **Staged ablative reconstruction**:

  - Syme's amputation (at age around 14 months). Combined bony and soft tissue stabilisation of the hip (at age 2–3 years). Physeal sparing or sacrificing knee fusion (at age 5–8 years). Initially, extension prosthesis is used; eventually the child progresses to an above-knee prosthesis. This is a sound option for severe femoral deficiency where the least number of surgeries and hospital time is a priority for the parents and where social, cultural and religious influences allow. In this strategy, a Syme's is performed early before any real attachment to the foot has developed in the infant (or parents). Effective and early hip reconstruction optimises hip biomechanics, which creates the proximal foundation for a more efficient gait. The important objective of achieving knee joints at the same level can only be achieved by fusing the unstable and proximally based native knee joint so as to achieve a stable femoro-tibial segment for prosthetic use. This must be timed and adapted (physeal sparing or sacrificing) so that by skeletal maturity, there is between 8 to 10 cm residual "thigh" segment shortening. This allows the use of a prosthesis with a knee component that is at the same height as the normal knee.

- **Staged limb reconstruction**:

  - Combined bony and soft tissue stabilisation of the hip (hip reconstruction at age 2–3 years). Knee cruciate ligament reconstruction (at age 5–7 years). Two episodes of staged and modest femoral lengthening procedures. Guided growth as needed. Planned and timed contralateral epiphyseodesis or acute femoral shortening at maturity as required.[3,4]
  - Staged limb reconstruction is a huge commitment by all parties throughout childhood. It is natural for a parent to desire reconstruction rather than ablation, especially when the tibial segment is virtually normal and the foot looks and functions normally. Removing functioning parts of your precious child is highly counter-intuitive. Nevertheless, the final functional outcome will be inverse to the amount of lengthening that is required. Many surgeries will be required, and complications will be encountered.
  - It is hard to predict whether an individual's final functional outcome will be better than it would have been with a prosthesis; however, function isn't everything, and appearance has traditionally ranked highly in social acceptance.

FACTORS THAT INFLUENCED THE CHOICE OF TREATMENT
• Age of the child
• Severity of limb length inequality
• Parents' acceptance or rejection of ablation of the foot as part of treatment
• Parents' acceptance or rejection of protracted multi-stage frame surgery

The choice of treatment based on these factors is shown in Table 32.1.

Table 32.1 Choice of Treatment Based on the Factors That Influenced the Decision

Factors		Treatment Implications
Age of the child	2 years	The age of the child is ideal for considering hip reconstruction and just beyond the optimal age for foot ablation. At 2 years of age, the prospect of ablative reconstruction is a little harder to accept.
Severity of limb-length inequality	Severe shortening (anticipated disparity at skeletal maturity is 27 cm)	The options are to avoid lengthening and provide a prosthesis after ablating the foot or to undertake staged lengthening combined with timed growth arrest of the opposite lower limb.
Parents' acceptance or rejection of foot ablation	Unacceptable	This decision excludes the option of staged ablative reconstruction.
Parents' acceptance or rejection of protracted multi-stage frame surgery	Acceptable	The decision is to plan and proceed with staged lengthening and reconstruction.

How Was This Boy Treated?

Since both ablative reconstruction and limb reconstruction options were appropriate for this boy, we had a dialogue with the family unit and enabled them to meet other children (and their parents) who are undergoing or have undergone either treatment pathway.[5]

Stage 1

This was a complex hip reconstruction,[6] using a technique akin to some extent to that described by Paley.[7]

The child was positioned supine on a radio-lucent table with a bolster under the left buttock to rotate the pelvis 30 to 40 degrees (to facilitate "AP" and "lateral" femoral neck and head imaging). Tranexamic acid was given, and the surgical sites were pre-infiltrated with local and adrenaline. Cell salvage was used intra-operatively.

First the adductors were released via a medial groin incision. Through a bikini incision, sartorius and rectus femoris were released from their origins, and the psoas tendon was divided over the pelvic brim. Care was taken not to breach the hip capsule. An abductor slide extraperiosteally off the outer table was performed to allow free adduction of the abducted proximal segment.

Then, through a lateral approach to the proximal femur, the gluteus maximus was released. The piriformis was released as internal rotation of the hip was restricted. An arthrogram was

performed and using the bulls-eye technique a guide wire was passed from the tip of the trochanter into the centre of the head.[2] A second guide wire was passed 45 degrees to this into the
head to guide reconstruction of a 130-degree neck-shaft angle using the Coventry screw and
plate system.

A trapezoidal wedge of bone was resected from the subtrochanteric region of the proximal
femur to correct the coxa vara and proximal femoral flexion deformities. Some shortening was
also performed to de-tension the reconstruction before the femoral retroversion was corrected
and the plate was applied to the shaft. A tension band wire construct was added for stability
(Figure 32.2a and 32.2b). Bone morphogenetic protein can also be used to stimulate ossification
of the femoral neck but was not used in this case.

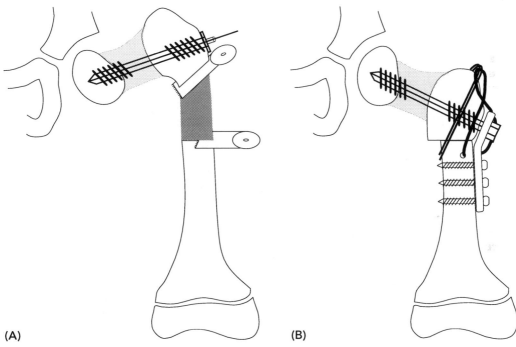

(A)   **(B)**

Figure 32.2a and **32.2b** Line drawings of proximal femoral osteotomy technique and fixation
using Coventry hip screw system and tension band wire construct with bone tunnel.

A Witt modification of the Dega acetabuloplasty was performed where the bone cut entered
the sciatic notch, which gave the freedom to locate the hinge for correction anteriorly or posteriorly by appropriate placement of the graft.[8] After this, the femoral reconstruction tension
was reassessed to see if further shortening was required. Wounds were closed, and a spica was
applied.

Post-Operative Management

Limited CT with reconstruction views and 3D rendering was performed while the child was
sleepy on the way back to the ward. Daily, the inpatient pain team reviewed and optimised analgesia. The spica was removed in clinic after six weeks and X-rays were obtained. Weight bearing
with an extension prosthesis was allowed after radiological union of osteotomy.

Regular follow up with plain films was continued to confirm maintenance of reconstruction,
identify loss of fixation and confirm ossification of the femoral neck (Figure 32.3).

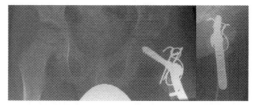

Figure 32.3 AP and lateral radiographs show left proximal femoral reconstruction using Coventry system and tension band wire construct. Note the healed Dega osteotomy with improved acetabular index and the non-ossified femoral neck.

Stage 2
The boy underwent his first lengthening aged 7 using the LRS system with extension across the knee as he was cruciate-deficient (Figure 32.4).

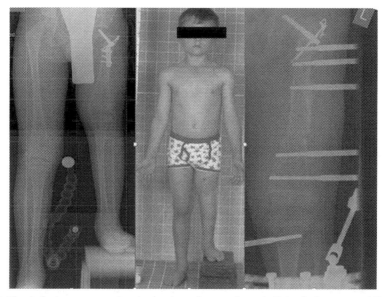

Figure 32.4 The left shows a mechanical axis radiograph and clinical photo aged 7 immediately before his first lengthening using the LRS system with cross-knee protection. The radiograph on the right is immediately after application of external fixator and osteotomy.

Stage 3
At age 9, he underwent his second lengthening using the same system (Figure 32.5).

Stage 4
Guided growth with axis correction and contralateral epiphyseodesis were performed.

Stage 5
He underwent a successful transphyseal cruciate reconstruction aged 15 and a half and is awaiting a final intramedullary lengthening nail technique of 5 cm to reduce his deficit to only 1 cm.

He needs to be followed till skeletal maturity following the final lengthening.

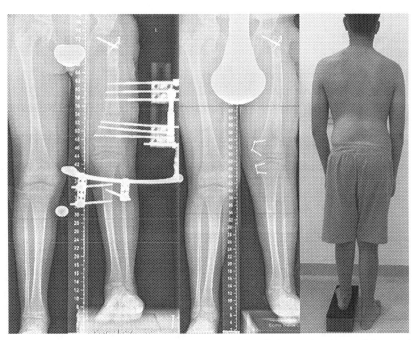

Figure 32.5 Shows a post-operative film immediately after application of frame for second lengthening and then a mechanical axis and posterior clinical photo after lengthening.

Comment

Early hip reconstruction in these cases is highly challenging and should be performed in units with expertise in limb reconstruction and neonatal hip dysplasias.[9] Whilst this has always been the first surgery in our limb reconstruction strategy for congenital femoral deficiency, cruciate ligament reconstruction prior to lengthening was introduced into our pathway three years ago and is now our standard practice. The timing and technique of first lengthening is dictated by completion of these first two stages and by the number of lengthening procedures intended. Our target for each lengthening episode in congenital femoral deficiency is more modest than some units in order to preserve adjacent joint function in a healthcare system where resources and allied health services such as physiotherapy and occupational therapy are less available. Evolving technologies for lengthening such as lengthening plates may facilitate earlier femoral lengthening episodes without having to use external fixation, which is often poorly tolerated by the patient and family.

References

1. Saldanha KA, Blakey CM, Broadley P, Fernandes JA. Defining patho-anatomy of the knee in congenital longitudinal lower limb deficiencies. *J Limb Lengthen Reconstr.* 2016;2:48–54.
2. Eidelman M, Jauregui JJ, Standard SC, Paley D, Herzenberg JE. Hip stability during lengthening in children with congenital femoral deficiency. *International Orthopaedics.* 2016;40(12):2619–25.
3. Cooper A, Fernandes JA. Lower limb deficiency syndromes. *Orthopaedics and Trauma.* 2016;30–6: 547–52.
4. Herring JA, Birch JG. *The child with a limb deficiency.* IL: American Academy of Orthopaedic Surgeons; 1998. ISBN13:9780892031757.
5. Simpson-White RW, Fernandes JA, Bell MJ. King's procedure for Aitken B/Paley 2a proximal femoral focal deficiency with 19-year follow-up: A case report. *Acta Orthopaedica.* 2012;84(3):323–5.

6. Dhital K, Giles SN, Fernandes JA. Combined bony and soft tissue stabilisation of the hip in congenital femoral deficiency. European Paediatric Orthopaedic Society Meeting. 2018 Apr 18. Oslo.

7. Paley D. SUPERhip and SUPERhip2 procedures for congenital femoral deficiency. In: Hamdy RC, Saran N, editors. *Paediatric pelvic and proximal femoral osteotomies*. New York: Springer Nature, 2018. pp. 287–356. ISBN 978-3-319-78033-7.

8. Witt AN, Jager M. Die Berechtigung und Indikation autoplastischer Spantransplantation in der heutigen orthopädischen Chirurgie. *Chir Plast Reconstr*. 1966;2:48–64.

9. National Institute for Health and Care Excellence. Combined bony and soft tissue reconstruction for hip joint stabilisation in proximal femoral focal deficiency (PFFD). NICE; 2009 [updated 2018]. (Interventional Procedures Guidance [IPG297]). Available from: www.nice.org.uk/guidance/ipg297.

Caroline M Blakey and James A Fernandes

Case

A 2-year-old boy born at term presented with significant leg length discrepancy (Figure 33.1). The short, left leg was externally rotated. The left foot reached the junction of the proximal and middle-third of the contralateral tibia. The shortening was from the femoral segment with a clinically normal leg and mild hypoplasia of the foot. There were fixed flexion and abduction deformities at the hip and 30° of fixed flexion of the knee with 40° of further flexion. The spine and the upper limbs were normal. Radiographs revealed mild acetabular dysplasia and Paley Type 4 distal diaphyseal femoral deficiency (Figure 33.2).[1] The distal femoral epiphysis was ossified.

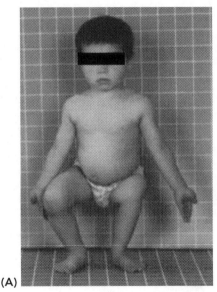 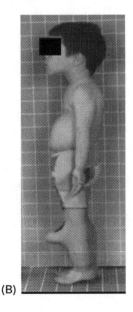

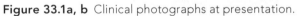

(A)   **(B)**

Figure 33.1a, b Clinical photographs at presentation.

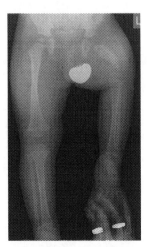

Figure 33.2 Lower limb AP radiograph at presentation.

Magnetic resonance imaging and an arthrogram of the knee confirmed absence of the distal femoral diaphysis with a mobile pseudarthrosis between the proximal diaphysis and the distal femoral epiphysis (Figure 33.3). The proximal tibia was cupola-shaped. The patella was hypoplastic, and the intercondylar notch was absent.

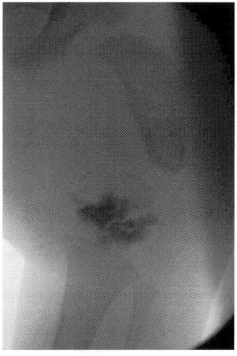

Figure 33.3 Arthrogram of left knee.

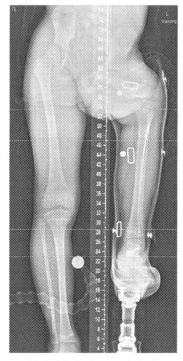

Figure 33.4 AP radiograph in extension prosthesis.

At the time of presentation, the child had been ambulating with an extension prosthesis (Figure 33.4).

Questions
- What are the problems that need to be addressed?
- What are the aims of treatment?
- What are the commonly available options for treatment?
- What are the factors that may influence your choice of treatment?
- What treatment would you recommend for this boy?
- How long would you follow-up this boy after treatment?

The Problems That Need to Be Addressed Are

- Significant limb length inequality
- Distal femoral pseudarthrosis
- Dysplastic knee joint with contractures
- Dysplastic hip joint with contractures

The Aims of Treatment in This Boy Were to

- Achieve equal leg length by maturity, with straight limbs
- Maintain functional joints which are pain-free
- Restore a near-normal gait

Options for Treatment

Options to equalise leg lengths:

- Biological reconstruction (osteosynthesis of the pseudarthrosis, multiple lengthening procedures +/– epiphyseodesis of the contralateral limb)
- Osteosynthesis of the pseudarthrosis, Van Nes rotationplasty and prosthetic fitting.
- Osteosynthesis of the pseudarthrosis, knee fusion and Syme's amputation

Options for stabilising joints:

- Hip—acetabular and/or femoral osteotomy
- Knee—cruciate ligament reconstruction

Options for correcting deformities:

- Release of soft tissue contractures

FACTORS THAT INFLUENCE THE CHOICE OF TREATMENT

- Age of the child
- Relationship between diaphysis and distal epiphysis
- Extent of limb length inequality
- Adjacent joint stability
- Range of movement of hip and knee
- Complexity and duration of treatment

The choice of treatment based on these factors in shown in Table 33.1.

Table 33.1 Factors that influenced the choice of treatment

Factors		Treatment Implications
Age of the child	2 years	The femur needs to be ossified before undertaking any lengthening procedure.[2]
		Amputation and knee fusion, or alternatively Van Nes rotationplasty would be good options if multiple limb-lengthening procedures are unacceptable.[3,4]
		Amputation performed early will allow the child maximum opportunity to become accustomed to the prosthesis.

(Continued)

Table 33.1 (Continued)

Factors		Treatment Implications
Relationship between diaphysis and distal epiphysis	Distal femoral pseudarthrosis Presence of distal femoral epiphysis	The femur is not amenable to lengthening before osteosynthesis of the pseudarthrosis. The presence of the distal femoral epiphysis has a favourable impact on severity of leg length discrepancy and on the normal development of the proximal tibia, which requires loading from the distal femoral condyles.
Adjacent joint stability	Hip—dysplastic acetabulum Knee—absence of the intercondylar notch	A minimum centre edge angle of 20° and neck shaft angle of 110° are considered necessary to reduce the risk of hip dislocation.[5] Instability is correlated to the severity of femoral deficiency.[6] Hypoplasia of the distal femur and intercondylar notch are associated with cruciate ligament deficiency[7] and pose a risk for knee subluxation during lengthening. Muscle releases and external fixation spanning the joint may be needed to prevent knee subluxation.
Range of movement of the hip and knee	Knee—30° fixed flexion deformity of the knee with 40° further flexion achievable Hip—fixed flexion and abduction contracture	Knee stiffness is common in distal femoral deficiencies with hypoplasia and contracture of muscles. Stiffness will increase with sequential lengthening procedures. A fixed flexion deformity of the knee will require correction by osteotomy, and a quadricepsplasty may be required to maintain functional knee flexion. Releases of rectus femoris, psoas and the hip abductor may be needed.
Extent of limb length inequality	24–25cm predicted LLD at maturity (i.e. > 20% discrepancy)	Since complications increase during lengthening of more than 20% length discrepancy, arresting growth or shortening of the contralateral limb may be required in this child. Shortening of the contralateral limb is less commonly accepted by parents especially if the final height of the child is likely to be low.
Complexity and duration of treatment	Foot ablation and knee fusion or rotationplasty and prosthetic fitting, versus biological reconstruction	Foot ablation and knee fusion with prosthetic fitting involves fewer procedures and early rehabilitation. A limb not suited for multiple lengthening or with severe knee stiffness can be treated with a rotationplasty. This entails rotating the limb externally by 180° via a mid-tibial osteotomy[8] or through the knee and allows the equivalent of a below-knee prosthesis. The procedure may, however, be considered cosmetically unacceptable to the family. Biological reconstruction requires multiple hospital admissions with interruption of schooling; this should be explained while discussing treatment options with the family as it will have an impact on the family including siblings. Long-term sequelae and potential complications need to be considered.

How Was This Child Treated?

The child underwent osteosynthesis of the femoral pseudarthrosis followed by reconstruction of the hip and first-stage femoral lengthening as outlined in Table 33.2.

Table 33.2 Staged Treatment Undertaken in This Child

Age	Problems to Be Addressed	Procedure Undertaken
4 years	Distal femoral pseudarthrosis	Wedge resection of left proximal femoral diaphysis to correct fixed flexion deformity. Distal epiphysis drilling with central excavation to allow the femoral diaphysis to be reduced into it. Fixation with K-wires supplemented by monolateral frame to proximal diaphysis and ring fixator distally. Inductos (BMP2) and autologous iliac crest grafting to hasten healing (Figure 33.5).
7 years	Left hip dysplasia at risk of instability with lengthening	Left hip surgery to ensure proximal stability prior to any planned femoral lengthening—psoas lengthening at the brim, abductor slide, Dega acetabuloplasty and application of spica cast (Figure 33.6).
10 years	Significant predicted leg length discrepancy 24–25cm	Left femoral corticotomy, acute correction of flexion deformity and Ilizarov lengthening with cross-knee protection and foot extension plate (Figure 33.7). Rectus and tensor facia lata lengthening.

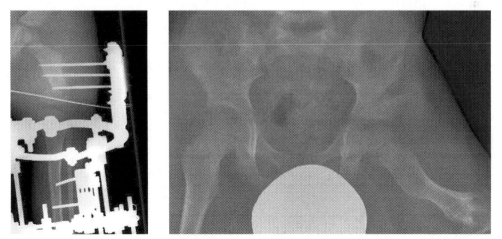

Figure 33.5, 33.6 Monolateral frame with cross-knee protection to supplement osteosynthesis of pseudarthrosis (A) and Dega acetabuloplasty (B).

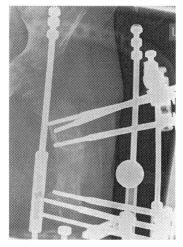

Figure 33.7 Ilizarov lengthening of the femur.

At age 12, options for ongoing treatment were discussed with the family. Biological reconstruction involving 4–5 lengthening procedures, correction of angular deformity, possible contralateral limb epiphyseodesis and the high chance of permanent knee stiffness were explained. Other options including ablative reconstruction and Van Nes rotationplasty were also discussed.

The boy, however, decided not to proceed with further surgery as he was very involved with wheelchair tennis at the national level and was keen to avoid interrupting his training. He walked with a painless Trendelenburg gait. He had a persistent 20° fixed flexion deformity at the hip which was abducted but could be adducted up to neutral. There was 30° fixed flexion deformity at the knee with further flexion to 90°. The ankle was mobile and stable. He wore an extension prosthesis modified to accommodate a plantar flexed foot to reduce the prominence at the foot under the trousers (Figure 33.8a–d).

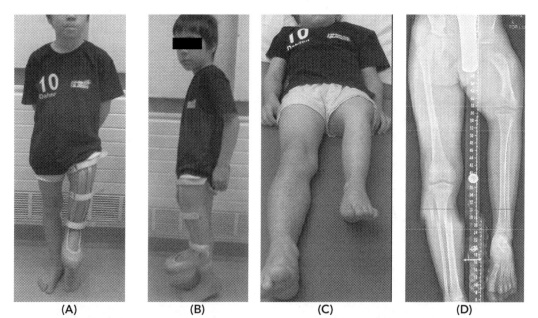

(A)　　　　　　　(B)　　　　　　　(C)　　　　　　　(D)

Figure 33.8A–C Clinical photographs at final follow-up. (D) Radiographs at final follow-up.

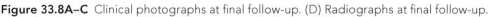

Comments

The function of the knee is a very important factor that influences the outcome following reconstruction of distal femoral deficiency. Due to the level of the foot, a bending prosthesis is not possible, making activities such as running and cycling difficult in early childhood. Limb lengthening is an option, but the knee will become progressively stiff with sequential lengthening. Quadricepsplasty can be attempted for the stiff knee, but the outcome associated with a dysplastic knee is unpredictable.

References

1. Paley D, Standard S. Treatment of congenital femoral deficiency. In: Flynn JM, Wiesel S, editors. *Operative techniques in pediatric orthopaedics*. Philadelphia: Lipincott William and Wilkins; 2010. p. 177.
2. Cooper A, Fernandes JA. Lower limb deficiency syndromes. *Orthop Trauma*. 2016;30(6):547–52.
3. Westin GW, Sakai D, Wood W. Congenital longitudinal deficiency of the fibula: Follow-up of treatment by Syme amputation. *J Bone Jt Surg Am*. 1976;58(4):492–6.
4. Fulp T, Davids J, Meyer L, Blackhurst D. Longitudinal deficiency of the fibula: Operative treatment. *J Bone Jt Surg Am*. 1996;78(5):674–82.
5. Suzuki S, Kasahara Y, Seto Y, Futami T, Furukawa K, Nishino Y. Dislocation and subluxation during femoral lengthening. *J Pediatr Orthop*. 1994;14(3):343–6.
6. Eidelman M, Jauregui J, Standard S, Paley D, Herzenberg JE. Hip stability during lengthening in children with congenital femoral deficiency. *Int Orthop*. 2016;40:2619–25.
7. Saldanha K, Blakey C, Broadley P, Fernandes JA. Defining patho-anatomy of the knee in congenital longitudinal lower limb deficiencies. *J Limb Lengthening Reconstr*. 2016;2(1):48–54.
8. Van Nes C. Rotation-plasty for congenital defects of the femur. *J Bone Jt Surg Br*. 1950;32B:12–16.

Nicholas Peterson, Christopher Prior, Selvadurai Nayagam

Case

A 10-month-old boy was referred with a deformity of the right upper limb present from birth. He had a short forearm with severe radial deviation of the wrist and the absence of two digits including the thumb (Figure 34.1).[1] Movements of the shoulder were normal, and elbow flexion was to 90 degrees. There were no anomalies in the other limbs, and there were no signs of systemic disease. Associated anomalies of the cardiovascular system, the haemopoietic system and the gastrointestinal and genitourinary tracts had been ruled out with appropriate investigations.

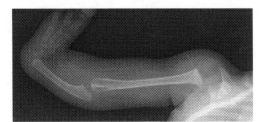

Figure 34.1 Radiograph demonstrating a Bayne & Klug type IV radial aplasia.

The x-ray showed a Bayne & Klug type IV radial aplasia where the entire radius was absent.

Questions
- What are the problems related to the right upper limb that need to be addressed in this infant?
- What are the aims of treatment?
- What are the commonly available options for treatment?
- What are the factors that may influence your choice of treatment?
- What treatment would you recommend for this infant?
- How long would you follow-up this boy after treatment?

The Problems That Need to Be Addressed Are

- The deformity—radial deviation and palmar flexion of the wrist with impaired hand function due to a biomechanically disadvantageous position of the hand
- Total absence of a thumb with consequent loss of prehension (ability to grip with fingers and thumb)
- Instability of the wrist 'joint' (a true synovial joint does not exist between the radial anlage and carpus)
- Unsightly appearance of the deformed and short limb

The Aims of Treatment Are to

- Improve hand function by correcting the radial deviation of the hand and repositioning the wrist centrally over the end of the forearm such that finger action is optimised.
- Stabilise the wrist over the end of the ulna so that grip power is maximised.
- Facilitate future pollicisation of a digit.
- Improve the appearance of the limb.

Options for Treatment to Fulfil Each Aim

- For correction of radial deviation

  - Acute correction through open releases, flaps and shortening ulnar osteotomies
  - Gradual correction with serial casts and splintage
  - Gradual correction with an external fixator

- Repositioning the wrist over the forearm

  - Radialisation
  - Ulnarisation
  - Centralisation

- Stabilisation of the wrist over the end of the ulna

  - Stabilisation of the wrist (ulna with carpus)
  - Construction of 'Y' ulna with micro-vascular transfer of a metatarsal
  - Tendon transfers to rebalance muscle forces around the wrist

FACTORS THAT INFLUENCED THE CHOICE OF TREATMENT
• The age of the child • Severity of the deformity and extent of deficiency • Range of motion of the elbow • Status of the opposite upper limb • Facilities and expertise

How these factors influenced the choice of treatment is outlined in Table 34.1.

Table 34.1 Factors Taken into Consideration While Planning Treatment

Factors		Treatment Implications
Age of the child	10 months	This is an optimal age to start treatment if staged surgery is planned.
Severity of deformity	Severe deformity	Not a candidate for serial casting (casting may be considered for mild deformity). Similarly, splinting may be suitable in Bayne & Klug type I deformities (a normal but short radius) but would not be appropriate in this case. Acute correction runs the risk of neurovascular compromise unless the already-short ulna is shortened even more. Gradual correction with an external fixator offers the ability to correct the most severe deformities safely.
Extent of deficiency	Complete agenesis of radius (type IV)	Radial lengthening alone might be considered for Bayne & Klug type I or II but clearly is not an option in cases of radial aplasia.
Range of motion of the elbow	Flexion to 90 degrees	Correction of radial deviation of the wrist in bilateral cases should be avoided if the elbow is stiff as the ability of the hand to reach the face will be compromised. In this infant with unilateral involvement and elbow flexion to 90 degrees, correction of the radial deviation is justified.
Status of the opposite upper limb	The opposite upper limb is normal	If both upper limbs have type IV deficiency, surgical correction may be contraindicated if the elbows are stiff in extension or if treatment has been delayed till the child has adapted to the deformed position of the limbs.
Facilities and expertise	Facilities and expertise to undertake microvascular anastomosis	Construction of a 'Y' ulna with free transfer of a metatarsal can only be undertaken if these facilities are available.

Decision-Making from the Options

- Radialisation and ulnarisation

  o The benefits of radialisation[2,3] and ulnarisation[4] are that both techniques provide a 'mobile' wrist in contrast to the stiff but stable wrist following 'centralisation'. However, the range of wrist movement following radialisation and ulnarisation is not normal—the joint created is not synovial but a 'pseudoarthrosis'. Radialisation has been associated with some risk of recurrence, and ulnarisation involves shortening the ulna in an already-short forearm with a need for subsequent forearm lengthening.

- Centralisation

  o Centralisation improves hand function by providing a stable wrist. Centralisation with internal fixation entails multiple surgeries to exchange the fixation rod as the child grows. Acute centralisation by open releases, ulnar osteotomy with shortening, tendon transfers and dorsal bi-lobed skin flaps—to make up for radial deficiency of skin—are performed less often since gradual correction by external fixation achieves correction without need for shortening.[5-7]

Pollicisation is the third stage of treatment, ideally performed early before the child establishes 'scissoring' movements as a method of picking objects up. This implies that the wrist should be re-aligned ideally by the age of 12–18 months.

How Was the Child Treated?

Stage 1: Soft Tissue Distraction and Deformity Correction

After induction of anaesthesia, the arteries were mapped using Doppler ultrasound (Figure 34.2) to plan safe corridors for wire insertion of the Ilizarov fixator. A three-ring Ilizarov circular external fixator was applied with the proximal ring on the distal humerus and the middle ring on the proximal ulna with the elbow in extension (Figure 34.3). The third ring was applied with wires through the metacarpals (Figure 34.4). The radial most digit was left free to have an unscarred digit available for pollicisation in the future. The anaesthetists avoided using paralytic agents to allow the surgeon to notice any nerve irritation during wire insertion.

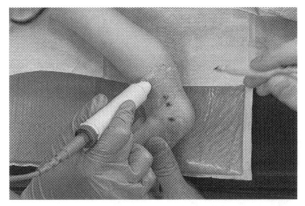

Figure 34.2 Doppler ultrasound mapping of the arterial supply to the hand.

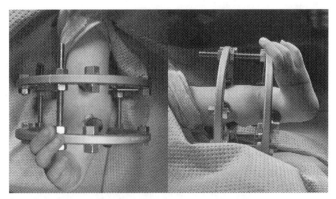

Figure 34.3 Distal humeral and proximal ulnar rings were applied with the elbow in extension (to protect against potential elbow subluxation during the process of gradual centralisation).

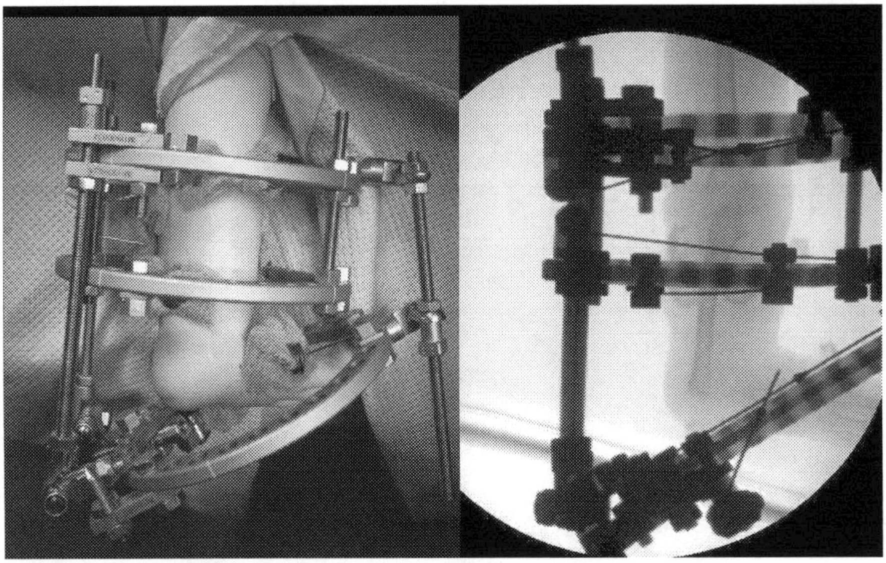

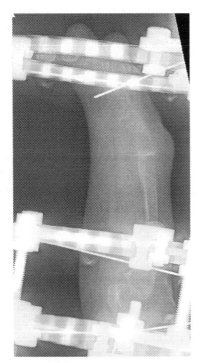

Figure 34.4 The third ring was applied with wires through the metacarpals.

Post-Operative Management after Stage 1

The immediate after-care consisted of pain management, pin-site care[8] and a period of adjustment by child and family to the presence of a circular fixator on the limb. Distraction was started on the third day after surgery. The correction rate was adjusted based on the tolerance of the soft tissues and patient comfort. The child was discharged on the fifth post-operative day. Distraction was continued until the desired alignment of the hand was achieved (Figure 34.5).

Figure 34.5 The deformity is sufficiently corrected to proceed with the second-stage surgery.

Stage 2: Centralisation over an Intramedullary Rod

Under general anaesthesia, the fixator was removed, and the limb was prepared for open surgery. The head of the chosen metacarpal, the head of the ulna and the carpus were exposed through two dorsal incisions. The fibrous 'capsule' was released on the radial and volar sides to allow the carpus to be transposed onto the end of the ulna. The intramedullary cavity of the ulna was reamed with 2.5 mm reamers. Under fluoroscopic guidance, a 2 mm Kirschner wire was passed from the head of the metacarpal, through the medullary cavity and across the carpus into the track prepared previously in the ulna. Since the ulna was bowed, a percutaneous osteotomy was performed at the apex of the bow, and the K-wire was brought out through the olecranon. The K-wire was then pulled proximally until its tip lay just beneath the articular cartilage of the metacarpal head distally (Figure 34.6a). The wire was bent and cut at the olecranon and was secured to prevent subsequent migration or backing out by a 2.0 mm plate (Figure 34.6b). An Ilizarov frame was applied with proximal ulnar and metacarpal wires to maintain the hand in its corrected position.

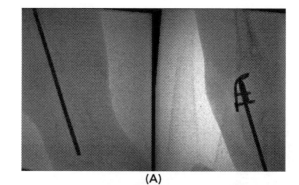

(A)

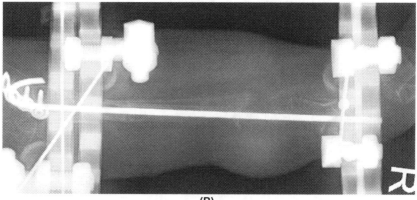

(B)

Figures 34.6a and **b** A 2.0 mm plate is used to prevent the wire from backing out, and an Ilizarov frame is applied with proximal ulnar and metacarpal wires to maintain the hand in its corrected position.

Post-Operative Management after Stage 2

The fixator was removed under anaesthesia after six to eight weeks. A plaster cast was applied and substituted soon after for a custom-made thermoplastic splint across the ulna and hand. Final images are shown in Figure 34.7.

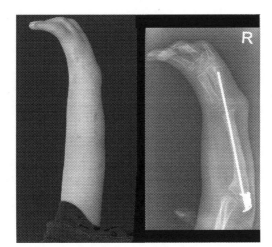

Figure 34.7 The wrist is now centralised on the distal ulna. Residual deformity is present in the fingers and may be addressed at the time of pollicisation.

Comment

Follow up is until skeletal maturity.

At around 18 months to 2 years after surgery, the metacarpal and ulna will have grown to the extent that the intramedullary-transcarpal wire will be too short. Leaving a short wire risks recurrence of the deformity and cut-out of the wire from the bone.[9] This necessitates exchanging the short wire for one of greater length and diameter at 18–24-month intervals. At the first exchange, a 2.8 mm wire is used, then a 3.2 mm wire before finally reaming with a 4 mm reamer and inserting a 3.5 mm Fassier-Duval telescopic rod (Figure 34.8). The telescopic rod can often be left in situ for three to five years, by which time, around the age of 11–12 years, a spontaneous carpal fusion occurs. At this point, no further external splintage will be required.[10]

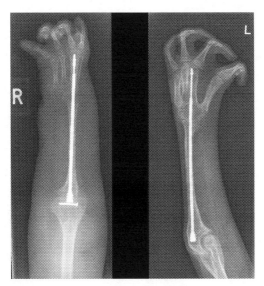

Figure 34.8 These images (from other patients) illustrate how a Fassier-Duval rod is left in situ until the wrist fuses and no longer requires splintage.

References

1. Skerik SK, Flatt AE. The anatomy of congenital radial dysplasia: Its surgical and functional implications. *Clin Orthop.* 1969 Oct;66:125–43.
2. Buck-Gramcko D. Radialization as a new treatment for radial club hand. *J Hand Surg.* 1985 Nov;10(6 Pt 2):964–8.
3. Buck-Gramcko D. Radialization for radial club hand. *Tech Hand Up Extrem Surg.* 1999 Mar;3(1):2–12.
4. Paley D. The Paley ulnarization of the carpus with ulnar shortening osteotomy for treatment of radial club hand. *SICOT-J.* 2017;3:5.
5. Sabharwal S, Finuoli AL, Ghobadi F. Pre-centralization soft tissue distraction for Bayne type IV congenital radial deficiency in children. *J Pediatr Orthop.* 2005 Jun;25(3):377–81.
6. Kessler I. Centralisation of the radial club hand by gradual distraction. *J Hand Surg Edinb Scotl.* 1989 Feb;14(1):37–42.
7. Bayne LG, Klug MS. Long-term review of the surgical treatment of radial deficiencies. *J Hand Surg.* 1987 Mar;12(2):169–79.
8. Davies R, Holt N, Nayagam S. The care of pin sites with external fixation. *J Bone Joint Surg Br.* 2005 May;87(5):716–19.
9. Kawabata H, Shibata T, Masatomi T, Yasui N. Residual deformity in congenital radial club hands after previous centralisation of the wrist: Ulnar lengthening and correction by the Ilizarov method. *J Bone Joint Surg Br.* 1998 Sep;80(5):762–5.
10. Goldfarb CA, Klepps SJ, Dailey LA, Manske PR. Functional outcome after centralization for radius dysplasia. *J Hand Surg.* 2002 Jan;27(1):118–24.

CASE 35: ULNAR CLUB HAND

Christopher Prior, Nicholas Peterson, Selvadurai Nayagam

Case

This 8-year-old boy presented with recurrent bowing of his left forearm. A deformity of his left forearm had been noted soon after birth, and a provisional diagnosis of mild longitudinal ulnar deficiency had been made. Whilst under observation for this problem, at the age of 2 years, he sustained a lateral condyle fracture that needed open reduction and fixation (Figures 35.1a, 35.1b). By the time he was reviewed again for the original problem, the deformity had worsened.

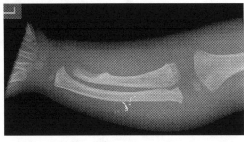 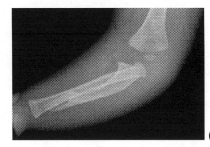

(A) (B)

Figures 35.1a, b Two views showing the lateral condyle fracture sustained by this child when aged 2 years whilst under observation for an ulnar dysplasia causing a club hand appearance.

Examination at the age of 5 years revealed a curvature to the left forearm and a prominence over the lateral aspect of the elbow. The hand was held in a position of ulnar deviation at the wrist. There was loss of the terminal range of elbow extension and a reduction in the arc of pronation-supination to 60% of the normal range. X-rays showed a deficiency of the distal ulna and bowing of both the radius and ulna, and the radial head was dislocated (Figures 35.2a–c).

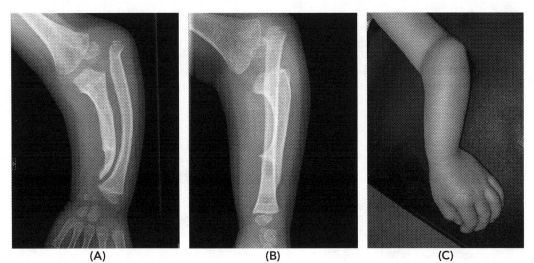

(A) (B) (C)

Figures 35.2a–c Radiographs and clinical photograph depicting the deformity caused by the curved radius and ulna, shortened ulna and dislocation of the radial head at the elbow.

Proximal ulnar lengthening and gradual relocation of the radial head using an Ilizarov fixator was successful (Figures 35.3a–d). In just over three years, the deformity recurred as did the dislocation of the radial head. At the age of 8 years, the clinical findings were similar to those at 5 years, with the exception of a greater curvature distally near the wrist (Figures 35.4a, 35.4b).

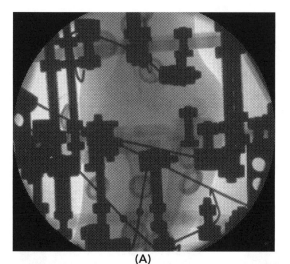
(A)

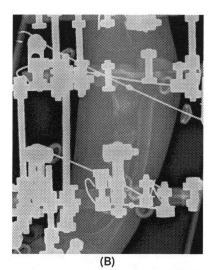
(B)

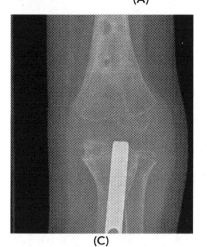
(C)

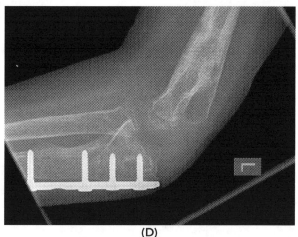
(D)

Figures 35.3a–d This was the child's first surgery when aged 5 years to increase the length of the ulna and reduce the radial head. A proximal ulnar lengthening was performed (A, B) and the regenerate column plated to shorten time in external fixation (C, D).

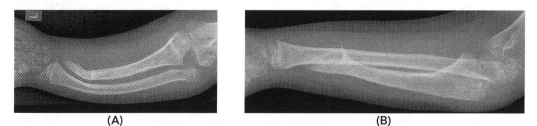
(A)   (B)

Figures 35.4a, b The recurrence of radial head dislocation at the age of 8 years and a greater curvature to the radius and ulna distally. The distal ulna remains dysplastic.

Questions

- What are the problems that need to be addressed in this boy?
- What are the aims of treatment?
- What are the available options for treatment?
- What are the factors that may influence your choice of treatment?
- What treatment would you recommend for this boy?
- How long would you follow-up this boy after treatment?

The Problems to Be Addressed

- Length discrepancy between the radius and ulna
- Dislocation of the radial head
- Curvature of the forearm bones
- Limitation of elbow and forearm motion
- Unsightly appearance of the limb

The Aims of Treatment

- Improve elbow extension by reduction of the posteriorly dislocated radial head
- Restore length relationships between radius and ulna
- Improve cosmesis by

  o Correcting the curvature of the radius and ulna
  o Reducing the dislocated radial head

- Improve forearm motion by correcting the curvature of the radius and ulna

Options for Treatment

- No intervention but continued observation
- Excision of the dislocated radial head and acute correction of forearm deformity through osteotomies of distal radius and ulna
- Lengthening of the ulna with correction of ulnar deformity and reduction of radial head with concurrent correction of radial bowing

---

FACTORS THAT INFLUENCED THE CHOICE OF TREATMENT

- Previous good compliance by the child and family for treatment using the Ilizarov method
- Successful restoration of radio-humeral joint congruity through ulnar lengthening previously
- Poor results from radial head excision in young children

How Was This Boy Treated?

The Ilizarov fixator was assembled with a wire and ring configuration such that distal osteotomies of both ulna and radius at the CORA of the deformities allowed for an acute correction and, without any changes to the assembled fixator, lengthening of the ulna was then carried out with gradual reduction of the radial head.

The fixator and wire configurations were as follows:

1. Proximal ring with crossed wires in the ulna only
2. Middle ring with crossed wires in the radius only
3. Distal ring with one wire in the radius and one in the ulna, and one wire across both bones
4. Hand ring with two crossed wires in metacarpals

Using percutaneous access, small drill holes were created at the levels of the planned osteotomies in the distal radius and ulna. The osteotomies were completed using an osteotome. Acute correction of the ulnar angulation of both radius and ulna was performed by manipulating the rings. The fixator was stabilised once the desired correction was obtained (Figures 35.5a–d).

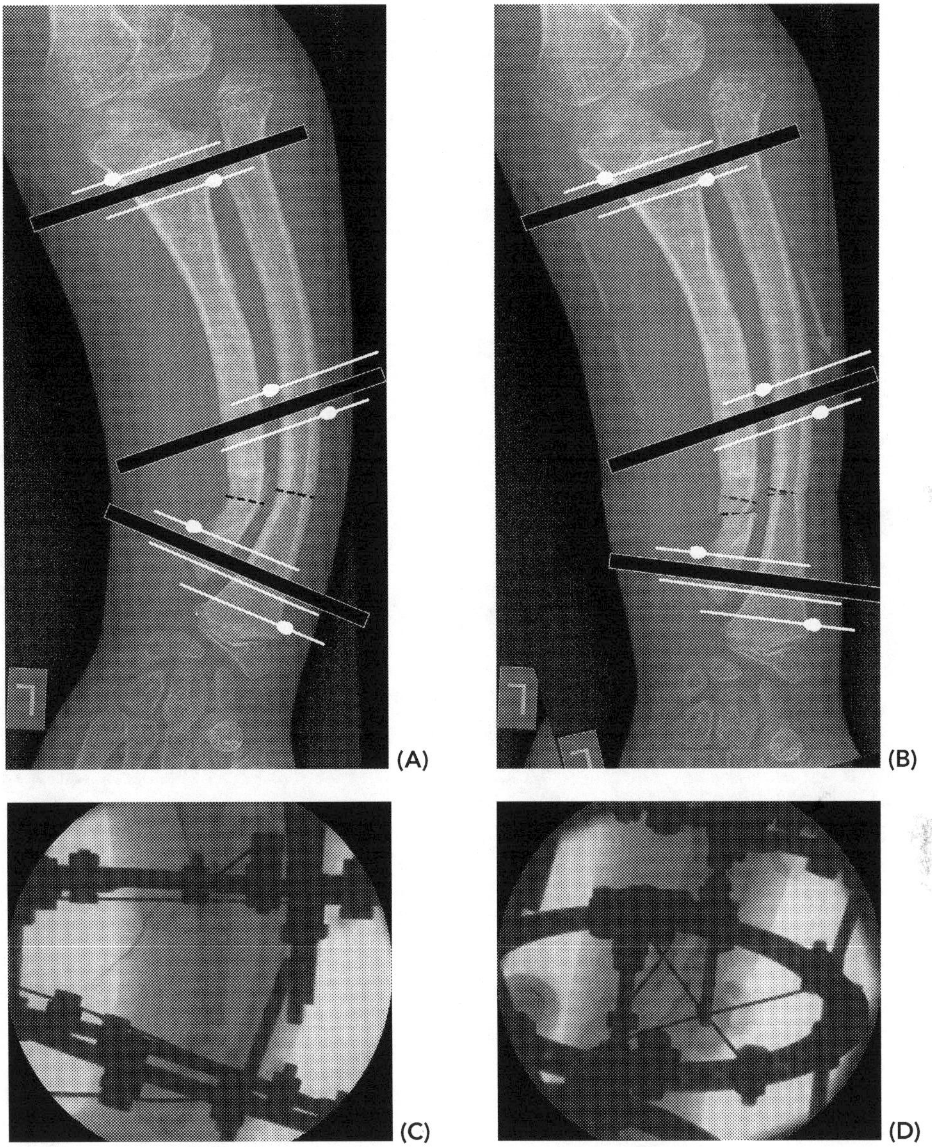

Figures 35.5a–d Figures 35.5a and 35.5b show the setup of the Ilizarov assembly. The proximal ring is attached to ulna only, the middle ring to radius only and the distal ring to both forearm bones. The simulated correction (b) improves the abnormal distal curvature of radius and ulna. Thereafter, gradual distraction commences between proximal and middle rings to lengthen the ulna and pull the whole radius distally. Figures 35.5c and 35.5d are intraoperative views of the distal osteotomies just prior to, and after, acute correction.

After a latency period of seven days, distraction was commenced between the proximal ring and the middle ring of the fixator at 0.75 mm per day divided into three parts. This separation of rings at this level achieved distraction osteogenesis at the level of the ulnar osteotomy, but as the radius was linked to both the middle and distal ulnar rings (and with the distance between these two rings unchanged), the radial head was advanced distally without separation of the osteotomy of the radius (Figures 35.6a–c).

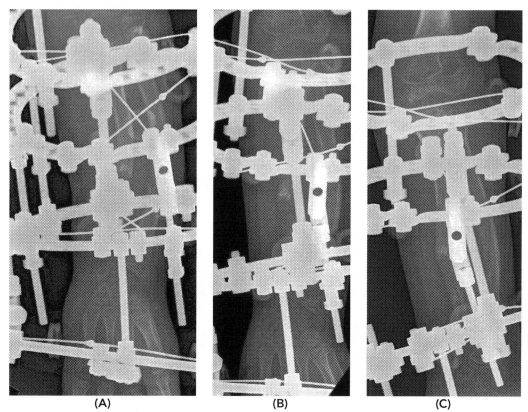

(A)   **(B)**   **(C)**

Figures 35.6a–c Post-operative sequence of x-ray images showing gradual lengthening of the distal ulna and a simultaneous axial translation of the entire radius with reduction of the radial head at the elbow.

Post-Operative Management

Regular physiotherapy to prevent joint stiffness, pin site care and pain control were followed throughout the period when the fixator was on.

Gradual reduction of the radial head occurred when the length of the ulna was such that the 'space' within the forearm was sufficient to accommodate the full length of the radius. The radio-capitellar joint was screened under x-ray image intensification to check the congruency of joint reduction. Minor adjustments to the regenerate column created in the distal ulna were made, and this enabled seating the radial head concentrically against the capitellum. No further adjustments to the fixator were done till the regenerate consolidated. Fixator removal was undertaken when x-rays confirmed consolidation of the regenerate column on both AP and lateral views (Figures 35.7a, b).

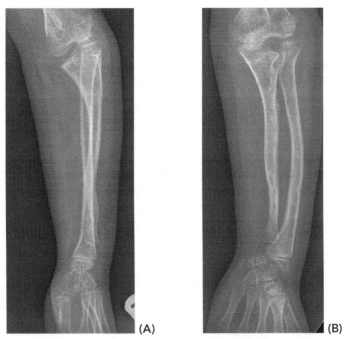

(A)　　　　　　　　　　　(B)

Figures 35.7a, b X-ray images taken at age 9 years, about 12 months after completion of previous treatment. The radial head remains reduced, and the ulnar length is improved.

Radiographs at the age of 14 years show the forearm shape is maintained, the length relationships between radius and ulna are normalised, and the radial head is articulating with the capitellum congruently (Figures 35.8a, b). The boy will be followed-up till he is skeletally mature.

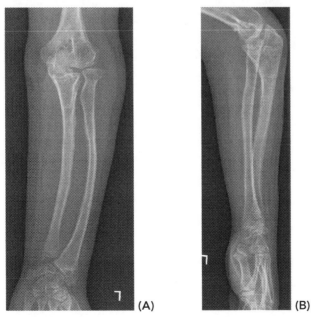

(A)　　　　　　　　　　　(B)

Figures 35.8a, b X-ray images taken at age 14 years. The focal fibrocartilaginous dysplasia has resolved spontaneously (as would be expected of the lesion), and the radial head remains in joint.

Comment

What Caused the Clinical Problem?

In this child, the ulnar deficiency was responsible for the length discrepancy between radius and ulna and a mismatch in growth. The slower growing ulna produced a tether to the growth of the radius.[1,2]

Ulnar club hand is the least common congenital limb aplasia and varies from slight under-development of the ulna to complete absence.[3,4,5] In moderate to severe categories, the proximal radius may be dislocated or fused at the elbow, and there is hypogenesis of digits. In milder degrees of ulnar underdevelopment, as in the case here, the problem lies in the mismatch of length between the two forearm bones leading to an increasing curvature of the radius and eventual dislocation of the radial head (if not dislocated at birth). An anlage of the ulna, often fibrocartilaginous, tethers the growing radius.[1] A similar type of ulnar club hand is acquired from conditions which interfere with longitudinal growth from the distal ulnar physis, e.g., nearby osteochondromas (in hereditary multiple exostoses) and even focal anomalies of the distal ulna.[2,6,7,8] In the event of increased radial bowing and loss of congruity at the radio-capitellar joint, the approach to treatment is very similar to that given here.

This case of ulnar club hand is even rarer as the ulnar dysplasia was caused by a focal fibrocartilaginous dysplasia.[1] This was chosen to illustrate the treatment principles that can be applied to an ulnar club hand arising from radius-ulna growth mismatch from a mild longitudinal deficiency or from hereditary multiple exostoses.

References

1. Carroll RE, Bowers WH. Congenital deficiency of the ulna. *J Hand Surg Am.* 1977;2(3):169–74.
2. Vogt B, Tretow HL, Daniilidis K, Wacker S, Buller TC, Henrichs M-P, et al. Reconstruction of forearm deformity by distraction osteogenesis in children with relative shortening of the ulna due to multiple cartilaginous exostosis. *Journal of Pediatric Orthopedics.* 2011;31(4):393.
3. Ogden JA, Watson HK, Bohne W. Ulnar dysmelia. *J Bone Joint Surg Am.* 1976;58(4):467–75.
4. Bauer AS, Bednar MS, James MA. Disruption of the radial/ulnar axis: Congenital longitudinal deficiencies. *J Hand Surg Am.* 2013;38(11):2293–302.
5. Swanson AB, Tada K, Yonenobu K. Ulnar ray deficiency: Its various manifestations. *J Hand Surg Am.* 1984;9(5):658–64.
6. Watts A, Ballantyne J, Fraser M, Porter D. The association between ulnar length and forearm movement in patients with multiple osteochondromas. *The Journal of Hand Surgery.* 2007;32(5):667–73.
7. Kazuki K, Hiroshima K, Kawahara K. Ulnar focal cortical indentation: A previously unrecognised form of ulnar dysplasia. *J Bone Joint Surg Br.* 2005;87(4):540–3.
8. Gottschalk HP, Light TR, Smith P. Focal fibrocartilaginous dysplasia in the ulna: Report on 3 cases. *J Hand Surg Am.* 2012;37(11):2300–3.

DISCREPANCIES OF LIMB LENGTH

Christopher Prior, Nicholas Peterson, Selvadurai Nayagam

Case

A 7-year-old female presented with a limb length discrepancy. She had neurofibromatosis Type 1 with a large plexiform tumour over the right thigh and gluteal region causing overgrowth of the right femur. She was using a 4 cm shoe raise, but there was concern that the discrepancy was increasing as she grew.

Clinical examination confirmed the leg length discrepancy and the difference in girth between right and left thighs. Her right hip had a 15-degree fixed flexion deformity and could not abduct beyond 30 degrees.

The standing full-length limb X-rays confirmed the localised gigantism of the femur and leg length discrepancy of 40 mm. MRI scans showed a large plexiform neurofibroma extending from the pelvis into the gluteal region and proximal thigh (Figure 36.1).

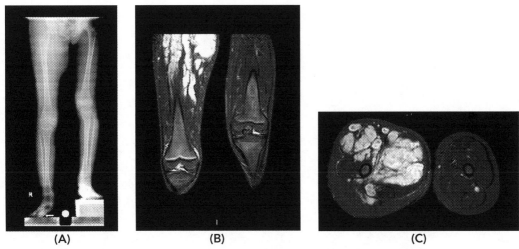

(A) (B) (C)

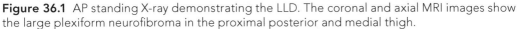

Figure 36.1 AP standing X-ray demonstrating the LLD. The coronal and axial MRI images show the large plexiform neurofibroma in the proximal posterior and medial thigh.

Questions

- What are the problems that need to be addressed in this girl?
- What are the aims of treatment?
- What are the commonly available options for treatment?
- What are the factors that may influence your choice of treatment?
- What treatment would you recommend for this girl?
- How long would you follow-up this girl after treatment?

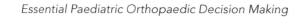

The Problems That Need to Be Addressed Are

- Limb length discrepancy (LLD) of the femur altering gait
- Risk of increase of LLD with age
- Impediments to surgical options by the large plexiform tumour in the thigh

The Aims of Treatment in This Child Are to

- Equalise limb lengths or at least decrease LLD sufficiently to avoid the need for a shoe raise
- Prevent further overgrowth of the femur, if possible
- Improve the appearance of the limb

Options for Treatment to Fulfil Each Aim

- Equalising limb lengths
  - Epiphyseodesis of the right femur
    - Temporary
    - Permanent
  - Acute shortening of the right femur
  - Gradual shortening of the right femur
  - Lengthening of left femur
- Preventing further overgrowth of the right femur
  - Permanent epiphyseodesis
- Improve the appearance of the limb
  - Debulk the plexiform tumour

> **FACTORS THAT INFLUENCED THE CHOICE OF TREATMENT**
>
> - The age of the child
> - Limitations of standard treatment methods in overgrowth syndromes
> - Effects of the plexiform tumour

The choice of treatment based on these factors is outlined in Table 36.1.

Table 36.1 Factors that influenced the choice of treatment

Factors		Treatment Implications
Age of the child	7 years	She has sufficient years of growth remaining to try guided growth as a means of decreasing LLD.
Limitations of standard treatment methods in overgrowth syndromes	Permanent epiphyseodesis	Permanent epiphyseodesis in young children with overgrowth may not achieve accurate equalisation of limb lengths.

Table 36.1 (Continued)

Factors		Treatment Implications
	Guided growth	Guided growth using 8-plates for equalisation of limb lengths can be controversial because there is uncertainty over the speed of growth reduction[1] and the technique can lead to coronal or sagittal plane deformities.[2]
	Acute	The right femur is, despite overgrowth, not amenable to large amounts of acute shortening in one operation owing to the defunctioning effect on the muscles[3] and the increase in the girth of the limb in the presence of the tumour. If shortening is done, the degree of shortening must be modest.
Effects of the plexiform tumour		Contractures, limitation of movement and pain contributing to abnormal gait may influence the surgical approach.

How Was This Child Treated?

The complexity of the clinical problem warranted a staged approach.

Stage 1: *Temporary epiphyseodesis of the right distal femur using 8-plates (at age 7).* This was performed with the rationale of slowing down the rate of increase in LLD with the option of removing the plates and allowing growth to continue in the future, if required.

Eight-plates were inserted on the medial and lateral aspects of the right distal femur. Care was taken to preserve the physis and perichondral ring, and to ensure that the plates were positioned in the centre of the growth plate to prevent a sagittal plane deformity (Figure 36.2).

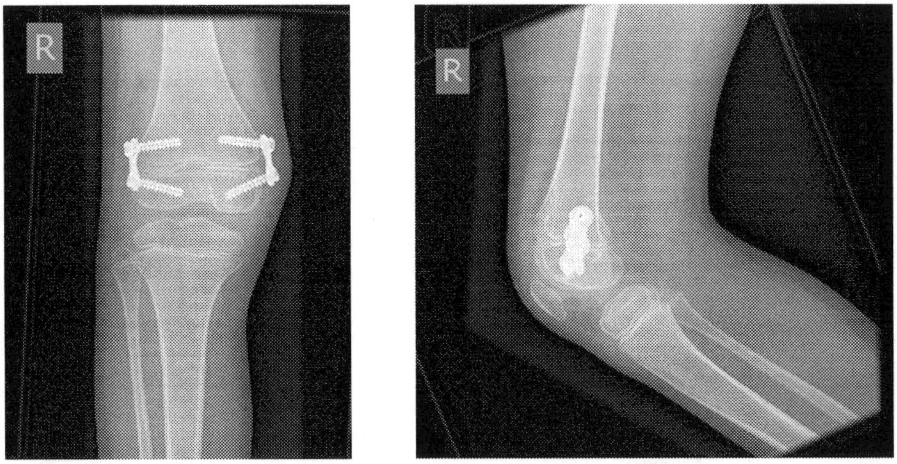

(A)   (B)

Figure 36.2 Medial and lateral 8-plates to the right distal femur for temporary epiphyseodesis.

Stage 2: *Debulking of the tumour in the proximal thigh and gluteal area to reduce pain and the localised mass effect.*

This was carried out by plastic surgeons over several sessions.

Stage 3: *Femoral shortening and derotation.*

At age 11, the LLD had reduced to 3 cm, but the gluteal neurofibroma had produced an external rotation contracture at the hip that led to a marked out-toeing gait.

MRI images of the femur showed that the tumour had not invaded the periosteum and that a 'window' for surgical access to the femoral shaft was present through the posterior aspect of the lateral compartment, away from the tumour (Figure 36.3).

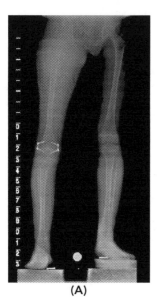
(A)

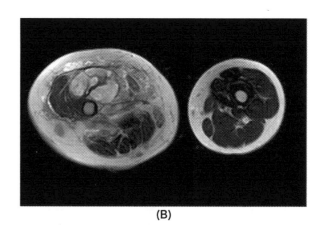
(B)

Figure 36.3 AP X-ray demonstrating the LLD at age 11 (A). Axial MRI demonstrating the plane through which the femur can be accessed behind normal muscle to avoid encountering the plexiform tumour (B).

Under general anaesthesia, the mid-shaft of the femur was exposed extra-periosteally via a lateral approach along the intermuscular septum (Figures 36.4a, 36.4b). A shortening derotation osteotomy was performed aided by a derotation arc used in conjunction with a rail external fixator. Half-pins were inserted anteriorly proximal and distal to the intended osteotomy site using external fixator rail clamps placed at 40 degrees to each other in the axial plane. (Figures 36.5a, 36.5b) Two low-energy osteotomies were performed 25 mm apart using drills and osteotomes, and the 25 mm segment of bone was removed. The fixator clamps were reduced on the rail to achieve the derotation while maintaining coronal and sagittal alignment (Figure 36.6a, 36.6b). The osteotomy ends were compressed using a compression unit on the rail.

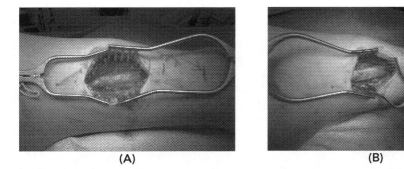

(A)   (B)

Figures 36.4a, b A submuscular and extra-periosteal approach under the mass of vastus late-ralis (as indicated on the MRI) in the middle of the femur avoided encountering the bulk of the neurofibroma.

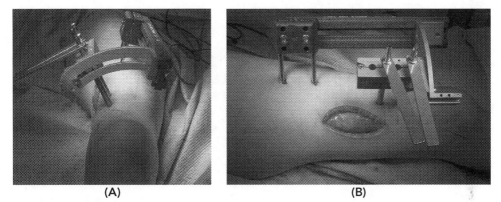

(A)   (B)

Figures 36.5a, 36.5b Half-pins are inserted anteriorly through two clamps set at 40 degrees apart in the axial plane. The use of a derotation arc template facilitated this correction with the rail fixator.

A large fragment locking plate was contoured to the femur with the aid of fluoroscopy. A sub-muscular plane was developed under the vastus lateralis along the lateral border of the femur. The contoured locking plate was passed retrograde and secured to the bone with locking screws, ensuring that the distal femoral physis was preserved. A cortical screw was passed up the femo-ral neck to reduce the risk of a femoral neck stress riser (Figure 36.7).

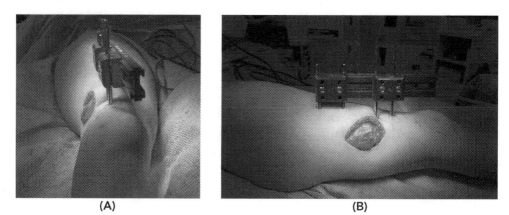

(A) (B)

Figures 36.6a, 36.6b After excision of a 25 mm segment of femur, the clamps fixed onto the same rail, thereby achieving the derotation without loss of coronal or sagittal plane alignment. The muscle bulge through the incision is due to the shortening performed.

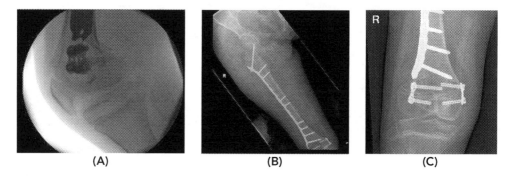

(A) (B) (C)

Figure 36.7 Intraoperative imaging demonstrating slightly more anterior placement of the distal femoral 8-plates. Post-operative X-rays demonstrating the lateral femoral submuscular plate in situ after the shortening and derotation osteotomy.

The 8-plates were revised at the same surgery to a slightly anterior position to offset a fixed flexion deformity of the knee that developed subsequent to the tumour affecting the hamstrings.

Post-Operative Management

A partial weight-bearing protocol was instituted before inpatient discharge. This was increased gradually by six weeks, advancing to full weight bearing. Union was evident on x-rays by three months, and full consolidation was confirmed at 12 months (Figure 36.8). Eighteen months after the shortening osteotomy, the submuscular plate was removed to enable serial MR imaging of the tumours.

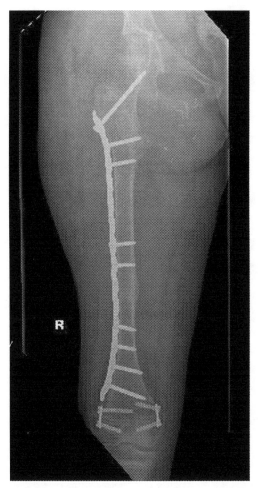

Figure 36.8 X-ray right femur taken 12 months post-procedure confirming union and consolidation of the osteotomy.

Bone age assessments suggested she had a skeletal immaturity of about two years behind her chronological age. When leg length equality was established, the femoral 8-plates were removed to avoid over-shortening. At the same time, a varus deformity at the knee, which had recently developed arising from the proximal tibia, was treated using guided growth (Figure 36.9). This surgery coincided with the patient starting a trial of MEK inhibitor therapy.[4]

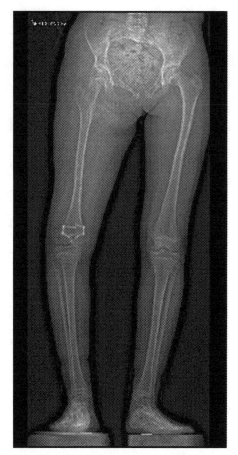

Figure 36.9 AP standing EOS X-ray demonstrating equal limb lengths. The varus deformity at the knee was found to arise from the tibia and subsequently treated by guided growth.

At 16, the alignment of the lower limbs was satisfactory and limb lengths were equal. Her pain had become reasonably well controlled. As there is unlikely to be much further growth owing to reaching skeletal maturity and the use of MEK inhibitor treatment, the current X-rays represent the final outcome (Figure 36.10).

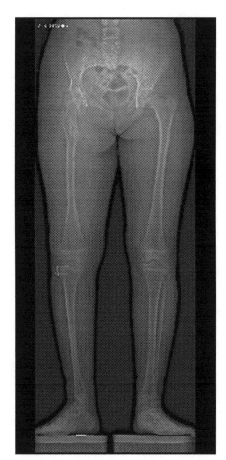

Figure 36.10 AP standing EOS X-ray at age 16. Equal leg lengths and satisfactory overall alignment.

References

1. Lauge-Pedersen H, Hägglund G. Eight plate should not be used for treating leg length discrepancy. *J Child Orthop.* 2013;7(4):285–8. doi: 10.1007/s11832-013-0506-7.
2. Lee WC, Kao HK, Yang WE, Chang CH. Tension band plating is less effective in achieving equalization of leg length. *J Child Orthop.* 2018;12(6):629–34. doi: 10.1302/1863-2548.12.170219.
3. Holm I, Nordsletten L, Steen H, Folleräs G, Bjerkreim I. Muscle function after mid-shaft femoral shortening: A prospective study with a two-year follow-up. *J Bone Joint Surg Br.* 1994 Jan;76(1):143–6.
4. Klesse LJ, Jordan JT, Radtke HB, Rosser T, Schorry E, Ullrich N, Viskochil D, Knight P, Plotkin SR, Yohay K. The use of MEK inhibitors in neurofibromatosis type 1-associated tumors and management of toxicities. *Oncologist.* 2020 Jul;25(7):e1109–16.

Nicholas Peterson, Christopher Prior, Selvadurai Nayagam

Case

A 12-year-old boy was referred for limb length discrepancy (LLD) following previous treatment in another institution. Meningococcal septicaemia at the age of 3 left him with physeal arrests in both tibiae. He presented with a limb length discrepancy of 7 cm and a shorter left lower limb. The left tibia had both proximal and distal physeal arrests with a loss of the normal proximal tibiofibular relationship due to continued growth of the fibula. The right tibia had a distal physeal arrest. Both ankles were in varus (Figure 37.1).[1] At the age of 7, he had undergone a proximal tibial metaphyseal osteotomy to correct a varus deformity.

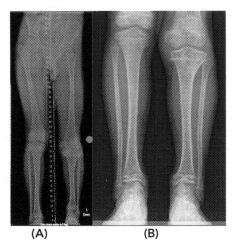

(A)   (B)

Figure 37.1 (A) Scanogram aged 12 showing a 7 cm limb length discrepancy arising from the left tibia, disproportionately short tibiae bilaterally and varus ankle deformities. (B) AP images of both tibiae aged 8. On the left side, proximal and distal tibial growth arrests are seen. On the right, only the distal physis has arrested. Both ankles have a varus deformity.

The tibia-to-femur length ratio was 0.5 on the left and 0.7 on the right (normal ratio ~ 0.8).[2]

With a further four years of growth remaining, Menelaus' rule of thumb was used to calculate the final length of the femur and determine the target length of both tibiae for equality and normal body proportions.[3] The left tibia required 14 cm of lengthening whilst the right required 7 cm, of which approximately 2.4 cm would come from normal growth of the right proximal tibial physis, assuming that the physis was not 'sick' (a 'sick physis' is a normal-looking physis on plain x-ray but one that does not contribute to predictable longitudinal growth).[4]

Questions

- What are the problems that need to be addressed in this boy?
- What are the aims of treatment?
- What are the available options for treatment?
- What are the factors that may influence your choice of treatment?
- What treatment would you recommend for this boy?
- How long would you follow-up this boy after treatment?

The Problems That Need to Be Addressed Are

- Limb length discrepancy
- Fibular overgrowth
- Varus ankles
- Abnormal limb proportions

The Aims of Treatment Are to

- Equalise limb lengths by skeletal maturity
- Correct left tibio-fibular relationship
- Correct bilateral ankle deformity
- Restore normal lower limb proportions

Options for Treatment to Fulfil Each Aim

- Equalising limb lengths

    o Tibial lengthening (bilateral)—staged or simultaneous using:

        □ Circular fixator
        □ Monolateral rail fixator
        □ Intramedullary lengthening nail (these devices can be used in children with physeal arrests; some newer implants demonstrate promising results)[5]

- Correcting left tibio-fibular relationship

    o Fibular transport

        □ Circular fixator with syndesmosis screw
        □ Monolateral rail fixator with syndesmosis screw
        □ Intramedullary lengthening nail with syndesmosis screw

    o Fibular shortening

- Correcting ankle deformity

    o Acute correction of deformity
    o External fixator assisted deformity correction with or without lengthening
    o Gradual correction of deformity with circular fixator

FACTORS THAT INFLUENCED THE CHOICE OF TREATMENT

- Age of the boy
- Pattern of limb shortening
- Physeal health

The factors that were taken into consideration in the choice of treatment are shown in Table 37.1.

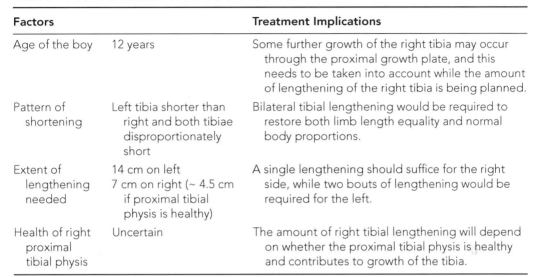

Table 37.1 Factors that influenced the choice of treatment

Factors		Treatment Implications
Age of the boy	12 years	Some further growth of the right tibia may occur through the proximal growth plate, and this needs to be taken into account while the amount of lengthening of the right tibia is being planned.
Pattern of shortening	Left tibia shorter than right and both tibiae disproportionately short	Bilateral tibial lengthening would be required to restore both limb length equality and normal body proportions.
Extent of lengthening needed	14 cm on left 7 cm on right (~ 4.5 cm if proximal tibial physis is healthy)	A single lengthening should suffice for the right side, while two bouts of lengthening would be required for the left.
Health of right proximal tibial physis	Uncertain	The amount of right tibial lengthening will depend on whether the proximal tibial physis is healthy and contributes to growth of the tibia.

Sequential, staged lengthening procedures were planned around the patient's school commitments. Acute deformity correction was planned for the bilateral ankle deformities at the same time as the lengthening procedures.[6]

How Was This Boy Treated?

At age 12, an acute correction of the left distal tibial varus deformity was performed through a supra-malleolar osteotomy, with a simultaneous diaphyseal osteotomy of the tibia. The fibula was osteotomised distally to accommodate the acute correction of the tibia. The fibula was not fixed proximally to enable a gradual descent of the fibular head with lengthening of the tibia and thus restore the normal tibio-fibular relationship (Figure 37.2). The desired lengthening of 7 cm to the left tibia was achieved and, after four months, a plate-after-lengthening (PAL) procedure using a submuscular tibial plate was performed to reduce frame time (Figure 37.3). Metalwork removal was performed in view of expected further bouts of lengthening. Long leg imaging at age 15 demonstrated disproportionately short tibiae, medial mechanical axis deviation on the right and a significant varus deformity to the right ankle (Figure 37.4).

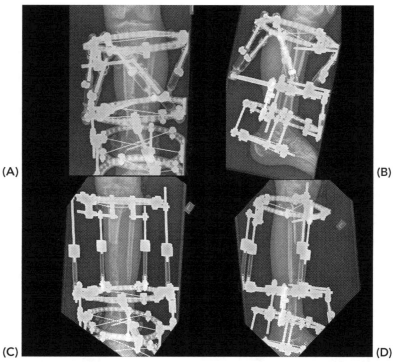

Figure 37.2a, b Immediate postoperative images after mid-diaphyseal osteotomy for lengthening and correction of the distal tibial varus. (C, D) Images at completion of lengthening (the hexapod struts have been exchanged for Ilizarov telescopic rods as the frame is now static).

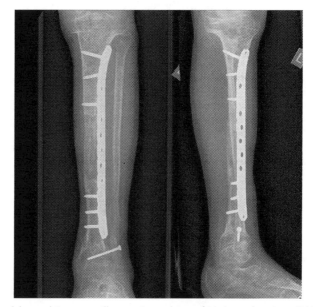

Figure 37.3 AP and lateral images illustrating plate-after-lengthening (PAL) of the left tibia. Note the normal proximal tibio-fibular relationship has been restored as well as the correct orientation of the ankle joint.

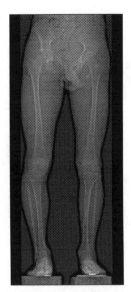

Figure 37.4 A long leg scanogram demonstrating limb length discrepancy, medial mechanical axis deviation on the right side and a right ankle varus deformity. Both tibiae were disproportionately short.

Tibial lengthening and deformity correction on the right tibia were next carried out. An external fixator-assisted corrective valgus osteotomy of the distal tibia was fixed with an anterior plate. This was followed by lengthening and deformity correction through a proximal tibial osteotomy using a medially applied rail fixator. The medial positioning of the rail fixator was to facilitate a subsequent PAL procedure (Figure 37.5).

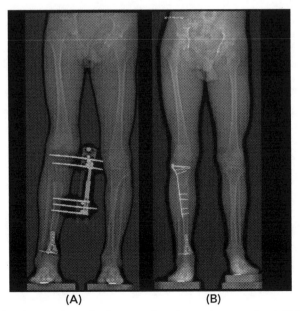

(A)   **(B)**

Figure 37.5a Lengthening and gradual correction through a proximal tibial osteotomy. Acute correction of distal tibial varus deformity. (B) A long leg image of the patient aged 16 with good final position of the mechanical axis and improvement in length proportions of femur to tibia. The PAL technique is shown. A 6 cm limb length discrepancy now remains to be addressed.

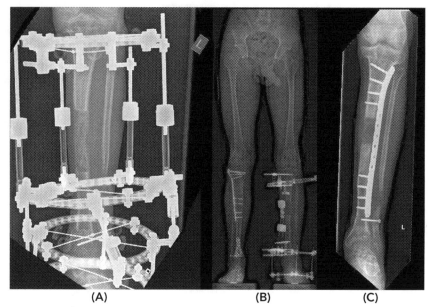

Figure 37.6a A further lengthening of the left tibia and fibula with a circular external fixator. (B) Long leg images at completion of lengthening and before a further PAL procedure. (C) Postoperative appearance of the lengthened left tibia and fibula following PAL.

The final lengthening of the left tibia and fibula was performed at age 16 using a circular external fixator. Some valgus deformity was noted during the lengthening process, and this was corrected using hinges prior to a final PAL procedure (Figure 37.6).

Postoperative Management

Each treatment episode of lengthening by external fixation required weekly attendance to a limb reconstruction clinic with its affiliated physiotherapy appointment. Compliance with the lengthening protocol and home physiotherapy programme was checked. Weight-bearing without restriction was allowed. Meticulous attention to pin-site care was provided through specialist nurses. After substitution of the external fixator by a plate, weight-bearing was reduced to 30% until the regenerate column was homogeneous and complete on x-ray. This was usually not more than four weeks. Thereafter, weight-bearing was increased again.

Comment

The patient was followed up for two years following his most recent procedure and requested metalwork removal. The final scanogram at skeletal maturity, demonstrated a limb length discrepancy of 8 mm, tibia-to-femur length ratios of 0.8 bilaterally and a central mechanical axis in both lower limbs. Both distal tibial varus deformities had been corrected, and the proximal tibiofibular relationship was normal (Figure 37.7).

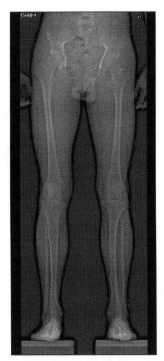

Figure 37.7 Final long leg images after metalwork removal. Normal tibia-to-femur ratios of 0.8 have been achieved. There is a radiologically measurable limb length discrepancy of 8 mm that is insignificant clinically.

He was discharged from follow-up at age 18 having no further issues and satisfied that all aims of surgery had been achieved.

References

1. Park DH, Bradish CF. The management of the orthopaedic sequelae of meningococcal septicaemia: Patients treated to skeletal maturity. *J Bone Joint Surg Br*. 2011 Jul;93(7):984–9.
2. Pietak A, Ma S, Beck CW, Stringer MD. Fundamental ratios and logarithmic periodicity in human limb bones. *J Anat*. 2013 May;222(5):526–37.
3. Westh RN, Menelaus MB. A simple calculation for the timing of epiphysial arrest: A further report. *J Bone Joint Surg Br*. 1981 Feb;63-B(1):117–19.
4. Eastwood DM, Sanghrajka AP. Guided growth: Recent advances in a deep-rooted concept. *J Bone Joint Surg Br*. 2011 Jan;93-B(1):12–18.
5. Helfen T, Delhey P, Mutschler W, Thaller PH. The correction of a 140 mm lower limb difference as a late complication of a childhood meningococcal sepsis with a fully implantable system. *J Pediatr Orthop B*. 2014 Jun;1.
6. Monsell FP, Barnes JR, Kirubanandan R, McBride AMB. Distal tibial physeal arrest after meningococcal septicaemia: Management and outcome in seven ankles. *J Bone Joint Surg Br*. 2011 Jun;93(6): 839–43.

CASE 38: DISCREPANCY OF THE LENGTH OF THE FIBULA

Caroline M Blakey and James A Fernandes

A 15-year-old boy was referred for activity-related pain and discomfort in his left ankle. There was a history of injury to this ankle, at the age of 7, treated by closed reduction and casting. He subsequently required cast wedging. Residual deformity was not apparent to the family, and he had remained asymptomatic until the time of presentation. He was now having difficulty with sports.

He had approximately 1 cm of shortening of the left lower leg but equal femoral segments. Examination of the left ankle revealed 10° valgus deformity and prominence of the medial malleolus. The tip of the lateral malleolus was proximally migrated. There was no localised tenderness. The range of movements of the ankle, subtalar joint and mid-tarsal joints were normal.

Plain radiographs of the ankle showed evidence of a healed fracture of the distal fibula. The distal fibular physis was fused, and the tip of the lateral malleolus was at a higher level than normal (Figure 38.1a, 38.1b, 38.1c). The distal tibial epiphysis was wedge-shaped with ankle valgus and lateral talar displacement.

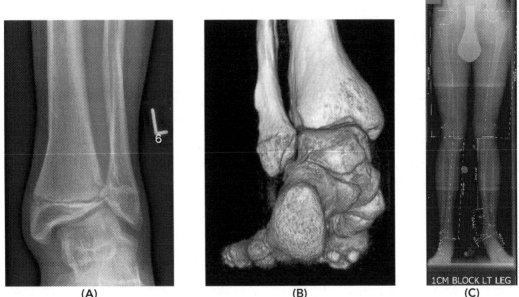

| (A) | (B) | (C) |

Figure 38.1 AP ankle radiograph at presentation (A); pre-operative CT 3D reconstruction demonstrating valgus malalignment (B); mechanical axis with pre-op planning (C).

Questions

- What are the problems that need to be addressed?
- What are the aims of treatment?
- What are the commonly available options for treatment?
- What are the factors that may influence your choice of treatment?
- What treatment would you recommend for this boy?

The Problems That Need to Be Addressed Are

The effects of premature distal fibular growth arrest

- Progressive deformity of the ankle
  - Distal tibial and ankle valgus
  - Talar displacement
- Limb length inequality
  - Left tibia shorter than right tibia
  - Fibula shorter than tibia on the left side

The Aims of Treatment in This Boy Are

- Correct deformity of the ankle
- Prevent progression of ankle deformity
- Equalise leg lengths and restore normal relative lengths of left tibia and fibula

Options for Treatment

Correcting valgus deformity of the ankle

- Supra-malleolar osteotomy of tibia (acute correction)
- Hemi-epiphyseodesis of distal tibia
- Gradual correction with external fixator

Preventing progression of ankle deformity and recurrence after correction

- Complete arrest of distal tibial growth plate
- Guided growth of distal tibial growth plate
- Langenskiold procedure creating synostosis between distal tibia and fibula[1]

Restoring normal relative lengths of fibula and tibia

- Lengthening of fibula
- Epiphyseodesis of tibia

Equalising limb lengths

- Insole raise
- Tibial lengthening

FACTORS THAT INFLUENCED THE CHOICE OF TREATMENT

- Age of the patient
- Presence of tibial deformity
- Status of the ankle joint
- Complexity and duration of treatment

The choice of treatment based on these factors in shown in Table 38.1.

Table 38.1 Factors that influenced the choice of treatment

Factors		Treatment Implications
Age	15 years	Insufficient growth remaining for guided growth of the distal tibia.
Distal tibial deformity	Present	Corrective osteotomy of the distal tibia will be required.
Status of the ankle joint	Normal painless range of movement with talar tilt	Loss of lateral ankle support from a normal lateral malleolus leads to talar tilt and displacement. Even mild talar tilt results in significant increase in joint contact pressures. Stiffness and chondral loss can ensue. This warrants early correction of the talar tilt.
Complexity and duration of treatment	Acute correction versus gradual correction	Reconstruction with a frame requires multiple admissions to hospital and can interrupt schooling.

How Was This Boy Treated?

The treatment of the boy is outlined in Table 38.2.

Table 38.2 Treatment Outline

Age	Problems to Be Addressed	Procedure Undertaken
16 years	Distal fibular growth arrest with shortening and loss of lateral strut with tilt of the ankle and talar shift	1st stage: Application of Taylor Spatial frame with two-ring construct. Talus gradually translated medially with an olive wire and arched tensioning to distract the ankle joint. Monolateral system added for fibular lengthening (Figure 38.2) after percutaneous osteotomy (Figures 38.3a, b).
	Secondary distal tibial deformity	2nd stage: Gradual correction with percutaneous tibial osteotomy and locking of distal tibiofibular joint transfixed with plain wire to distal ring (Figure 38.4). Locking of the tibiofibular joint is critical to avoid proximal migration.[2]
	Distal fibular poor regenerate	Bone grafting of fibula with frame in situ.
18 years	Developmental spasmodic peroneal flat foot	EUA left ankle and Botox injection to left peronei and EDL.
18 years	Lateral subtalar coalition with narrowed subtalar joint and pain	Left subtalar fusion, iliac crest graft and fixation.

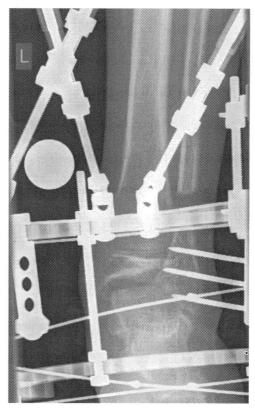

Figure 38.2 AP radiograph demonstrating fibular lengthening prior to second-stage procedure.

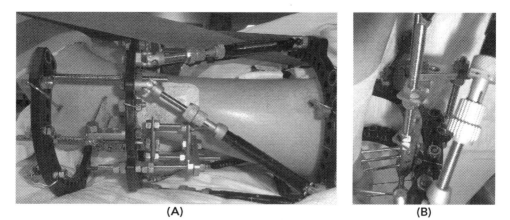

(A)   (B)

Figure 38.3a, b Clinical photographs demonstrating circular frame with incorporated monolateral lengthening rail.

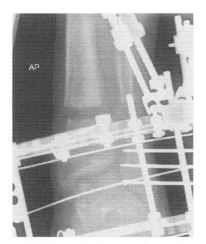

Figure 38.4 AP radiograph post tibial osteotomy and deformity correction with locking of ankle syndesmosis.

Post-Operative Management

The TSF protocol involved initial distraction for seven days followed by angular correction with translation and lengthening. Delayed consolidation of the fibular regenerate was seen, and cortico-cancellous bone graft facilitated union.

At completion of treatment, the calcaneum was well aligned under the tibia. Features of spasmodic flat foot were seen. Ankle movements were satisfactory: 15° dorsiflexion and 25° plantar flexion. There was no detectable subtalar movement, and there was 10° fixed valgus deformity. Further investigation revealed impingement of the talar process and markedly narrowed subtalar joint. A decision was made to fuse the subtalar joint.

At final follow-up, the patient had 25° dorsiflexion, 35° plantar flexion, no pain and symmetrical gait. The hindfoot alignment is normal (Figure 38.5a–c and Figure 38.6a, b). He had resumed all normal activity and had no problem even while surfing (Figure 38.6c).

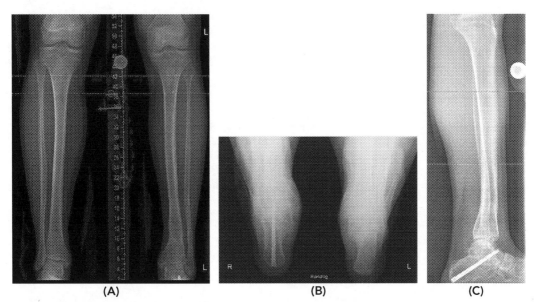

(A)   (B)   (C)

Figure 38.5a–c Radiographs at final follow-up.

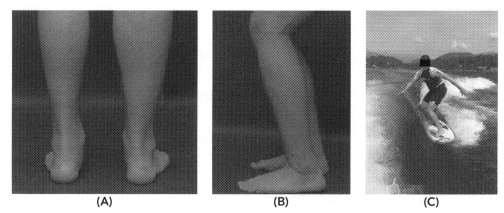

(A)   (B)   (C)

Figure 38.6a–c Clinical photographs at final follow-up.

Comments

The distal fibula acts as a lateral strut for the ankle,[3] and a short fibula will impact talar stability with resultant increased joint contact pressures.[4] During normal gait, the fibula moves distally with weight-bearing.[5] When growth arrest of the distal fibula occurs in young children, as in the case presented, the talus will tilt laterally with resultant valgus deformity. Pain secondary to increased joint pressures and arthritis may ensue.[6] Post-traumatic growth arrest of the distal fibula can lead to lateral wedging of the distal tibial epiphysis.[7,8]

The Langenskiold procedure, where a synostosis is created between the distal fibula and tibia, may provide maintenance of the lateral strut but needs to be considered early before significant proximal migration and deformity has occurred.[1]

References

1. Längenskiold A. Pseudarthrosis of the fibula and progressive valgus deformity of the ankle in children: Treatment by fusion of the distal tibia and fibular metaphyses: A review of three cases. *J Bone Jt Surg Am.* 1967;49(3):463–70.
2. Rozbruch S, DiPaola M, Blyakher A. Fibula lengthening using a modified ilizarov method. *Limb Lengthening News*; 2011.
3. Yablon I, Heller F, Shouse L. The key role of the lateral malleolus in displaced fractures of the ankle. *J Bone Jt Surg Am.* 1977;59(169–173).
4. Ramsey P, Hamilton W. Changes in tibiotalar area of contact caused by lateral talar shift. *J Bone Jt Surg Am.* 1976;58(3):356–7.
5. Kärrholm J, Hansson L, Selvik G. Changes in tibiofibular relationships due to growth disturbances after ankle fractures in children. *J Bone Jt Surg Am.* 1984;66(8):1198–210.
6. Brodie I, Denham R. The treatment of unstable ankle fractures. *J Bone Jt Surg Br.* 1974;56(2):256–62.
7. Kang S, Rhee S, Song S, Chung J. Ankle deformity secondary to aquired fibular segmental defect in children. *Clin Orthop Surg.* 2010;2:179–85.
8. Dias L. Valgus deformity of the ankle joint: Pathogenesis of fibular shortening. *J Pediatr Orthop.* 1985; 5:176–80.

Caroline M Blakey and James A Fernandes

Case

A 14-year-old premenarcheal girl was referred with long-standing pain and discomfort in her left foot and a short fourth toe which was present from birth. She was very conscious of the cosmetic appearance of her foot and disliked going without shoes. She was born at term and reached normal developmental milestones, and there was no family history of congenital abnormalities. There was no history of trauma.

She described pain on the dorsum of her foot, worse with activity but also at rest. She was able to carry out daily activities but had reduced her sporting activity and had modified her shoe wearing.

On examination, there was significant shortening of the fourth metatarsal with elevation of the toe. The fourth metatarsophalangeal joint was otherwise normal (Figure 39.1). The skin of the toe was healthy with no corns or plantar callosities. There was a subtle plantar ridge between the third and fifth rays distally.

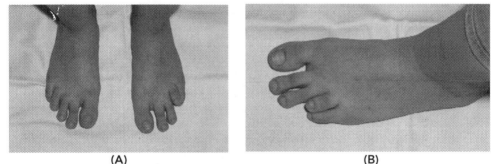

(A)   (B)

Figure 39.1a, b Clinical photographs at presentation.

Plain radiographs revealed 15 mm of shortening of the fourth metatarsal in comparison to the contralateral foot (Figure 39.2a, b). Pedobarography demonstrated normal plantar pressure levels (Figure 39.3).

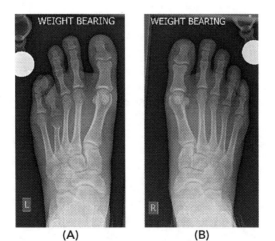

(A)   (B)

Figure 39.2a, b Weight bearing AP radiographs of (A) left and (B) right foot.

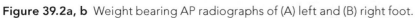

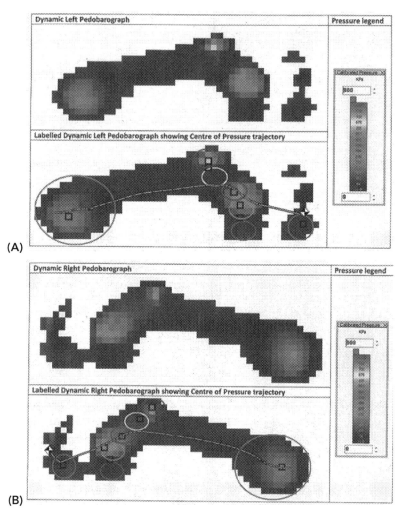

Figure 39.3a, b Pedobarographic images.

Questions

- What are the problems that need to be addressed?
- What are the aims of treatment?
- What are the commonly available options for treatment?
- What are the factors that may influence your choice of treatment?
- What treatment would you recommend for this girl?

The Problems That Need to Be Addressed Are
- Short fourth metatarsal with pain and elevated fourth toe
- Cosmetic deformity

The Aims of Treatment in This Girl Are
- Relieve pain
- Improve cosmesis

Options for Treatment

Relieve pain

○   Trial of accommodative shoe wear

Improving cosmesis and pain:

○   Metatarsal lengthening

  □   Acute lengthening with intercalary bone graft
  □   Gradual lengthening with external fixator

FACTORS THAT INFLUENCED THE CHOICE OF TREATMENT
- Age of the child
- Severity of symptoms
- Degree of shortening
- Abnormal loading of the metatarsals
- Cosmetic concerns
- Complexity of treatment

The factors that influenced the treatment are shown in Table 39.1.

Table 39.1 Factors influencing the choice of treatment

Factors		Treatment Implications
Age of the child	14 years	Operative treatment is generally reserved for children close to maturity to allow completion of growth.[1]
Severity of symptoms	Pain	Brachymetatarsia most often does not require treatment but can cause symptoms. The short metatarsal may cause deformity of the toe, with the stretched metatarsal ligament forcing the phalanx of the affected ray dorsally between adjacent metatarsal heads.[2] This cocked-up toe can be cosmetically unsightly, make shoe wear difficult and cause corns or skin breakdown. Transfer metatarsalgia of the adjacent toes could also develop. The dorsal subluxation can cause pain at the metatarsophalangeal joint.
Degree of shortening	15 mm	When the phalanx remains distal to adjacent metatarsal heads, it is less likely to cause a cocked toe. Shortening of less than 10 mm is usually asymptomatic.[3]

(Continued)

Table 39.1 (Continued)

Factors		Treatment Implications
Altered foot mechanics	Normal pedobarograph	Metatarsalgia may result from transfer of load to the adjacent metatarsal heads. The pedobarograph was normal in this case; many surgeons would suggest that surgery is not indicated.
Cosmetic concerns	The patient was very concerned about the appearance	Surgery may be considered but the patient must understand the risks associated with the procedure and that one cannot guarantee improvement in symptoms or cosmesis.
Complexity of the treatment		Metatarsal lengthening, whether acute or with gradual distraction, has associated risks, and these should be fully understood by the family before embarking on treatment.
		Osteotomy and gradual distraction may reduce risk of associated stiffness of the metatarsophalangeal joint. Stabilisation with a pin through the phalanges into the metatarsal head is critical.[4] Gradual lengthening reduces the risk of over-lengthening with metatarsalgia. There is no donor site morbidity with gradual lengthening, and greater length disparities can be corrected without risk of neurovascular injury.[4] However, pin site infection, regenerate fracture and premature consolidation can occur.

How Was This Child Treated?

Fourth metatarsal lengthening was performed with the Orthofix mini-rail external fixator and cross-joint stabilisation of the fourth metatarsophalangeal joint (Figures 39.4a, b).

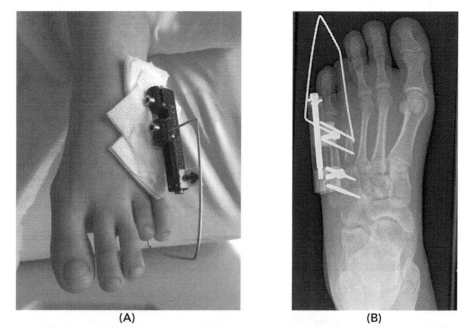

(A)   (B)

Figure 39.4a, b Orthofix mini-rail in situ; (B) clinical photograph, (B) AP radiograph

Post-Operative Management

The lengthening protocol was carefully planned with gradual distraction and regular radiographs (Figure 39.5). Regular pin site care was given, and she remained partial weight bearing during the period of lengthening. The external fixator was removed in the clinic six months post-surgery on consolidation of the regenerate.

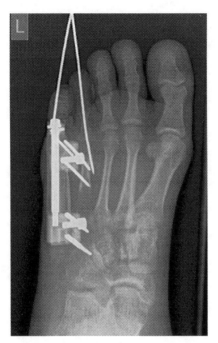

Figure 39.5 Distraction osteogenesis in progress.

At final follow-up, the patient was satisfied with the outcome. She was happy with the cosmetic appearance of her foot and had no pain. The fourth toe sits in an excellent position and has good range of movement (Figure 39.6, 39.7). There is a broken wire end in situ, but this causes no problem.

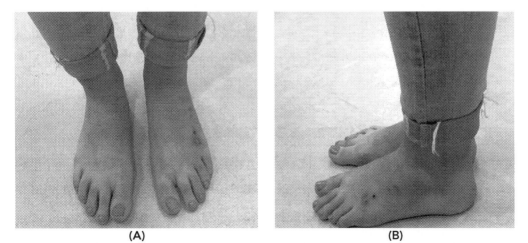

(A)   (B)

Figure 39.6a, b Clinical photographs at final follow-up.

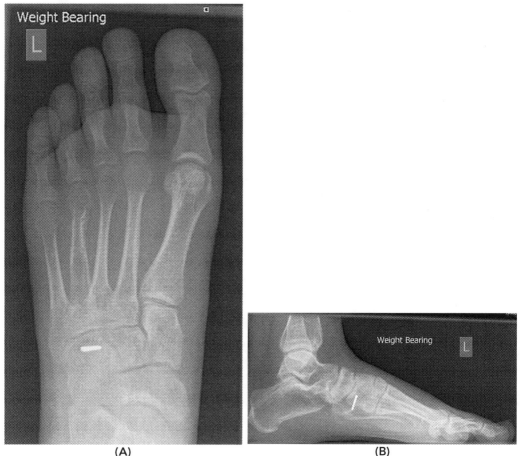

(A)   **(B)**

Figure 39.7a, b Radiographs at final follow-up.

References

1. Giannini S, Faldini C, Pagkrati S, Miscione M, Luciani D. One-stage metatarsal lengthening by allograft interposition: A novel approach for congenital brachymetatarsia. *Clin Orthop Relat Res.* 2010;468(7):1933–42.
2. Davidson R. Metatarsal lengthening. *Foot Ankle Clin.* 2001;6(3):499–518.
3. Lee K-B, Park H-W, Chung J-Y, Moon E-S, Jung S-T, Seon J-K. Comparison of the outcomes of distraction osteogenesis for first and fourth brachymetatarsia. *J Bone Jt Surg Am.* 2010;92:2709–18.
4. Levine S, Davidson R, Dormans J, Drummond D. Distraction osteogenesis for congenitally short lesser metatarsals. *Foot Ankle Int.* 1995;16(4):196–200.

Christopher Prior, Nicholas Peterson, Selvadurai Nayagam

Case

A 12-year-old boy with a background of autistic spectrum disorder (ASD) and attention deficit hyperactive disorder (ADHD) presented with chronic wrist pain and an unsightly deformity of the wrist with a prominence on the medial side. At the age of 7, he had sustained a low-energy Salter-Harris II fracture which was managed with closed manipulation and immobilisation in a cast (Figure 40.1). He was discharged from the service after the fracture had healed, and re-presented five years later with pain and deformity.

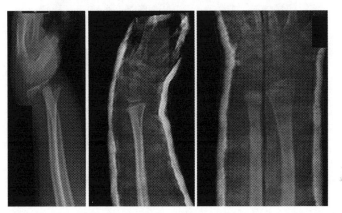

Figure 40.1 Salter Harris II fracture of the right distal radius with significant displacement and subsequent post-manipulation images.

On examination, the forearm was short, the wrist was radially deviated, and the head of the ulna was unduly prominent. Ulnar deviation of the wrist and pronation and supination were reduced. X-rays confirmed relative shortening of the radius, loss of radial inclination of the distal articular surface and a physeal bar. CT images revealed an accessible central physeal bar of the distal radius involving 20% of the physis (Figure 40.2).

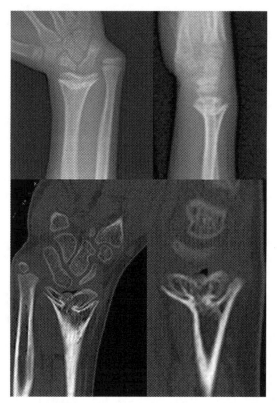

Figure 40.2 Radial shortening with evidence of central physeal bar formation on CT. Note the patient had an incidental luno-triquetral synostosis.

Bone age was estimated from a PA radiograph of the contralateral hand and wrist with software interpretation (BoneXpert) reporting both Tanner-Whitehouse II and Greulich-Pyle scores.[1] The bone age was assessed as being similar to the chronological age. This indicated that four years of growth was remaining. The contralateral normal wrist had a negative ulnar variance of 3 mm. This meant the right ulna would require to be shortened by 19 mm in order to achieve a comparable ulnar variance.

Questions

- What are the problems that need to be addressed?
- What are the aims of treatment?
- What are the available treatment options to fulfil these aims?
- What are the factors that may influence your choice of treatment?
- Based on these points, what treatment would you recommend for this child?
- How long would you follow-up this child after treatment?

The Problems That Need to Be Addressed Are

- Distal radial physeal arrest
- Progressive nature of deformity and propensity for recurrence
- Radio-ulnar length discrepancy resulting in:
    - Ulnar abutment of the carpus
    - Reduced movements of the wrist and forearm
- Pain
- Cosmetic concerns

The Aims of Treatment in This Child Are to

- Remove the physeal tether and facilitate resumption of normal physeal growth of the radius
- Correct the deformity of the wrist
- Restore the normal relative lengths of radius and ulna
- Relieve pain, improve cosmesis

Options for Treatment to Fulfil Each Aim

- Removing physeal tether and resuming normal physeal growth

    - Resection of bony bar (epiphysiolysis)

- Correction of wrist deformity and correcting radio-ulnar length discrepancy

    - Acute shortening of the ulna
    - Gradual radial lengthening by distraction osteogenesis
    - Distal ulnar epiphyseodesis

- Relieve pain and improve cosmesis by previously listed measures

FACTORS THAT INFLUENCED THE CHOICE OF TREATMENT

- Age of the boy and skeletal growth remaining before skeletal maturity
- Size and location of bony bar
- Extent of disparity between radial and ulnar lengths
- Psychological and social factors

The choice of treatment based on these factors is shown in Table 40.1.

Table 40.1 Factors that influenced the choice of treatment

Factors		Treatment Implications
Age & growth remaining	12-year-old with four years of growth remaining	If insufficient time remains for growth, then an epiphysiolysis (removal of the bony bar to restore growth) is not indicated. In this child, there is sufficient growth remaining to attempt bar resection.
Size and location of the bar	Bar involves 20% of the area of the growth plate, and it is located in an accessible site	Physeal bar resection can be undertaken as the area and location of the bar are favourable criteria for this option.

(*Continued*)

Table 40.1 (Continued)

Factors		Treatment Implications
Extent of length disparity between radius & ulna	19 mm of shortening of the ulna is required to normalise relative lengths of radius and ulna.	Acute shortening of the ulna by 19 mm may be potentially too much to achieve with an intact interosseous membrane. Epiphyseodesis of the distal ulna is an option for minimising the length disparity between the radius and ulna.
Psychological and social factors	Autism spectrum and ADHD	The child may not be able to co-operate with the demands of distraction osteogenesis with an external fixator over a protracted period.

How Was This Boy Treated?

In light of the patient's ASD and ADHD, the treatment plan included a combination of techniques:

- Acute shortening of the ulna and temporary distal ulnar epiphyseodesis (if the epiphysiolysis was successful and the length regained at the radius sufficient, the ulnar epiphyseodesis could be reversed by removal of the screw).
- Epiphysiolysis of the distal radius to allow the final mismatch of length to be corrected over time.

Step 1: Epiphysiolysis of Distal Radius

With the tourniquet inflated, access to the volar distal radius was made using a modified Henry's approach. The physis and the position of the bar were identified using fluoroscopy. A trap-door flap was cut in the periosteum, and a small window was made in the volar cortex just proximal to the physis using a 2 mm drill and osteotomes (Figures 40.3a–d).

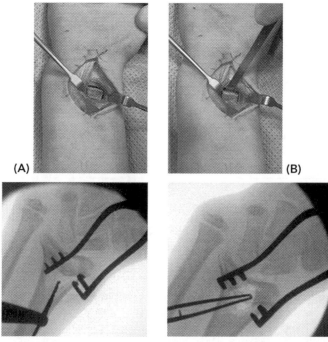

(A)   (B)   (C)   (D)

Figures 40.3a–d Henry's approach to the volar surface of the distal radius is used. A trap-door is elevated in the juxtaphyseal region over the location of the bar as determined by preopera-

Using a small curette and a dental burr with cool saline irrigation and suction, cancellous bone was removed until a continuous rim of physis was seen all around the edges of the cavity (Figure 40.4a, b). Bone wax and a strip of the flexor carpi radialis and fat were used as graft to fill the void and prevent reformation of a bony bar. The periosteum and pronator quadratus were repaired to hold the graft in place.

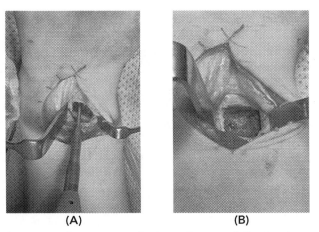

(A)   (B)

Figure 40.4a, b A burr is used to remove the bony bar carefully. Suction and irrigation aid in preventing thermal necrosis and allowing visualisation of the rim of normal physis when the bar is excised.

Step 2: Acute Ulnar Shortening

Through a dorsal incision, the distal ulna was exposed extra-periosteally, and a 2.7 mm locking compression plate was placed on the distal ulna, avoiding damage to the distal ulnar physis and perichondral ring. Distal holes through the plate were pre-drilled, and the plate was removed to plan the shortening osteotomy.

A transverse osteotomy was made using a sagittal saw on low power with cool saline lavage to prevent thermal necrosis. A second osteotomy was made 10 mm proximally and the segment removed. The tension from shortening was assessed to ensure good coaptation of the cut surfaces before a further 3 mm of bone was removed. The plate was applied in compression mode, and contact, alignment and stability were confirmed (Figure 40.5a).

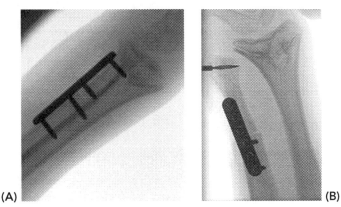

(A)   (B)

Figures 40.5 (A) A mini-fragment plate based on 2.7 mm screws was used in compression mode to hold the acutely shortened ulna. (B) Fluoroscopy-guided drilling and placement of a screw across the distal ulnar physis completed the procedure.

Step 3: Distal Ulnar Temporary Epiphyseodesis
A mini fragment cortical screw was passed retrograde across the physis through a small incision (Figure 40.5b).

Post-Operative Management

The forearm was splinted for four weeks in a cast (Figure 40.6).

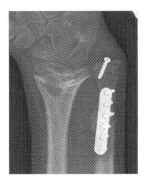

Figure 40.6 Four weeks after acute ulnar shortening and epiphysiolysis of distal radius.

At six months post-procedure, CT images indicated that the radial epiphysiolysis had not been successful in restoring growth (Figure 40.7). Further acute shortening of the ulna of 14 mm and permanent drill epiphyseodesis of the distal ulna were carried out after removing the transphyseal screw.

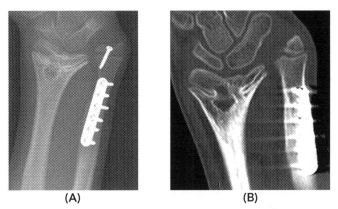

(A)   (B)

Figure 40.7 At six months post-procedure, the distal ulna has continued to grow. Failure of the epiphysiolysis may be due to bridge recurrence at the edges of the previous surgical excision or the formation of secondary tethers.[2]

Ten months later, the patient was pain-free and had recovered a full range of movement. There was no significant residual angular deformity of the distal radius (Figure 40.8).

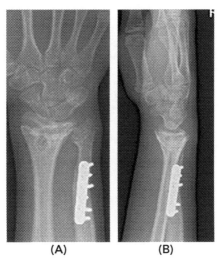

(A)   (B)

Figure 40.8 Final radiographic appearance.

Follow-up to skeletal maturity is required to ensure no significant deformity recurs.

Comment

Though other treatment options were available, the treatment modalities chosen were tailored to the child's and family's circumstances.

Failure of epiphysiolysis may be due to incomplete excision of the bar due to difficulty in visual confirmation of complete removal. This can be aided by regular washing out and suction. Use of a wrist arthroscope to see all around the cavity at the end of the procedure may be helpful. Other potential causes of failure include bony bridge recurrence and the creation of secondary tethers.[2]

References

1. Roche AF, Davila GH, Eyman SL. A comparison between Greulich-Pyle and Tanner-Whitehouse assessments of skeletal maturity. *Radiology*. 1971 Feb;98(2):273–80. doi: 10.1148/98.2.273. PMID: 4322351.
2. Hasler CC, Foster BK. Secondary tethers after physeal bar resection: A common source of failure? *Clin Orthop Relat Res*. 2002 Dec;(405):242–9. doi: 10.1097/00003086-200212000-00031. PMID: 12461380.

DECREASED JOINT MOBILITY

Nicholas Peterson, Christopher Prior, Selvadurai Nayagam

Case

A 12-year-old right hand–dominant female presented with difficulties using her left hand especially when two-handed activities were involved. This problem had been present since early childhood but had become more noticeable in adolescence owing to the changing nature of activities and her increasing need for independence.

Examination of the right arm and hand was normal. The left arm had a stable elbow and normal flexion and extension, but the forearm and hand were held in a position of excessive pronation (20 degrees beyond the normal position of full pronation) (Figure 41.1). Any passive attempt to supinate the forearm produced some movement at the radio-carpal joint but not between the forearm bones.

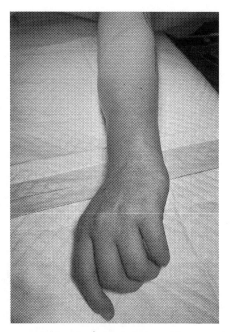

Figure 41.1 Clinical photograph showing the left hand in a position of over-pronation by 20 degrees.

The hand was held in such over-pronation that adaptive movements at the shoulder and elbow were not able to bring the hand into a near-neutral position. As a consequence, in two-handed activities, this nondominant hand was unable to position an object suitably to allow the contralateral normal hand to manipulate the object with fine dexterity.

Forearm x-rays and CT scans confirmed the presence of a proximal radio-ulnar synostosis (Figures 41.2a, b).

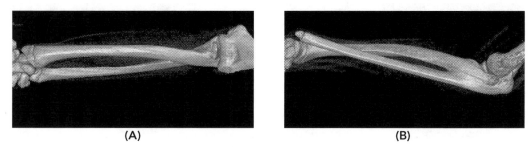

(A) **(B)**

Figures 41.2 3D CT scan–reconstructed images depicting the proximal radio-ulnar synostosis and fixed position of the wrist in pronation.

Questions
- What are the problems that need to be addressed in this girl?
- What are the aims of treatment?
- What are the commonly available options for treatment?
- What are the factors that may influence your choice of treatment?
- What treatment would you recommend for this girl?
- How long would you follow-up this girl after treatment?

The Problems to Be Addressed

- The poor functional position of the nondominant hand

  - Inability to compensate using adaptive shoulder and elbow positions
  - Loss of coordinated two-handed activities

The Aims of Treatment

- Re-position the hand to allow for greater function either in single or double-handed activities
- Choose a hand position that allows for an effective useful range aided by compensation from shoulder and elbow movements

Options for Treatment

- Resection of synostosis
- Derotation of the forearm to place hand in a more functional position without taking down the synostosis

  - Through radius and ulna[1,2]
  - Through the synostosis[3]

Most published reports on attempts to take down a congenital synostosis and re-establish pronation and supination describe poor results.[4] The sole exception is that described by Kanaya et al which involves removing the synostosis and the use of a free vascularised adipose-fascial interposition graft.[5,6] There are, as yet, no results other than those of the originator to compare with. Recently Nakasone et al suggested that return of movement is not only dependent on the manner of removal of the synostosis and interposition but the correction of deformities within the radius and ulna.[7]

FACTORS THAT INFLUENCED THE CHOICE OF TREATMENT

A derotation through the synostosis was selected in this case for the following reasons:

- Single incision approach that is cosmetically advantageous.
- Avoiding a mismatch of the osteotomised ends of the ulna once the radius and carpus are derotated (the axis of rotation is usually closest to the axis of the radius).
- The age and gender of the patient (12 years, female) suggest that natural remodelling potential has decreased.

Treatment

A position of 20 degrees pronation from the neutral position would allow continued prone hand activities (comfortable use of a mouse or keyboard) and, with some shoulder and elbow position adaptation, a neutral hand position to be of greater use in coordinated two-handed activities.[3] As the patient's hand was held in a position of 20 degrees beyond the position of full pronation, this derotation arc would amount to 90 degrees.

Through a curved incision starting at the lateral edge of the insertion of triceps tendon and extending distally along the subcutaneous border of the ulna (Figure 41.3a), two fascio-cutaneous flaps were elevated to reveal the anconeus (Figure 41.3b). The anconeus, supinator and the entire common extensor origin were elevated sharply off bone to reveal the fusion mass (Figure 41.3c). Forceful retraction was avoided, preventing posterior interosseous nerve injury.

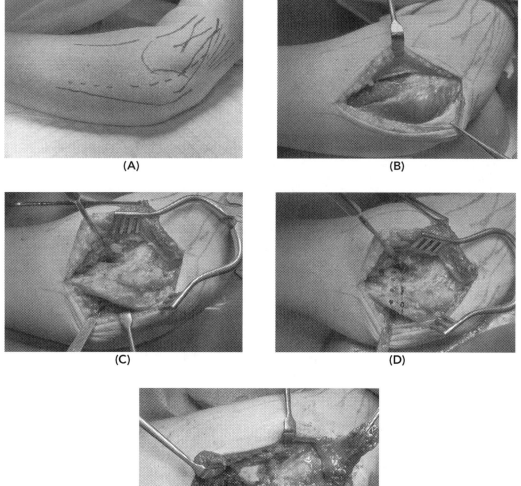

Figures 41.3 Palpation allows surface anatomy to be marked and the skin incision drawn just before surgery (A). Reflection of skin with fascia exposes anconeus and extensor carpi ulnaris (B). Both muscles and the extensor origin are elevated sharply off bone to reveal the synostosis and radial head (C). The proposed segment to be removed is marked by drill holes (D). The segment is removed, shortening performed before derotation, and deflation of the tourniquet to ensure satisfactory return of circulation before fixation with plate and screws (E).

The central portion of the synostosis, identified on x-ray, had the 10 mm segment of bone to be removed marked with drill holes (Figure 41.3d). The segment was removed carefully.

The forearm was then shortened to avoid soft tissue tension before being gently derotated. A contoured small fragment plate was used to fix the fragments under compression. The tourniquet was deflated and the distal circulation confirmed to be satisfactory before all screws were inserted in the plate (Figure 41.3e). The wound was closed in layers and a plaster-of-Paris long-arm back slab applied and maintained for six weeks.

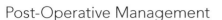

Post-Operative Management

Physiotherapy was commenced at six weeks after some signs of early bone healing were visible on x-ray (Figures 41.4 a, b). A year later, the appearance and function had improved, and the girl was quite pleased with the outcome. Further follow-up was not deemed necessary.

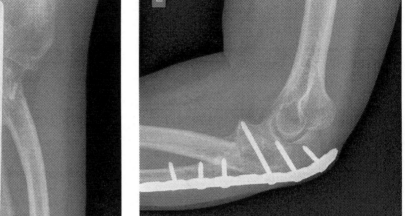

(A)   (B)

Figures 41.4a, 4b Post-operative x-ray images confirming union of the derotation and shortening osteotomy through the synostosis.

Comment

Surgery is needed only in a few cases and usually for a fixed over-pronation of the hand. The optimal position to achieve will depend on whether the condition is unilateral or bilateral and whether the treated hand is dominant. Specific recommendations on the final hand position are less useful than a careful consideration of the specific functional problems the presenting fixed hand position causes the patient and working out the optimum position that will allow those disabilities to be overcome.

It is important to note the following key points of performing a derotation through the synostosis:

- Tension is produced in the neurovascular structures when derotating the forearm. A shortening osteotomy should be incorporated to reduce this tension.
- Deflation of the tourniquet to confirm return of vascularity should precede wound closure. In the event of poor vascularity, the amount of derotation should be reduced or further shortening performed.

References

1. Ramachandran M, Lau K, Jones DHA. Rotational osteotomies for congenital radioulnar synostosis. *Journal of Bone and Joint Surgery British Volume*. 2005;87(10):1406–10.
2. Hung NN. Derotational osteotomy of the proximal radius and the distal ulna for congenital radioulnar synostosis. *Journal of Children's Orthopaedics*. 2008;2(6):481–9.
3. Simcock X, Shah AS, Waters PM, Bae DS. Safety and efficacy of derotational osteotomy for congenital radioulnar synostosis. *J Pediatr Orthop*. 2015;35(8):838–43.
4. Wood VE. Congenital radio-ulnar synostosis. In: Buck-Gramcko D, editor. *Congenital malformations of the hand and forearm*. 1st ed. New York: Churchill Livingstone; 1998. pp. 487–515.

5. Kanaya F. Mobilization of congenital proximal radio-ulnar synostosis: A technical detail. *Tech Hand Up Extrem Surg.* 1997;1(3):183–8.
6. Kanaya F, Ibaraki K. Mobilization of a congenital proximal radioulnar synostosis with use of a free vascularized fascio-fat graft. *J Bone Joint Surg Am.* 1998;80(8):1186–92.
7. Nakasone M, Nakasone S, Kinjo M, Murase T, Kanaya F. Three-dimensional analysis of deformities of the radius and ulna in congenital proximal radioulnar synostosis. *J Hand Surg Eur.* 2018;43(7):739–43.

CASE 42: TARSAL COALITION

Leo Donnan

Case

A previously healthy 11-year-old girl presented with a three-month history of pain in the left foot that has not responded to a period of rest in a stiff boot.

She walked with an antalgic gait. The medial longitudinal arch was lower on the left side than on the right. When she stood on tip toes, her left heel did not swing into varus, and the arch did not get restored as much as on the right (Figure 42.1a). The gastroc-soleus was mildly tight, and passive motion of the subtalar joint was reduced. Tenderness was elicited just anterior to the lateral malleolus. Rapid inversion of the forefoot produced pain and demonstrable spasm of the peroneal muscles (Figure 42.1b). A provisional diagnosis of a tarsal coalition was made.

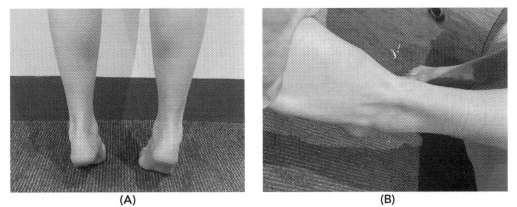

(A)   (B)

Figure 42.1 Appearance of the feet when standing on tip toes. Reduced hind foot movement into varus when compared with right (A) and spasm of the peroneal tendons on rapid inversion (B).

Plain radiographs of the foot confirmed the presence of a calcaneo-navicular coalition (Figure 42.2a), best seen on the oblique view (Figure 42.2b). A CT scan was done to exclude any other coalition not visualised on the plain radiographs (Figure 42.3).

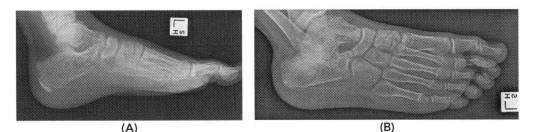

(A)   (B)

Figures 42.2a and b Radiographs showing the presence of a calcaneo-navicular synchondrosis.

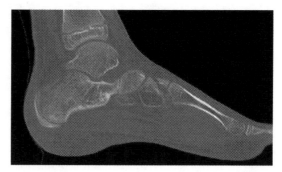

Figure 42.3 CT scan confirming an isolated calcaneo-navicular coalition.

Questions

- What are the problems that need to be addressed in this girl?
- What are the aims of treatment?
- What are the available treatment options to fulfil these aims?
- What are the factors that may influence your choice of treatment?
- Based on these points, what treatment would you recommend for this girl?
- How long would you follow-up this child after treatment?

The Problems That Need to Be Addressed Are
- Pain and peroneal spasm
- Hind foot stiffness
- Planovalgus deformity

The Aims of Treatment in This Girl Were to
- Relieve foot pain and muscle spasm
- Restore subtalar motion
- Improve the medial longitudinal arch
- Improve the gait pattern

Options for Treatment to Achieve These Aims
- Non-operative treatment
  - Orthotic management
  - Immobilisation in a walking cast for six weeks in isolation or combined with sub-talar joint injection with steroid and local anaesthetic
- Surgical treatment
  - Excision of the coalition
    - Open[1]
    - Arthroscopic[2]
  - Prevent recurrence with interposition of:
    - Extensor digitorum brevis muscle
    - Wax
    - Fat graft
  - Correct residual deformity
    - Hind foot osteotomy for residual valgus following excision of the coalition
    - Lengthening of the heel cord, if tight
  - Triple fusion

FACTORS THAT INFLUENCED THE CHOICE OF TREATMENT
• Severity of symptoms
• The age of the girl
• Presence of fixed deformities and severity and rigidity of the deformities
• Presence of other coalitions[3]
• Presence of arthritic changes

The choice of treatment based on these factors is outlined in Table 42.1.

Table 42.1 Factors That Influenced the Choice of Treatment

Factors		Treatment Implications
Severity of symptoms	Pain is severe enough to be forced to limit physical activity	This justifies surgical intervention if conservative treatment fails.
Age of the girl	11 years	Surgical intervention is likely to be less effective as the child gets older, and hence surgery, if required, should not be delayed.
Presence of fixed deformity and severity and rigidity of the deformity	Mild planovalgus deformity	As the deformity is mild, there is scope for an attempt at conservative treatment which can be effective in 30–50% of cases with relief of symptoms.
	The deformity is moderately rigid and peroneal spasm is present	Excision of the coalition is justified. If hindfoot deformity is not corrected, then calcaneal osteotomy may be indicated.
Presence of other coalitions	Solitary calcaneo-navicular coalition	Excision of coalition is justified.
Presence of arthritic changes	No clinical or radiologic features of arthritis	Options that avoid stiffening of joints are preferred in the absence of arthritis (no justification for performing triple arthrodesis).

The final plan of treatment for this girl is excision of the coalition with interposition fat graft[4] since conservative treatment failed.

How Was This Child Treated?

The patient was placed in the supine position with a wedge under the buttock. An oblique incision was used taking care to identify and isolate the branches of the superficial peroneal nerve at the medial end of the wound (Figure 42.4).

The coalition was exposed by elevating the extensor brevis muscle from the anterior process of the calcaneum just above the peroneal sheath with a diathermy on low power (Figure 42.5). Once the coalition was exposed, a hypodermic needle was used to mark the most medial part to be excised and checked with fluoroscopy. Flat bone levers were placed on either side of the coalition, and a bone block of around 0.8 to 1 cm was excised, being very careful not to damage the cartilage of the talar head in doing so. The coalition was much deeper than appreciated from the imaging, and the deeper recesses were carefully cleared. Fluoroscopy was used to check that a clear space had been achieved (Figure 42.6). The resultant defect was filled with a small fat graft harvested from the medial thigh (Figure 42.7). The wounds were closed in a standard fashion and the foot and ankle placed in a removable back slab.

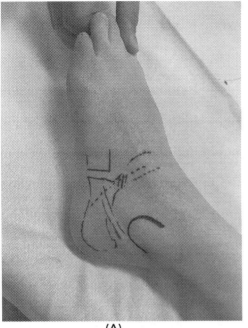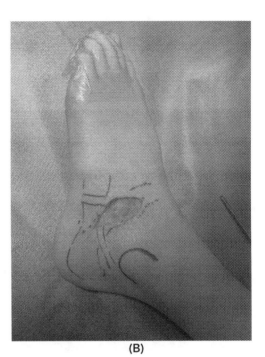

(A)   (B)

Figure 42.4 Surface anatomy and making the surgical incision.

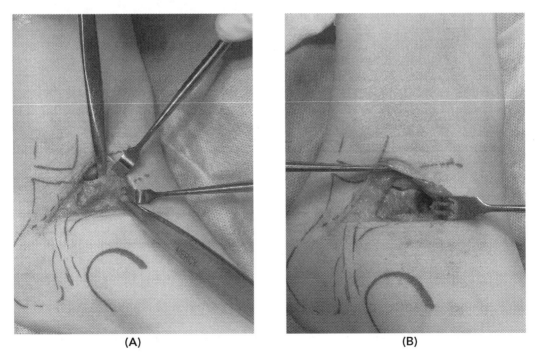

(A)   (B)

Figure 42.5 Exposure and excision of the coalition.

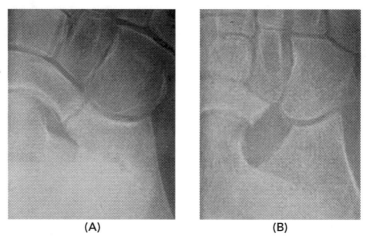

(A)   (B)

Figure 42.6 Fluoroscopy confirming the position of the coalition and completeness of excision.

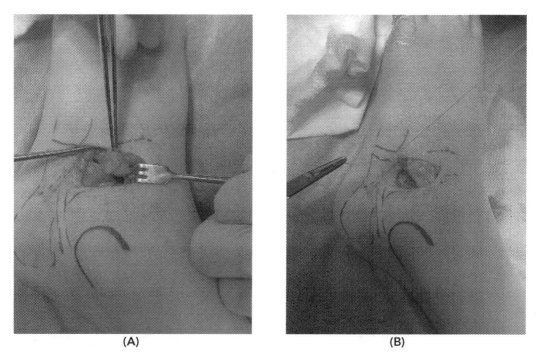

(A)   (B)

Figure 42.7 Fat grafting of defect and coverage with extensor brevis muscle.

Post-Operative Management

The patient remained non–weight bearing for two weeks and then transferred into a moon boot for progressive mobilisation. Range-of-motion exercises were started at this point of time, focusing on inversion, eversion and calf stretching. Normal activity was permitted after eight weeks.

At the last follow-up, she had no pain in the foot, the range of motion of the subtalar and mid-tarsal joints had improved, and she was pleased with the outcome.

Comment

Following excision of calcaneo-navicular coalition, restoration of subtalar movement is often less than expected, and occasionally a patient may experience some ongoing ache in the foot and for that reason the patient should be followed-up till skeletal maturity.

References

1. Carli A, Leblanc E, Amitai A, Hamdy RC. The evaluation and treatment of pediatric tarsal coalitions. *JBJS Rev.* 2014 Aug 12;2(8):01874474-201408000-00002. doi: 10.2106/JBJS.RVW.M.00112.
2. Bonasia DE, Phisitkul P, Amendola A. Endoscopic coalition resection. *Foot Ankle Clin.* 2015;20(1):81–91.
3. Docquier P-L, Maldaque P, Bouchard M. Tarsal coalition in paediatric patients. *Orthop Traumatology Surg Res.* 2019;105(1):S123–31.
4. Masquijo J, Allende V, Torres-Gomez A, Dobbs MB. Fat graft and bone wax interposition provides better functional outcomes and lower reossification rates than extensor digitorum brevis after calcaneonavicular coalition resection. *J Pediatr Orthop.* 2017;37(7):e427–31.

Benjamin Joseph and Hitesh Shah

Case

A 12-year-old boy presented with complaints of a deformity of the right knee and inability to flex the knee. In early childhood, he had osteomyelitis of the right femur. The deformity and knee stiffness developed following this, over a short period of time, but have not progressed appreciably over the last few years. On examination, there was a puckered, depressed scar on the lateral aspect of the upper third of the thigh. There was a genu recurvatum deformity of 30 degrees of the right knee (Figure 43.1), and no passive flexion was possible (i.e., ankylosis of the knee in hyper-extension). The patella was mobile and not stuck down to the femur. He walked with a stiff-knee gait with circumduction of the right lower limb during the swing phase. He sat awkwardly on a chair with his right leg sticking out in front.

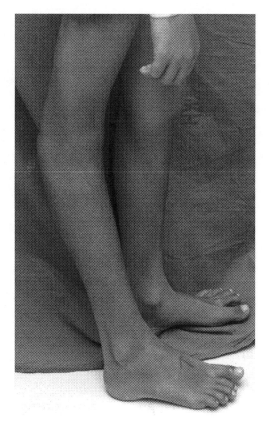

Figure 43.1 Genu recurvatum of the right knee.

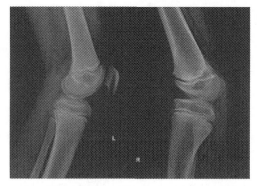

Figure 43.2 Lateral radiographs of both knees. The femoral condyles are flattened on the right side, but the joint space and the alignment of the femoral and tibial growth plates are normal.

X-rays of the knees showed flattening of the femoral condyles of the right femur (Figure 43.2) and genu recurvatum. The growth plates of the distal femur and the proximal tibia were normal, and the joint space was also normal.

Questions

- What are the problems that need to be addressed?
- What are the aims of treatment?
- What are the available treatment options?
- What are the factors that may influence your choice of treatment?
- What treatment would you recommend for this boy?
- How long would you follow-up this boy after treatment?

The Problems That Had to Be Addressed Are

- Genu recurvatum of 30 degrees
- Extra-articular ankylosis of the knee in hyper-extension with contracture of the quadriceps muscle
- Stiff-knee gait with circumduction during the swing phase of gait
- Risk of weakening the quadriceps muscle excessively by over-zealous surgery

The Aims of Treatment in This Boy Are

- Correct the genu recurvatum deformity
- Restore about 90 degrees of knee flexion to enable him to sit on a chair comfortably and to improve his gait pattern
- Avoid weakening the quadriceps muscle excessively

Options for Treatment

- Proximal quadricepsplasty
- Distal quadricepsplasty

FACTORS THAT INFLUENCED THE CHOICE OF TREATMENT

- Type of ankylosis (extra-articular versus intra-articular)
- Site of the recurvatum deformity
- The site of the previous infection
- Age of the child
- Surgical approach
- Surgical technique

The choice of treatment based on these factors is outlined in Table 43.1.

Table 43.1 Factors That Influenced the Choice of Treatment

Factors		Treatment Implications
Type of ankylosis (extra-articular versus intra-articular)	Since the radiograph of the knee shows a normal joint space, it suggests that the ankylosis is extra-articular.	Release of the quadriceps contracture should be done to see if the deformity will correct and knee flexion can be restored.
Site of the recurvatum deformity	Knee joint (not in the distal femur or the proximal tibia)	Since there is no deformity of the distal femur or the proximal tibia, surgery on the femur or tibia is not required to correct genu recurvatum.
Site of previous bone infection	Proximal third of the femur	Since the original infection affected the proximal shaft of the femur, it seems likely that the site of maximum fibrosis will be in this area. A proximal quadricepsplasty is indicated.

(Continued)

Table 43.1 (Continued)

Factors		Treatment Implications
Age of the child	12 years	It would have been desirable to perform the quadricepsplasty at a younger age before flattening of the femoral condyles developed. Flattening of the femoral condyles could persist if the surgery was further delayed, and this could compromise the result.
Surgical approach	Lateral versus anterior approach	A lateral approach is preferred as it will enable excision of the scar and direct access to the vastus lateralis. Another advantage of the lateral approach over an anterior approach is that there is minimal tension on the incision once the knee is flexed.
Surgical technique	Thompson (distal release) versus the Judet quadricepsplasty (proximal release)	Most surgeons prefer the Judet technique with some modifications.[1-4]

How Was This Boy Treated?

The boy underwent a proximal quadricepsplasty through a lateral approach. The depressed scar was excised (Figure 43.3), and the underlying vastus lateralis muscle was identified. The scarred and fibrotic upper fibres of the vastus lateralis were erased from the lateral surface of the femur, the lateral inter-muscular septum and the linea aspera. Some passive flexion of the knee was now possible.

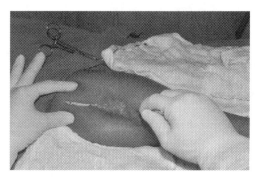

Figure 43.3 Puckered scar on the lateral upper one-third of the thigh.

In order to decide if further release of the vastus lateralis was needed, two fingers were placed deep to the vastus lateralis, and the knee was passively flexed (Figure 43.4). The fingers got pinched between the taut vastus lateralis and the femur, indicating that further release of the muscle was required.

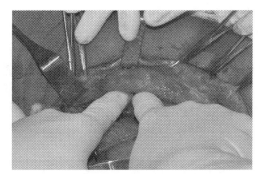

Figure 43.4 Two fingers are placed deep to the vastus lateralis, and an attempt is made to flex the knee. If the muscle is contracted, the fingers will get pinched between the femur and the taut muscle.

Further release of the vastus lateralis was performed progressing distally till no further tightness was noted. Attention was now given to the vastus intermedius muscle; the tight fibrotic fibres were released right down to the distal femur (Figure 43.5). The rectus femoris was contracted, and it was released from its origin. The vastus medialis was not released as 80 degrees of passive flexion was achieved (i.e., 110 degrees of correction) at this point. The wounds were closed over a suction drain.

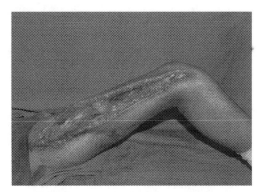

Figure 43.5 Extent of release needed to obtain 80 degrees of knee flexion.

Post-Operative Management

The knee was held in 80 degrees of flexion in a plaster cast for a period of four weeks. Intensive quadriceps-strengthening exercises and active knee flexion exercises were encouraged for six months after cast removal. Protected weight bearing with crutches was permitted after removal of the cast, and the crutches were discarded after the quadriceps power of Grade 4 (MRC grade) was restored.

Nine years later, there was no residual genu recurvatum (Figure 43.6); the knee could be flexed to 80 degrees (Figure 43.7). The quadriceps power was Grade 4 (MRC) with a 5-degree extension lag. The femoral condyles had remodelled and were not flat as before (Figure 43.8). His gait was normal, and he sat well on a chair. The lateral incision had healed exceedingly well (Figure 43.9).

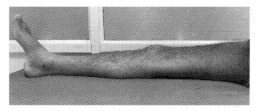

Figure 43.6 At the final follow-up, there is no recurvatum deformity.

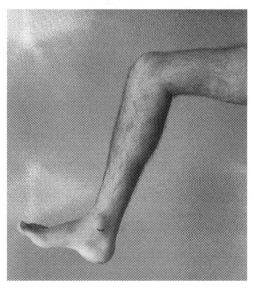

Figure 43.7 Knee flexion of 80 degrees has been maintained.

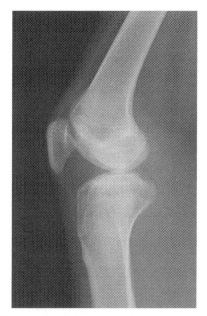

Figure 43.8 Some re-modelling of the shape of the femoral condyles has occurred.

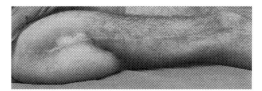

Figure 43.9 Well-healed scar of the lateral incision.

Follow-Up

The boy was followed beyond skeletal maturity to see if loss of correction would occur, and we also wanted to see to what extent the femoral condyles would remodel. Though the young man on his last visit requested us to do further surgery in order to enable him to squat, we did not comply as in all likelihood further release would result in significant weakness of the quadriceps.

Comment

Quadriceps contracture following injection fibrosis is far more localised, and such an extensive release as done in this boy is rarely required.

The two main techniques for treating an acquired quadriceps contracture are the Judet proximal quadricepsplasty and the Thompson distal quadricepsplasty. Weakness of knee extension and persistence of an extension lag are more frequently encountered following the distal release. In this instance, on account of the severe contracture, extensive muscle release was anticipated. We opted for a proximal release to minimise the risk of an extension lag.

References

1. Jackson AM, Hutton PA. Injection-induced contractures of the quadriceps in childhood: A comparison of proximal release and distal quadricepsplasty. *J Bone Joint Surg Br.* 1985;67(1):97–102.
2. Persico F, Vargas O, Fletscher G, Zuluaga M. Treatment of extraarticular knee extension contracture secondary to prolonged external fixation by a modified Judet quadricepsplasty technique. *Strategies in Trauma and Limb Reconstruction.* 2018;13:19–24. https://doi.org/10.1007/s11751-017-0302-x.
3. Holschen M, Lobenhoffer P. Treatment of extension contracture of the knee by quadriceps plasty (Judet Procedure). *Oper Orthop Traumatol.* 2014;26(4):353–60. doi: 10.1007/s00064-013-0286-8.
4. Blanco CE, Leon HO, Guthrie TB. Endoscopic quadricepsplasty: A new surgical technique. *Arthroscopy.* 2001;17(5):504–9. doi: 10.1053/jars.2001.24062.

Binu P Thomas

Case

A 10-year-old boy developed a compartment syndrome of the right forearm following treatment of a fracture of the ulna by traditional bone setters. He underwent a fasciotomy and debridement of necrotic muscles elsewhere at a local hospital.

He presented two years later with a grossly atrophied limb, flexion deformity of the wrist, flexion deformity of fingers and an adducted thumb (Figure 44.1). The Volkmann's sign was positive, and the flexion deformity of the wrist of 70 degrees was not passively correctible. The adducted thumb was stiff and could not be passively abducted. No active finger flexion was present while a jog of finger extension was present, and the intrinsic muscles of the hand were also not working. Sensations were lost distally from the mid-forearm. The radial pulse was palpable. The features were indicative of severe Volkmann's ischaemic contracture (VIC). An x-ray of the forearm showed that the bones were osteoporotic; the deformities of the wrist and hand were evident, and there were no signs of the original fracture (Figure 44.2).

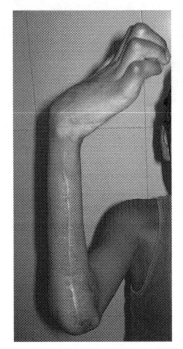

Figure 44.1 The grossly atrophied limb, flexion deformity of the wrist, flexion deformity of fingers and hyperextension at the metacarpophalangeal joints characteristic of severe VIC are all clearly evident. The old scar of previous surgery is also visible.

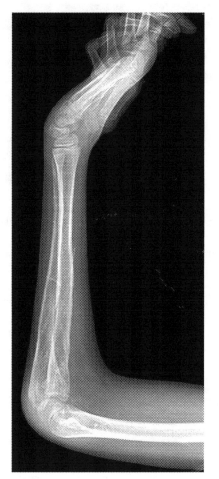

Figure 44.2 The x-ray of the forearm and hand demonstrating the classical deformities and gross osteoporosis.

Questions

- What are the problems that need to be addressed in this boy?
- What are the aims of treatment?
- What are the available treatment options?
- What are the factors that may influence your choice of treatment?
- What treatment would you recommend for this boy?

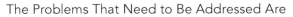

The Problems That Need to Be Addressed Are

- Deformities

    o Severe flexion deformity of the wrist and fingers
    o Adduction contracture of the thumb

- Loss of motor function

    o Absence of active finger and thumb flexion
    o Weak finger and wrist extension

- Loss of sensation

    o Glove type of anaesthesia below the middle of the forearm

- Total loss of hand function due to all these problems

The Aims of Treatment in This Boy Are

- Correct the deformities of the wrist, fingers and thumb
- Provide active finger and thumb flexion
- Improve the power of finger extension
- Provide a stable wrist and thumb
- Improve the sensation of the hand and restore protective sensibility
- Provide a reasonably cosmetic and functional hand by all of the previous measures.

Options for Treatment to Fulfil Each Aim

- Correcting wrist and finger deformity

    o Prolonged aggressive hand therapy
    o Excision of the contracted flexor tendons and atrophied flexor muscles
    o Proximal row carpectomy
    o Prolonged splinting in the corrected position

- Correcting thumb adduction contracture

    o Thumb web stretching and splinting
    o Thumb web release
    o Thumb web release and first carpometacarpal joint fusion

- Providing active finger and thumb flexion

    o Tendon transfers using the wrist extensors to restore finger and thumb flexion
    o Free functioning muscle transfer

- Improving weak finger and wrist extension

    o Physiotherapy and muscle strengthening
    o Extensor tenolysis

- Providing a stable thumb and wrist

    o Tendon transfers to provide muscle balance
    o First carpo-metacarpal fusion
    o Wrist fusion

- Restoring sensations in the hand

    o Neurolysis of the ulnar and median nerves

FACTORS THAT INFLUENCED THE CHOICE OF TREATMENT

- Severity of deformities
- Power of muscles that have not been affected
- Willingness of the child and parents to accept multi-staged surgery and prolonged rehabilitation

The factors that influenced treatment are shown in Table 44.1.

Table 44.1 Factors that influenced the treatment choice

Factors		Treatment Implications
Severity of deformities	Severe wrist flexion deformity	Deformities are very unlikely to improve appreciably with physiotherapy alone.
	Severe finger flexion deformity	Deformities are likely to improve following release of contracted tissues but unlikely to get fully corrected.
	Severe thumb adduction deformity	Additional bony surgery likely to be needed to obtain complete correction of deformities.
Power of muscles that have not been affected	All muscles of the flexor compartment are paralysed	Since no flexor or extensor muscle has Grade 5 muscle power, tendon transfers to restore hand function cannot be considered. A free muscle transfer is the only available option.
	Muscles of the extensor compartment are not paralysed but are very weak	The power of extensor muscles may improve by a Grade or two once the flexion deformities of wrist and fingers are corrected. Tendon transfers that could potentially provide dynamic stability of the wrist and thumb are not possible, and so these joints need to be stabilised by arthrodesis.
Willingness of the child and parents to accept multi-staged surgery and prolonged rehabilitation	Child and parents are willing for staged surgery and rehabilitation	3-stage surgery spanning two years planned.

How Was This Boy Treated?

The child was initially started on hand therapy by serial stretching of the contracted fingers and wrist. However, as anticipated, the improvement was negligible, and hence the first-stage surgery was undertaken.

Stage 1

The contracted atrophied flexor muscles were excised, and tendons of the flexor digitorum superficialis were also excised. The tendons of the flexor digitorum profundus were tenolysed to get passive finger flexion. The passive wrist extension improved, and the wrist could be brought to the neutral position after this soft tissue release. The hand was splinted in maximum correction.

Stage 2

Following wound healing and splinting in the corrected position, the next-stage surgery was done. The median nerve was identified and neurolysed. The anterior interosseous nerve was identified and isolated. A free gracilis myo-cutaneous flap was harvested and transferred to the forearm. The proximal end of the muscle was sutured to the medial epicondyle and remnant of the common flexor origin. The distal end was woven into the ends of the flexor digitorum profundus and flexor pollicis longus tendons under optimum tension (Figure 44.3). The nerve to gracilis was anastomosed to the anterior interosseous nerve, and the vessels were anastomosed to the brachial vessels in an end-to-side fashion. The perfusion of the transferred skin flap was carefully monitored (the appearance of the flap on the fifth postoperative day is shown in Figure 44.4).

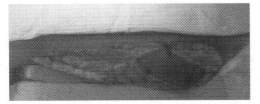

Figure 44.3 The intraoperative photograph showing the myo-cutaneous gracilis flap being inset in the forearm.

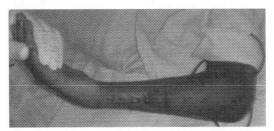

Figure 44.4 The fifth postoperative day photograph showing the viable myo-cutaneous gracilis flap inset in the forearm.

Stage 3

Good active flexion of the thumb and fingers were restored by the transferred gracilis, but persistent flexion deformity of the wrist and adduction deformity of the thumb were noted. The thumb deformity was corrected by arthrodesis of the carpometacarpal joint of the thumb using a tension band technique holding the thumb in the optimum position of function (Figure 44.5). Since there was no recovery of power of the wrist extensors, an arthrodesis of the wrist with a proximal row carpectomy as described by Anderson[1] was performed (Figure 44.6). The final appearance of the forearm and hand is shown in Figure 44.7.

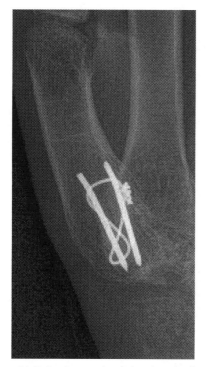

Figure 44.5 Radiograph of the thumb showing the technique of the first CMC joint arthrodesis.

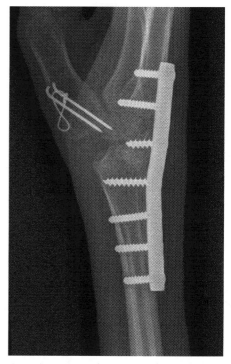

Figure 44.6 Radiograph of the forearm and wrist showing the technique of wrist arthrodesis.

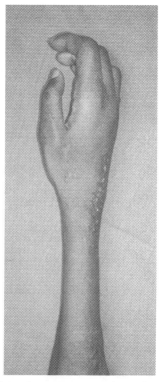

Figure 44.7 Final appearance of the forearm and hand.

Postoperative Management

Following the free muscle transfer, a splint that held the wrist in extension and fingers in the functional position was used for six weeks. Gentle range of motion exercises were commenced. Electrical stimulation was given to the transferred muscle till contractions were observed, after which strengthening exercises were begun. A thermoplastic splint was given for long-term use to prevent recurrent contractures.

Follow-Up

The boy was followed up for six years from the first surgery and three years from the third-stage surgery.

At the most recent follow-up, he had Grade 4 power of the transferred muscle with a total active finger flexion of 100 degrees. The thumb and wrist were stable in functional positions allowing prehensile function of the hand. Protective sensibility was present in the territory of the median nerve. Hand function had improved significantly.

Comment

Acute compartment syndrome following treatment by native bone setters still occurs in developing countries.[1] Early diagnosis and urgent fasciotomy are mandatory if a Volkmann's ischaemic contracture is to be prevented. The management of severe ischaemic contracture is quite difficult, and intensive hand therapy and prolonged splinting followed by surgery are essential for a good outcome.[2] A functioning free muscle transfer is used when the residual muscle power is poor or absent as illustrated in this case.[3] Severe flexion deformity of the wrist with capsular contractures warrants a proximal row carpectomy and wrist fusion[4] in the functional position.

References

1. Anderson GA. The child's hand in the developing world. In: Gupta A, Kay SPJ, Scheker LR, editors. *The growing hand*. London: Mosby; 2000. pp. 1097–114.
2. Botte MJ, Keenan MA, Gelberman RH. Volkmann's ischemic contracture of the upper extremity. *Hand Clin*. 1998;14(3):483–97.
3. Oishi SN, Ezaki M. Free gracilis transfer to restore finger flexion in Volkmann ischemic contracture. *Tech Hand Up Extrem Surg*. 2010;14(2):104–7. doi: 10.1097/BTH.0b013e3181d4459d.
4. Anderson GA, Thomas BP. Arthrodesis of flail or partially flail wrists using a dynamic compression plate without bone grafting. *J Bone Joint Surg Br*. 2000;82-B(4):566–70. doi: 10.1302/0301-620X.82B4.0820566.

LOWER MOTOR NEURON PARALYSES

CASE 45: THE PARALYSED KNEE

Benjamin Joseph and Hitesh Shah

Case

An 18-year-old male presented with deformities of the right hip, knee and foot and weakness of the right lower limb. They were present since early childhood when he had acute flaccid paralysis preceded by a febrile episode suggestive of poliomyelitis. Some recovery did occur initially, but since the last 10 years there was no appreciable change in muscle strength. The deformities developed over time. He complained that his right knee buckled when he walked on uneven ground or while he negotiated stairs or slopes.

On examination, the right thigh and calf were wasted. He had 15° fixed flexion and 15° fixed abduction deformities of the hip, 20° flexion deformity of the knee and severe equino-cavus deformity of the right foot (Figure 45.1, 45.2). The power of muscles of the lower limb are shown in Table 45.1. His sensations were normal. The ilio-tibial band, hamstrings, gastroc-soleus and plantar fascia were contracted. On account of the abduction deformity of the hip and the severe equinus, there was apparent lengthening of the right lower limb when, in fact, there was true shortening of the right lower limb of 3 cm. He walked on level ground in an awkward manner, vaulting over the plantarflexed right foot. He walked with a right hand-on-thigh gait while walking up or down a slope.

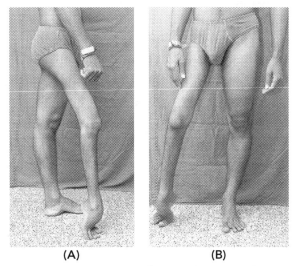

(A)   (B)

Figure 45.1 Wasting of the right thigh and calf and deformities of the hip, knee and ankle are clearly evident.

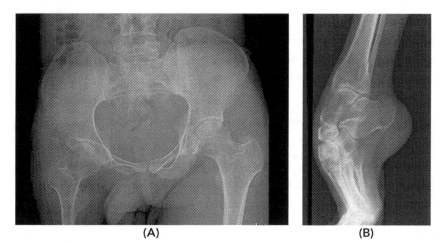

(A)   **(B)**

Figure 45.2 AP radiograph of the pelvis shows a hypoplastic right hemipelvis, pelvic obliquity due to hip abduction deformity and forward tilt of the pelvis due to hip flexion deformity (A). Lateral radiograph of the foot and ankle shows the severe equino-cavus (B).

Table 45.1 Power of Muscles in the Right Lower Limb

Joint	Muscle Group	Power (MRC scale)
Hip	Flexors	Grade 4
	Extensors	Grade 3
	Abductors	Grade 3
	Adductors	Grade 3
	Internal rotators	Grade 3
	External rotators	Grade 4
Knee	Extensor (Quadriceps femoris)	Grade 0
	Flexors (Hamstrings)	Grade 3+
Ankle	Dorsiflexors	Unable to test reliably due to severe equinus deformity
	Plantarflexors	Grade 5
Subtalar joint	Invertors	Grade 5
	Evertors	Grade 5

Questions

- What are the problems that need to be addressed?
- What are the aims of treatment?
- What are the available treatment options to fulfil these aims?
- What are the factors that may influence your choice of treatment?
- Based on these points, what treatment would you recommend for this young man?

The Problems That Need to Be Addressed Are
- Deformities of the right hip, knee and ankle
- Limb length inequality
- Instability of the knee

The Aims of Treatment Are to
- Facilitate a more normal gait
- Abolish knee instability
- Equalise limb lengths

Options for Treatment to Fulfil Each Aim
- Facilitating a more normal gait
  - Correct deformities that are contributing to the aberrant gait
    - Knee flexion deformity
      - Soft tissue release
      - Distal femoral osteotomy
    - Equino-cavus
      - Soft tissue release
      - Mid-tarsal osteotomy
      - Lambrinudi type of triple arthrodesis
  - Provide knee stability
- Abolishing knee instability
  - Bracing
    - Knee-ankle-foot orthosis (KAFO)
    - Floor-reaction orthosis (FRO)
  - Dynamic stabilisation by hamstring tendon transfer
  - Static stabilisation by creating 10° hyper-extension of the knee by a femoral supracondylar extension osteotomy
- Equalising limb lengths
  - Limb lengthening

FACTORS THAT INFLUENCED THE CHOICE OF TREATMENT
<ul><li>The age of the patient</li><li>The power of muscles</li><li>The effect of deformities on hip and knee stability</li><li>Preference of the patient</li></ul>

The choice of treatment based on these factors is outlined in Table 45.2.

Table 45.2 Choice of Treatment Based on the Factors That Influenced the Treatment

Factors		Treatment Implications
Age of the patient	18 years (skeletally mature)	Techniques of deformity correction and limb-length equalisation involving growth modulation are not feasible as the growth plates are fused.
		A supra-condylar extension osteotomy in order to create 10° hyperextension at the knee is justifiable since the patient is skeletally mature. Remodelling of the osteotomy and loss of correction seen in the skeletally immature is unlikely to occur.[1]
Power of muscles	The power of the hamstrings and gluteus maximus is less than Grade 5	For a hamstring transfer to effectively restore the power of knee extension, the hamstrings, hip extensor and gastroc-soleus must have Grade 5 power.[2]
Effect of deformities on hip and knee stability	Abduction deformity of the hip	Despite having a weak hip abductor, Trendelenburg gait is prevented by the abduction deformity.
	Flexion deformity of the knee	Flexion deformity of the knee is a major cause of knee instability; it is responsible for the knee buckling as the deformity makes the ground reaction force (GRF) to pass posterior to the axis of the knee.
	Equinus deformity of the ankle	An equinus deformity helps in extending the knee through the "plantarflexor–knee extensor couple". It is desirable to have a mild equinus deformity if the quadriceps is paralysed.
Preferences of the patient		The patient did not want any form of bracing and also did not want to undergo limb lengthening.

How Was This Young Man Treated?

It was decided to restore knee stability during stance by a femoral supra-condylar osteotomy and to partially correct the equino-cavus deformity to improve appearance. We opted to retain some equinus to contribute to knee stability during stance and also to compensate partly for the shortening of the limb. The abduction deformity was not corrected to avoid a Trendelenburg gait.

Through a vertical incision, the Achilles tendon was exposed and lengthened by a coronal z-plasty. The posterior capsule of the ankle joint was exposed after retracting the flexor hallucis longus along with the neuro-vascular bundle. A liberal posterior capsulotomy of the ankle was performed, and the posterior talo-fibular ligament was divided. The ankle was passively dorsiflexed; considerable improvement of the hindfoot equinus was achieved. Release of the plantar fascia from the calcaneum was done through an incision along the inferior border of the calcaneum on the medial aspect of the foot. Modest improvement of the cavus deformity was achieved. We opted not to proceed with a mid-tarsal osteotomy so as to maintain some equinus and also to compensate for the shortening.

Through an anteromedial incision on the thigh just proximal to the patella, the fibres of the vastus medialis were retracted, exposing the periosteum of the supracondylar region of the femur. The periosteum was incised longitudinally, and the femur was exposed. The planned anteriorly based bone wedge to be resected was marked with drill holes. The anterior cortex of the proximal fragment was fashioned into a "V"-shaped spike (Figure 45.3). The wedge of bone between the drill holes was removed with nibblers and a small osteotome. The posterior cortex was weakened with multiple drill holes and broken gently by extending the knee. Care was taken to ensure that the cortical bone spike on the end of the proximal fragment sank into the cancellous bone of the distal fragment as the knee was hyperextended by 10°.[3] The wound was closed in layers, and a long leg cast was applied holding the knee in 10° hyperextension and the ankle and foot in maximal dorsiflexion (Figure 45.4).

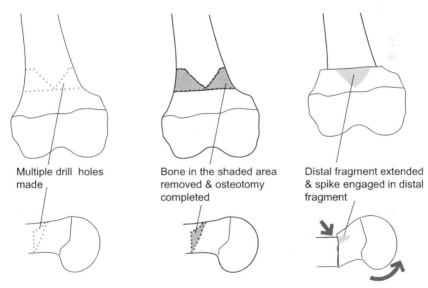

Multiple drill holes made

Bone in the shaded area removed & osteotomy completed

Distal fragment extended & spike engaged in distal fragment

Figure 45.3 Technique of spike osteotomy. (Reproduced from Figure 13.4, *Paediatric Orthopaedics—A system of decision-making* 2nd Edition.)

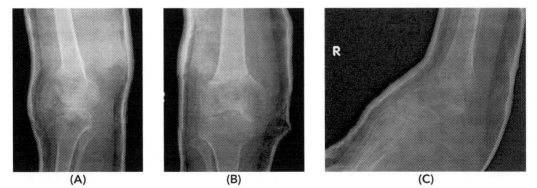

(A)   (B)   (C)

Figure 45.4 Completed spike osteotomy (A, B) with 10° hyperextension of the knee and residual equinus following soft issue release (C).

Post-Operative Management

The cast was removed at six weeks and the knee mobilised; weight-bearing was permitted after the x-rays showed sound union of the osteotomy (Figure 45.5).

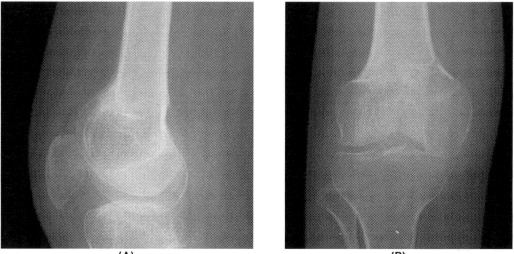

(A)   (B)

Figure 45.5 Radiograph at final follow-up showing sound union of the femoral osteotomy.

Follow-Up

He was followed-up for three years, at which time he was walking in a more acceptable fashion without having to resort to hand-to-thigh gait even while walking on uneven ground.

References

1. Joseph B, Watts H. Polio revisited: Reviving knowledge and skills to meet the challenge of resurgence. *J Child Orthop.* 2015 Oct;9(5):325–38. doi: 10.1007/s11832-015-0678-4. Epub 2015 Sep 11. PMID: 26362170; PMCID: PMC4619376.
2. Patwa JJ, Bhatt HR, Chouksey S, Patel K. Hamstring transfer for quadriceps paralysis in post polio residual paralysis. *Indian J Orthop.* 2012 Sep;46(5):575–80. doi: 10.4103/0019-5413.101044. PMID: 23162153; PMCID: PMC3491794.
3. Dietz FR, Weinstein SL. Spike osteotomy for angular deformities of the long bones in children. *J Bone Joint Surg Am.* 1988 Jul;70(6):848–52. PMID: 3392081.

Hitesh Shah and Benjamin Joseph

Case

A 5-year-old girl presented with progressive deformity of the right foot. She had low-level spina bifida with patchy neurologic deficit involving the right lower limb. Her bowel and bladder function were normal, and she did not have symptoms suggestive of sensory loss on her feet.

On examination, it was noted that the right lower limb was 1 cm shorter than the left (Figure 46.1a). The girth of her right calf was also less than the left. She had hind foot varus, forefoot adduction, an accentuated medial longitudinal arch and claw toes in the right foot. The ankle could be passively dorsiflexed up to the neutral position only (Figure 46.1b, c); all other deformities could be fully passively corrected. The clawing of the toes could be corrected by exerting upward pressure under the metatarsal heads. This indicated that the claw deformity was supple, and for the same reason early clawing was less obvious on weight-bearing. She walked with a foot drop and varus of the hind foot during the swing phase. The lateral border of the foot made initial contact with the ground, and in mid-stance the forefoot and the heel rested on the ground. The power of muscles around the foot and ankle are shown in Table 46.1 and in Figure 46.2. There was hypoaesthesia on the sole of the foot, but she had protective sensation.

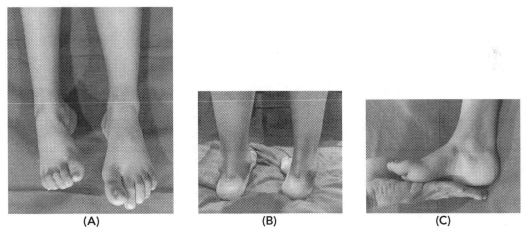

| (A) | (B) | (C) |

Figure 46.1 (A) Forefoot adduction and hindfoot varus of the right foot in a child with low-level spina bifida. The right lower limb is shorter and the foot is smaller than the left, and the girth is also less on the right. (B) Hind foot varus is seen on the right. (C) The ankle can be passively dorsiflexed up to neutral. Claw toes and cavus are evident when the foot is not bearing weight.

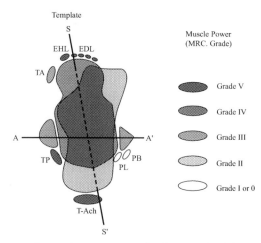

Figure 46.2 Muscle power of muscles acting on the foot and ankle.

Table 46.1 Power of Muscles Acting on the Foot and Ankle

Joint	Muscle	Power (MRC Scale)	Consequence
Ankle	Tibialis anterior	Grade 3-	Foot drop during swing
	Gastroc-soleus	Grade 5	Muscle imbalance between dorsiflexors and plantarflexors of the ankle leading to early contracture of the Achilles tendon
Subtalar joint & mid-tarsal joints	Tibialis anterior	Grade 3-	Forefoot adduction
	Tibialis posterior	Grade 5	Hindfoot varus
	Peroneus longus	Grade 0	Muscle imbalance between invertors and evertors
	Peroneus brevis	Grade 0	
Toes	Intrinsic muscles	Grade 0	Claw toes
	Flexor digitorum longus Flexor hallucis longus	Grade 5	Cavus Muscle imbalance between the intrinsic and extrinsic muscles acting on the toes
	Extensor digitorum longus Extensor hallucis longus	Grade 5	

Questions

- What are the problems that need to be addressed?
- What are the aims of treatment?
- What are the available treatment options to fulfil these aims?
- What are the factors that may influence your choice of treatment?
- Based on these points, what treatment would you recommend for this child?
- How long would you follow-up this child after treatment?

The Problems That Need to Be Addressed Are
- Deformities
  - Hindfoot varus
  - Forefoot adduction
  - Cavus
  - Claw toes

- Muscle imbalance across the ankle and subtalar axes
- Abnormal gait pattern
  - Poor ankle dorsiflexion in the swing phase
  - Varus deviation of the foot during the entire gait cycle

The Aims of Treatment in This Child Are to
- Correct deformities
- Restore muscle balance

Options for Treatment to Fulfil Each Aim
- Correcting deformities
  - Release structures contributing to the deformity (e.g., tibialis posterior)
  - Osteotomies

- Restoring muscle balance
  - Tendon transfer
  - Tendon release

FACTORS THAT INFLUENCED THE CHOICE OF TREATMENT

- The age of the child
- The severity and suppleness of the deformities
- Power of the muscles of the foot and ankle

The choice of treatment based on these factors is outlined in Table 46.2.

Table 46.2 Factors That Influenced the Choice of Treatment

Factors		Treatment Implications
Age of the child	5-year-old	Rebalancing of muscle power at this age can prevent progression of the deformity and also prevent the deformity from becoming rigid. The child may just be old enough to co-operate with rehabilitation after a tendon transfer.
Severity and suppleness of deformities	The deformities are supple and not severe	Soft tissue release should enable deformity correction; there is no role for osteotomies at this stage.

(Continued)

Table 46.2 (Continued)

Factors		Treatment Implications
Power of muscles around the foot and ankle	As shown in Table 46.1	Since the tibialis posterior has Grade 5 power it is suitable for transfer.[1] Furthermore, the tibialis posterior is the major deforming force contributing to the hindfoot varus; transferring it will remove this force and facilitate deformity correction. The choice of tendon transfer and the point of attachment of the transferred tendon will be determined by the muscle power of opposing muscles (Figure 46.3).[2]

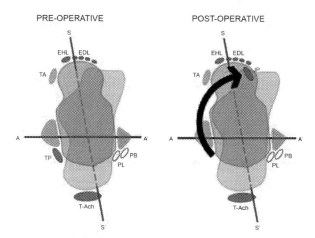

Figure 46.3 Restoring muscle balance across the ankle and subtalar axes by transfer of the tibialis posterior.

How Was This Child Treated?

The child was treated with a tibialis posterior transfer to the dorsum of the foot. Under general anaesthesia with a tourniquet inflated, the foot was examined. It was noted that the ankle could be dorsiflexed to 10 degrees beyond neutral, and hence lengthening of the gastroc-soleus was not done. A short incision was made, centred over the tuberosity of the navicular. The tendon of the tibialis posterior was detached from the navicular bone, and all the slips to other tarsals were divided. The tendon was tagged with a stay suture. A second incision was made on the medial aspect of the leg at the junction of the distal fourth and the proximal three-fourths of the leg, and the free end of the tibialis posterior tendon was drawn into the wound. A third incision was made on the dorso-lateral aspect of the foot. The tendon of the tibialis posterior was tunnelled in the subcutaneous plane and withdrawn into the third wound. Osteo-periosteal flaps were raised at the site chosen for attaching the transferred tendon. The foot was held in eversion with the ankle in 10 degrees of dorsiflexion, and the tibialis posterior tendon was anchored under the osteo-periosteal flaps under tension with non-absorbable sutures. The wounds were closed, and a below-knee cast was applied with the foot dorsiflexed and everted.

Post-Operative Management

The cast was retained for six weeks. After cast removal, physiotherapy aimed at re-educating the transferred muscle was commenced. A soft-lined ankle-foot orthosis (AFO) was worn when she was ambulant. At three months, the foot was plantigrade with no hindfoot varus. The cavus and clawing of the toes were no longer evident on weight-bearing (Figure 46.4).

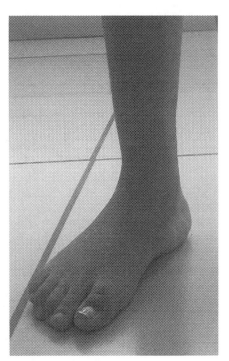

Figure 46.4 The foot is plantigrade, and the deformities have been well corrected.

Follow-Up

This child will be followed up till skeletal maturity to monitor the foot for early signs of recurrence of the hindfoot varus deformity.

References

1. Westin GW. Tendon transfers about the foot, ankle, and hip in the paralyzed lower extremity. *J Bone Joint Surg Am*. 1965 Oct;47(7):1430–43. PMID: 5837646.
2. Joseph B, Watts H. Polio revisited: Reviving knowledge and skills to meet the challenge of resurgence. *J Child Orthop*. 2015 Oct;9(5):325–38. doi: 10.1007/s11832-015-0678-4. Epub 2015 Sep 11. PMID: 26362170; PMCID: PMC4619376.

Hitesh Shah

Case

A 10-year-old boy presented with difficulty in getting his hand to his mouth to feed himself. He was born by a difficult vaginal delivery; there was history suggestive of shoulder dystocia. Soon after birth, there was no spontaneous voluntary movement of the right upper limb; however, he recovered significantly over time. At the age of 10, his hand function including grasp and release was normal. Muscle power at the elbow, wrist and hand were normal. Shoulder abductor, internal rotator and flexor power was good. He had a severe internal rotation contracture of the shoulder. He could raise his arm completely with the arm in internal rotation (Figure 47.1a), but he could not externally rotate his shoulder at all or take his hand to the back of the neck (Figure 47.1b). While attempting to get his hand to his mouth, he displayed a severe trumpet sign (Figure 47.1c).

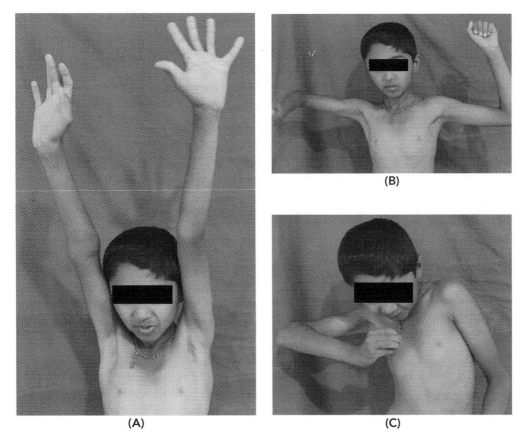

(A)

(B)

(C)

Figure 47.1 The boy can raise both his arms above his head; the right arm is internally rotated. The right upper limb is shorter than the left (A). External rotation of the right shoulder is not possible (B), and on attempting to get his hand to his mouth the shoulder abducts and a severe trumpet sign develops (C).

The medial border of the scapula became prominent on attempted passive external rotation (positive Putti sign). The humeral head was palpable posteriorly and became more prominent on internally rotating the shoulder passively; radiographs confirmed posterior subluxation of the right shoulder.

Questions

- What is this boy's shoulder function on the Mallet scale?
- What are the problems that need to be addressed?
- What are the aims of treatment?
- What are the available treatment options to fulfil these aims?
- What are the factors that may influence your choice of treatment?
- Based on these points, what treatment would you recommend for this child?
- How long would you follow-up this boy after treatment?

Shoulder Function on the Mallet Scale

The function in this boy fits into Mallet Grade 2 with the exception of active abduction which is near normal.[1]

- Mallet Grade 2:
    - Active abduction ≤30°
    - Zero degrees of external rotation
    - Hand to back of neck impossible
    - Hand to back impossible
    - Hand to mouth with marked trumpet sign

The Problem That Needs to Be Addressed Is
- Inability to get his hand to his mouth without having to abduct his shoulder

The Aim of Treatment in This Boy Is to
- Enable him to get his hand to his mouth without having to abduct his shoulder by improving external rotation of the shoulder

Options for Treatment to Fulfil This Aim
- Correction of internal rotation deformity
    - Release of internal rotator contracture
    - Release of internal rotator contracture and latissimus dorsi and teres major transfer to infraspinatus
    - External rotation osteotomy of the proximal humerus

FACTORS THAT INFLUENCED THE CHOICE OF TREATMENT

- Age of the child
- Severity of internal rotation deformity of the shoulder
- Presence of posterior instability of the shoulder

The choice of treatment based on these factors is shown in Table 47.1.

Table 47.1 Factors Influencing the Choice of Treatment

Factors		Treatment Implications
Age of the child	10 years old	Contracture release and tendon transfers performed in a young child may prevent dysplastic changes in the shoulder from developing or progressing.[2] This child is 10 years old, and the shoulder is already dysplastic; this favours an external rotation osteotomy of the humerus.[3,4]

(Continued)

Table 47.1 (Continued)

Factors		Treatment Implications
Severity of internal rotation deformity of the shoulder	Severe deformity	A severe deformity may not get fully corrected by release of contracted soft tissues alone, in which case additional surgery on the humerus may be needed. Since any degree of internal rotation contracture can be corrected by a humeral derotation osteotomy, this is the preferred option.
Presence of posterior instability of the shoulder		Tendon release and transfer are indicated before shoulder instability develops. Since the child is already 10 years old with established shoulder instability, tendon surgery may not be effective.

How Was This Boy Treated?

The boy was treated with an external rotation osteotomy of the humerus. The osteotomy was performed proximal to the deltoid insertion; the distal fragment was rotated 45° externally and fixed with a dynamic compression plate (Figure 47.2). The adequacy of rotational correction was checked before wound closure by moving the draped hand to the mouth over the drapes with the arm at his side.

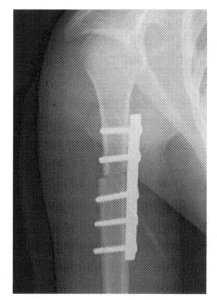

Figure 47.2 Derotation osteotomy of the humerus has been performed and fixed with a plate and screws.

Post-Operative Management

The arm was immobilised in a shoulder sling for six weeks. After union of the osteotomy, range-of-motion exercises were started.

Follow-Up

He was reviewed one year after surgery. He was able to raise his arms above his shoulders (Figure 47.3a), get his hands to the back of the head (Figure 47.3b) and take his hand to his mouth without a trumpet sign (Figure 47.3c). The child needs to be followed up till he is skeletally mature.

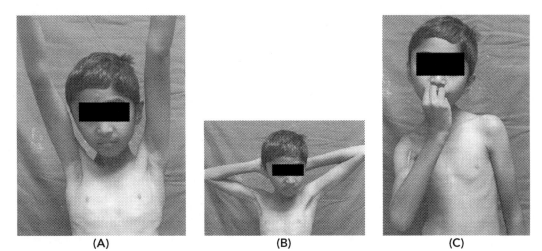

(A)　　　　　　　　**(B)**　　　　　　　　**(C)**

Figure 47.3 One year following surgery, he can raise his arms (A), take his hands to the back of his head (B) and get his hand to his mouth without a trumpet sign (C).

Comment

One indication to opt for a derotation osteotomy of the humerus over tendon transfers is the presence of glenoid dysplasia and distortion of the humeral head confirmed with CT or MRI scans.

Scans were not done in this boy as a decision to perform a humeral derotation osteotomy was taken irrespective of the status of the glenoid and the humeral head, on account of the severity of the internal rotation deformity of the shoulder.

References

1. Al-Qattan MM, El-Sayed AA. Obstetric brachial plexus palsy: The Mallet grading system for shoulder function-revisited. *Biomed Res Int*. 2014;2014:398121. doi: 10.1155/2014/398121.
2. Waters PM, Bae DS. Effect of tendon transfers and extra-articular soft-tissue balancing on glenohumeral development in brachial plexus birth palsy. *J Bone Joint Surg Am*. 2005;87:320–5.
3. Waters PM, Bae DS. The effect of derotational humeral osteotomy on global shoulder function in brachial plexus birth palsy. *J Bone Joint Surg Am*. 2006;88:1035–42.
4. Hultgren T, Jönsson K, Roos F, Järnbert-Pettersson H, Hammarberg H. Surgical correction of shoulder rotation deformity in brachial plexus birth palsy: Long-term results in 118 patients. *Bone Joint J*. 2014;96:1411–8.

CASE 48: THE PARALYSED ELBOW – MANAGEMENT OF EXTENSOR PARALYSIS

Binu P Thomas

Case

A 4-year-old girl presented with inability to actively extend her right elbow since birth and progressive flexion deformity of the elbow. She had brachial plexus birth palsy and had previously undergone surgery (a modified Hoffer's procedure) at the age of two years with good improvement of active shoulder abduction and external rotation. Her parents noticed that the child was reluctant to abduct her shoulder.

On examination, the Horner's sign was negative, and the radial pulse was normal. The right upper limb was hypoplastic (Figure 48.1), and there was a flexion deformity of the elbow of 20 degrees. The power of muscles of the upper limb is shown in Table 48.1.

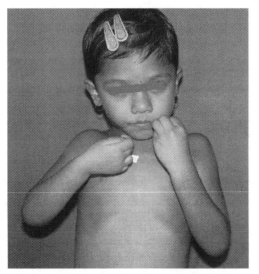

Figure 48.1 Preoperative photograph of a 4-year-old child with right-sided brachial plexus birth palsy showing active elbow flexion when she attempts to bring the hand to the mouth.

Table 48.1 Power of the Muscles of the Right Upper Limb

Region	Muscle	Power (MRC Grade)
Scapulo-thoracic	Trapezius	4
	Rhomboids	4
Shoulder	Pectoralis major	4
	Supraspinatus	4
	Infraspinatus	4
	Deltoid	4

(Continued)

Table 48.1 (Continued)

Region	Muscle	Power (MRC Grade)
Elbow	Biceps	4
	Brachialis	4
	Brachioradialis	3
	Triceps	0
Wrist	Wrist flexors	3
	Wrist extensors	3
Extrinsic muscles of hand	Finger flexors	3
	Finger extensors	3
Intrinsic muscles of hand		4

When asked to abduct both her shoulders, she was reluctant to abduct her right shoulder fully (Figure 48.2); following repeated requests, she did abduct the shoulder, but the elbow dropped into uncontrolled flexion with the hand almost hitting her face.

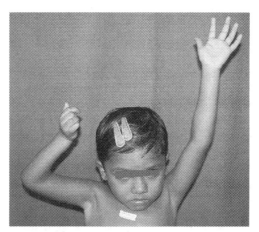

Figure 48.2 Photograph of the same patient as she attempts to extend the elbow for overhead activity shows the weakness of elbow extension.

Questions

- What are the problems that need to be addressed in this girl?
- What are the aims of treatment?
- What are the available treatment options to fulfil these aims?
- What are the factors that may influence your choice of treatment?
- Based on these points, what treatment would you recommend for this child?
- How long would you follow-up this child after treatment?

The Problems Related to the Limb That Need to Be Addressed in This Young Girl Are

- Instability of the elbow and weakness of extension (resulting in the child's reluctance to actively abduct shoulder above 90 degrees for fear of the hand hitting her face with uncontrolled elbow flexion)
- Inability to perform bilateral overhead activity
- Progressive flexion deformity of the elbow

The Aim of Treatment in This Child Is to

- Enable overhead activity by:
  - Providing active extension of elbow
  - Providing elbow stability during overhead activity

Options for Treatment to Fulfil Each Aim

- Restoring active elbow extension

  - Tendon transfer

    - Latissimus dorsi transfer to triceps
    - Deltoid to triceps transfer
    - Biceps to triceps transfer

  - Free muscle transfer
  - Nerve transfer

- Stabilisation of elbow

  - Restoring power of elbow extension
  - Elbow arthrodesis

FACTORS THAT INFLUENCED THE CHOICE OF TREATMENT

The factors that influenced the choice of treatment of the nerve injuries were:

- Age of the child
- The interval between the injury and intervention
- The nature of previous surgery
- Degree of flexion deformity of the elbow
- Functional impairment and potential complications of the surgical procedure

The choice of treatment based on these factors is shown in Table 48.2.

Table 48.2 Factors Influencing the Choice of Treatment

Factors		Treatment Implications
The age of the child	4 years old	By the age of 4 years, flexion deformity of the elbow of 20 degrees has developed; this is likely to progress unless muscle balance across the elbow is restored. An arthrodesis of the elbow could damage the growth plates of the distal humerus and proximal ulna, and this would result in significant shortening as there are almost 10 years of growth remaining.
Interval between nerve injury and intervention	4 years	As four years have elapsed since the nerve injury, any procedure that restores nerve continuity will not improve muscle power as the motor end plates would have degenerated.
The nature of previous surgery and muscles available for transfer	Modified Hoffer procedure done previously and now the biceps and brachialis are functioning well	The latissimus dorsi was transferred to restore external rotation of the shoulder and hence is no more available for transfer. The biceps can be transferred;[1-3] this would decrease the deforming force at the elbow and improve muscle balance.
Degree of flexion contracture of the elbow	Mild deformity	The options for tendon transfers in the presence of mild flexion contracture include the deltoid-to-triceps transfer (Moberg) and a biceps-to-triceps transfer.[4] The latter procedure is simpler.
Functional impairment and potential complications of surgical procedure	Permanent elbow stiffness Growth plate damage	Arthrodesis of the elbow is not a good option as it produces a stiff elbow and could affect the growth of the arm as well.

How Was This Child Treated?

Using a medial longitudinal incision, the biceps tendon was dissected (Figure 47.3). The branch of the musculocutaneous nerve to the biceps was identified and protected. The biceps tendon was then tenotomised.

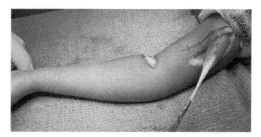

Figure 48.3 Intraoperative photograph showing the harvest of the biceps tendon using two incisions—a transverse incision at the elbow flexion crease for disinserting the biceps tendon, and a second incision at the medial arm for retrieving the biceps tendon and carefully dissecting the muscle, ensuring a relatively straight line of transfer to the triceps insertion. The nerve

Another incision was made on the posterior aspect of the elbow and triceps tendon, and insertion was identified (Figure 48.4). The biceps tendon was retrieved through this incision and sutured to the triceps insertion with osteo-periosteal sutures (Figure 48.5).

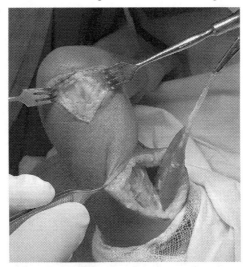

Figure 48.4 A posterior incision is made at the insertion of the triceps on the olecranon, and the biceps muscle is subcutaneously tunnelled from the medial arm incision.

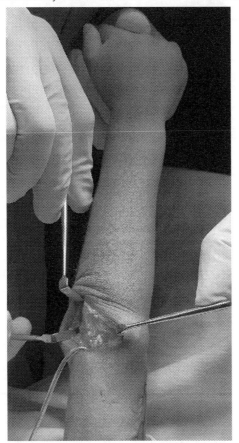

Figure 48.5 The biceps tendon is woven through the triceps using a Pulvertaft weave and osteo-periosteal non-absorbable sutures with the elbow in maximum extension and optimum tension.

The wound was closed, and an above-elbow posterior splint was applied with the elbow in extension.

Post-Operative Management

The splint and sutures were removed at four weeks, and gentle active extension and guarded flexion commenced. A thermoplastic splint was fabricated and continued for a further period of four weeks while the child was undergoing physiotherapy.

Follow-Up

The patient demonstrated very good active extension of the elbow with improvement of active shoulder movements. She was able to abduct the shoulder with the elbow in extension to perform overhead activities (Figure 48.6).

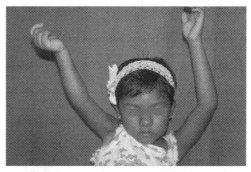

Figure 48.6 Post-operative follow-up photograph of the patient demonstrating good elbow extension and improved shoulder abduction.

Comment

The transfer of biceps to triceps contravenes the laws of tendon transfers as it is a non-phasic transfer.[5] Despite this, the transfer restored active extension of the elbow while the brachialis could actively flex the elbow in this child.

This procedure has been described in management of tetraplegia,[1] but is also a useful tendon transfer in treating birth palsies, particularly when flexion deformity at the elbow is negligible.

References

1. Kozin SH. Biceps-to-triceps transfer for restoration of elbow extension in tetraplegia. *Tech Hand Up Extrem Surg.* 2003;7(2):43–51.
2. Zancolli E. Surgery for the quadriplegic hand with active, strong wrist extension preserved: A study of 97 cases. *Clin Orthop.* 1975;(112):101–13.
3. Moberg E. Surgical treatment for absent single-hand grip and elbow extension in quadriplegia: Principles and preliminary experience. *J Bone Jt Surg.* 1975;57(2):196–206.
4. Sebastian S, Chung K. Reconstructive strategies for recovery of hand function. In: Chung K, Yang LJS, McGillicuddy J, editors. *Practical management of paediatric and adult brachial plexus palsies.* Philadelphia: Elsevier, 2012. pp. 114–42.
5. Anderson GA. The child's hand in the developing world. In: Gupta A, Kay SPJ, Scheker LR, editors. *The growing hand.* London: Mosby; 2000. pp. 1097–114.

Binu P Thomas

Case

A 7-year-old boy child sustained a right traumatic brachial plexus palsy following a fall from a tractor. His right upper limb was completely paralysed initially but over the course of two years had some patchy recovery with some return of shoulder and elbow function. He was seen at our hospital two years after the injury with weakness of the limb and very poor upper limb function. His ability to perform normal activities of daily living was severely compromised.

The power of all muscle groups of the upper limb was tested by manual muscle testing and recorded (Table 49.1).

Table 49.1 Power of the Muscles of the Right Upper Limb

Region	Muscle	Power (MRC Grade)
Scapulo-thoracic	Trapezius	5
	Rhomboids	5
Shoulder	Pectoralis major	3
	Supraspinatus	4
	Infraspinatus	4
	Latissimus dorsi	2
	Deltoid	4
Elbow	Biceps	3
	Triceps	0
Wrist	Wrist flexors	0
	Wrist extensors	3
Extrinsic muscles of hand	Finger and thumb flexors	0
	Finger and thumb extensors	0
Intrinsic muscles of hand		0

Partial recovery of the deltoid and biceps brachii enabled abduction of the shoulder and elbow flexion (Figure 49.1 and 49.2). The Horner's sign was negative, and the radial pulse was normally palpable. Hypoaesthesia was present in C5 to T1 dermatomes.

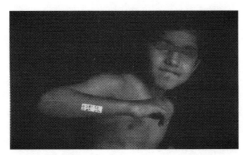

Figure 49.1 Photograph of a child with traumatic brachial plexus injury showing partial recovery of abduction of the shoulder and elbow flexion.

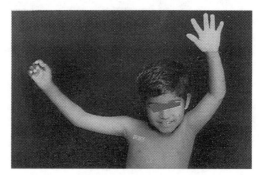

Figure 49.2 The child recovered enough to hold the limb in 90 degrees of shoulder abduction and elbow flexion by the functioning deltoid and biceps. There is no active elbow extension.

Questions
- What are the problems that need to be addressed in this boy?
- What are the aims of treatment?
- What are the available treatment options to fulfil these aims?
- What are the factors that may influence your choice of treatment?
- Based on these points, what treatment would you recommend for this child?

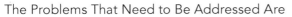

The Problems That Need to Be Addressed Are

- Lack of active elbow extension
- Instability of the wrist and the thumb
- Grasp and release not possible due to:
  - Lack of active wrist and finger flexion
  - Lack of active finger and thumb extension

The Aims of Treatment in This boy Are to

- Restore active elbow extension
- Enable grasp and release by:
  - Providing a stable thumb and wrist
  - Restoring finger flexion and
  - Restoring finger and thumb extension

Options for Treatment to Fulfil Each Aim

- Restoring active elbow extension
  - Moberg transfer of posterior deltoid to triceps with a fascia lata graft
  - Biceps to triceps transfer

- Stabilising the thumb and wrist
  - Tendon transfers to stabilise thumb and wrist
  - First carpo-metacarpal fusion and wrist fusion

- Restoring finger flexion
  - Free functioning muscle transfer with proximal reinnervation
  - Biceps to flexor digitorum profundus (FDP) transfer via fascia lata graft

- Restoring finger and thumb extension
  - Transfer of one of the wrist extensors to restore finger and thumb extension

---

FACTORS THAT INFLUENCED THE CHOICE OF TREATMENT

- Interval between injury and reconstructive surgical intervention
- Functioning muscles available for transfers

The choice of treatment based on these factors in outlined in Table 49.2.

Table 49.2 Factors That Influenced the Choice of Treatment

Factors		Treatment Implications
Interval between injury and reconstructive surgical intervention	Two years	Further spontaneous recovery cannot be expected beyond two years after the injury. Surgery on the brachial plexus to restore its continuity is not justified as motor end plate degeneration of the paralysed muscles would have occurred by two years.

(Continued)

Table 49.2 (Continued)

Factors		Treatment Implications
Functioning muscles available for transfers	Only rhomboids and the trapezius have Grade 5 power on the MRC scale	Ideally, muscles that are transferred to restore function should have Grade 5 power. Weaker muscles may be transferred as a means of restoring muscle balance or to act as a tenodesis. For such extensive paralysis as in this boy, a combination of joint fusions, tenodesis and free muscle transfers will be needed.

How Was This Child Treated?

Staged reconstructive procedures were planned and discussed with the boy's parents. They were willing to cooperate with the protracted treatment, and so we proceeded with the first stage.

Stage 1

The posterior part of deltoid muscle was isolated and by a fascia lata graft was transferred to the triceps tendon (Figure 49.3) to provide elbow extension (Moberg procedure).[1]

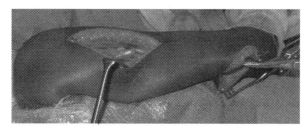

Figure 49.3 Intraoperative photograph showing the transfer of half of the deltoid muscle to the triceps using a fascia lata graft.

Stage 2

A sural nerve free graft was harvested and neurotised to 2, 3 and 4 intercostal nerves (Figure 49.4). The nerve graft was tunnelled subcutaneously across the axilla up to the elbow on the medial aspect and tagged and left for anastomosing to the nerve of the free muscle transfer at the next stage.

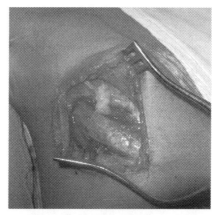

Figure 49.4 Intraoperative photograph showing the harvest of the intercostal nerves from the chest and extended with a sural nerve graft.

Stage 3

The boy was carefully followed up at six monthly intervals. When the Tinel's sign was detected at the distal free end of the sural nerve graft at the elbow, we proceeded with the next stage of reconstruction.

The gracilis muscle[2] was harvested with its neurovascular pedicle and transferred to the forearm. The proximal end was sutured to the common flexor origin at the medial epicondyle and distal end to the flexor digitorum profundus (FDP) and flexor pollicis longus (FPL) tendons to provide finger flexion (Figure 49.5a, 5b and 49.6).

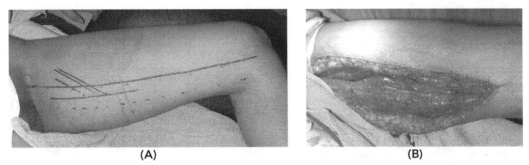

(A) **(B)**

Figure 49.5 (A) Intraoperative photograph showing the skin marking for the gracilis free muscle harvest. Note the markings for the neurovascular bundle entering the muscle about four finger breadths from the pubic tubercle. (B) Intraoperative photograph showing the harvest of the gracilis muscle from the medial aspect of the thigh.

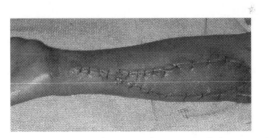

Figure 49.6 Intraoperative photograph showing the inset of the gracilis in the forearm. The gracilis is attached to the common flexor origin proximally and to the flexor digitorum profundus and flexor pollicis longus distally.

Stage IV

The carpometacarpal joint of the thumb was arthrodesed to provide a stable thumb in abduction using two parallel K-wires.[3]

Stage V

The extensor carpi radialis longus, though weak, was transferred to extensor digitorum and extensor pollicis longus to provide finger extension or at least to provide a tenodesis effect. This may not be in accordance with the rules of tendon transfers,[4] but since no other options were available, this surgery was done.

Postoperative Management

Each stage required intensive supervised physical therapy in the post-operative period.

Follow-Up

The reconstructive procedures were done over a span of nine years to avoid too much disruption of his schooling.

At the final follow-up, the patient had reasonable function of the right upper limb including elbow extension, finger and thumb flexion and grasp (Figures 49.7 and 49.8). Videos demonstrate progressive improvement and final function.

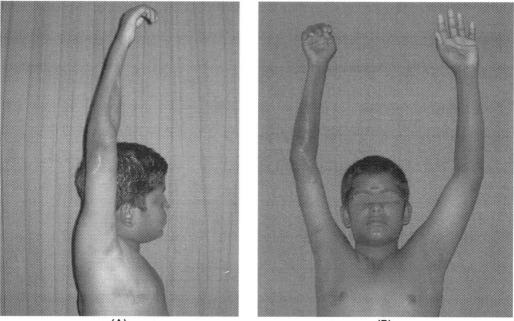

(A)   (B)

Figure 49.7 The follow-up photographs showing the full elbow extension following the Moberg transfer.

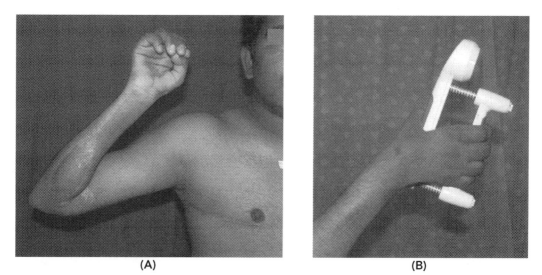

(A)   (B)

Figure 49.8 The follow-up photographs showing finger and thumb flexion and the ability to hold objects (the dynamometer). Note the scar over the chest from where the intercostal nerves were harvested and the gracilis flap in the forearm.

References

1. Moberg E. Surgical treatment for absent single-hand grip and elbow extension in quadriplegia: Principles and preliminary experience. *J Bone Jt Surg.* 1975;57(2):196–206.
2. Madura T, Doi K, Hattori Y, Sakamoto S, Shimoe T. Free functioning gracilis transfer for reanimation of elbow and hand in total traumatic brachial plexopathy in children. *J Hand Surg Eur Vol.* Published online 2018 Mar 16. doi: 10.1177/1753193418762950.
3. Coulet B, Waitzenegger T, Teissier J, et al. Arthrodesis versus carpometacarpal preservation in key-grip procedures in tetraplegic patients: A comparative study of 40 cases. *J Hand Surg.* 2018;43(5):483.e1–9. doi: 10.1016/j.jhsa.2017.10.029.
4. Sammer DM, Chung KC. Tendon transfers Part I: Principles of transfer and transfers for radial nerve palsy. *Plast Reconstr Surg.* 2009;123(5):169e–77e. doi: 10.1097/PRS.0b013e3181a20526.

Binu P Thomas

Case

A 5-year-old girl presented with history of having fallen onto a sharp object and lacerated her right wrist three months ago. The wound was initially treated at a local clinic, where it was cleaned and sutured. She complained of difficulty in using her right hand with loss of sensation on the palm.

On examination, there was a 4 cm long healed transverse scar on the flexion crease of the wrist. There was a total claw hand deformity with all four digits hyperextended at the metacarpo-phalangeal (MCP) joints and flexed at the inter-phalangeal (IP) joints. The thumb was adducted and supinated. There was wasting of both the thenar and hypothenar eminences (Figure 50.1). The power of the flexor digitorum superficialis (FDS) and the flexor digitorum profundus (FDP) was Grade 4 on the MRC scale. Power of all the intrinsic muscles of the hand was Grade 0. There were no sensations on the entire palm.

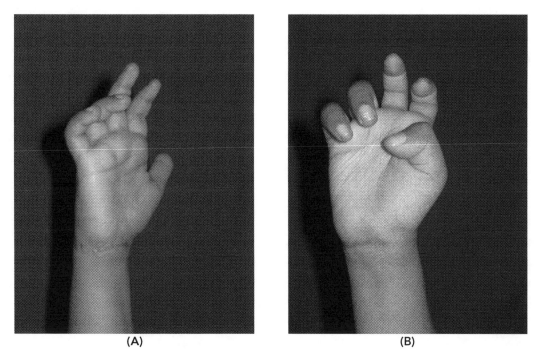

(A)   (B)

Figure 50.1 (A) Active flexion of the interphalangeal joints of the fingers and thumb indicating that the long flexor tendons are intact. (B) Clawing of the fingers and the scar over the wrist are clearly seen.

Questions

- What are the problems that need to be addressed in this girl?
- What are the aims of treatment?
- What are the commonly available options for treatment?
- What are the factors that may influence your choice of treatment?
- What treatment would you recommend for this girl?
- How long would you follow-up this girl after treatment?

The Problems Related to the Hand That Need to Be Addressed Are

- Deformity
  - Total claw hand
  - Adducted supinated thumb
- Loss of sensation of:
  - Median nerve area
  - Ulnar nerve area
- Loss of intrinsic power of:
  - Radial two lumbricals and thenar intrinsics innervated by median nerve
  - Hypothenar intrinsics, interossei, adductor pollicis and medial two lumbricals supplied by ulnar nerve

The Aims of Treatment in This Child Are to

- Correction of deformities of the fingers and thumb
- Restore intrinsic muscle power
- Restore protective sensation in the palm of the hand

Options for Treatment to Fulfil These Aims

- Correction of the deformity of the fingers and hand
  - Claw correction by tendon transfers
  - Claw correction by static procedures
  - Opponensplasty
  - 1st carpo-metacarpal joint (CMC) joint fusion
- Restore intrinsic muscle power and sensation by reconstruction of the injured nerves
  - Nerve repair
  - Nerve grafting
  - Neurotisation of branches of superficial radial nerve for critical sensation in thumb and index pulp

---

FACTORS THAT INFLUENCED THE CHOICE OF TREATMENT

The factors that influenced the choice of treatment of the nerve injuries were:

- The age of the child
- Time elapsed from the date of the injury
- The nature of injury
- Presence of associated loss of sensation

The choice of treatment based on these factors is shown in Table 50.1.

Table 50.1 Factors Influencing the Choice of Treatment

Factors		Treatment Implications
Age of the child	5 years old	Nerve recovery following nerve repair or grafting is very good in young children.[1]
Time elapsed from the date of the injury	3 months	Three months after the injury, direct neurorrhaphy will not be possible; a nerve graft will be needed to bridge the gap after excision of neuroma and glioma for both nerves.[2] Tendon transfers or other static procedures should be considered only if nerve procedures are not feasible or when it has crossed the critical limit of delay.
The nature of injury	Laceration by a sharp object	Since it was an open laceration with a sharp object resulting in neurotmesis and not a neurapraxia or axonotmesis, there is no point in anticipating natural recovery.[3]
Presence of associated sensory loss	Loss of both median and ulnar nerve sensation in the hand	Since sensation can be restored only by nerve repair procedures, nerve reconstruction is the preferred option rather than tendon transfers.

How Was This Girl Treated?

Using a curvilinear incision, the wrist was explored. The median and ulnar nerves were found to be transected, with proximal neuromas and distal gliomas and a gap of about 5 cm between the cut ends.

The neuromas and gliomas were excised. The sural nerve was harvested from the left leg, and the nerve defects were grafted with four cables ensuring fascicular alignment[4,5] under the operating microscope using 10-0 sutures.

Post-Operative Management

A below-elbow plaster-of-Paris splint was given with the wrist in 30-degree flexion for four weeks followed by gentle range of motion exercises and active intrinsic exercises. She was given a custom-made knuckle bender splint, and she wore it till she was able to hold the fingers actively in the lumbrical position.[6]

Follow-Up

Good recovery of the intrinsic muscles occurred by nine months (Figure 50.2). The sensation recovered till she had a two-point discrimination of 4 mm in the autonomous areas of the ulnar and median nerve. She had no residual deformity on follow-up after nine years. Further follow-up was not considered necessary.

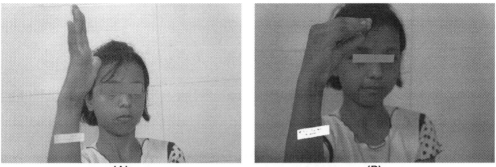

(A)   (B)

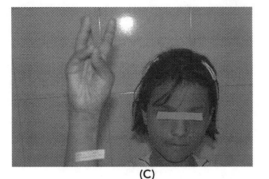

(C)

Figure 50.2 Hand function at follow-up showing that the clawing has been corrected (A). She can actively hold the hand in the lumbrical position, indicating that active flexion of the MCP joints and active extension of the IP joints have been restored (B). She can oppose the thumb (C).

References

1. Rolf Birch B, Achan PA. Peripheral nerve repairs and their results in children. *Hand Clin.* 2000; 16(4):579–95.
2. Anderson GA. The child's hand in the developing world. In: Gupta A, Kay SPJ, Scheker LR, editors. *The Growing Hand.* London: Mosby; 2000. pp. 1097–114.
3. Birch R, Quick T. Nerve injury & repair. In: *Green's Textbook of Operative Hand Surgery.* Vol 2. 7th ed. Philadelphia, PA: Elsevier.
4. Williams HB, Jabaley ME. The importance of internal anatomy of the peripheral nerves to nerve repair in the forearm and hand. *Hand Clin.* 1986;2(4):689–707.
5. Jabaley ME, Wallace WH, Heckler FR. Internal topography of major nerves of the forearm and hand: A current view. *J Hand Surg.* 1980;5(1):1–18. doi: 10.1016/s0363-5023(80)80035-9.
6. Anderson GA, Thomas BP, Pallapati SCR, Santoshi JA. Peripheral nerve injuries: Part 1 current aspects of PNI, effects of injury and evaluation. *Asian J Orthop Rheumatol.* 2006; 3(3):30–9.

UPPER MOTOR NEURON PARALYSIS

David A Spiegel

Case

An 11-year-old girl with a diagnosis of left hemiplegic cerebral palsy (GMFCS 1) presented for evaluation and treatment of a progressive deformity of the left foot. She was ambulating independently with an articulated ankle-foot orthosis (AFO), and was receiving physical therapy at school two to three times per week and once a month in the hospital as an outpatient. Previous treatment had included physical therapy involving a home stretching program, Botox injections, and serial casting.

She was concerned that her foot was turning in, that she was walking up on her toes, and that she often trips and falls. She had recently developed brace intolerance with pain and skin irritation over the dorso-lateral aspect of her left hindfoot, over the talar head and the anterior process of the calcaneus. There was also pain related to her knee bending backwards during ambulation.

On physical examination, she had equinovarus deformity of the left foot (Figure 51.1) which was moderately rigid; the foot could be passively abducted only to neutral. On the Silfverskiold test, her dorsiflexion was −10° with the knee flexed and −25° with the knee extended. There was mild mid-foot cavus with contracture of the plantar fascia. The muscle tone in the gastrocsoleus, tibialis anterior, and tibialis posterior was graded as a 1 on the Modified Ashworth Scale. She had good distal motor control. The muscle strength of the invertors was MRC grade 4+, while the power of evertors was grade 3. The left leg was 2 centimetres shorter than the right.

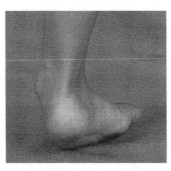

Figure 51.1 Clinical photo showing the equinovarus deformity of the left foot.

On observational gait analysis while walking barefoot, she had a left drop foot during the swing phase which was compensated by flexing more at the hip and knee to achieve clearance. Her left foot was supinated during both the swing and stance phases of gait. Initial contact was made on the lateral border of the forefoot in the region of the distal fifth metatarsal. During stance, she rolled onto the lateral border of her foot. Instrumented gait analysis showed that the tibialis anterior muscle was active throughout the gait cycle (i.e. during both the swing and stance phases).

Questions

- What are the problems that need to be addressed?
- What are the aims of treatment?
- What are the commonly available options for treatment?
- What are the factors that may influence your choice of treatment?
- What treatment would you recommend for this girl?
- How long would you follow-up this girl after treatment?

The Problems That Need to Be Addressed Are

- Contracture of the soft tissue structures on the postero-medial aspect of the ankle and foot and the plantar fascia that prevent passive correction of the deformity
- Muscle imbalance between strong invertors and weak evertors that contribute to the deformity and predispose to recurrence following correction of deformity
- Difficulty with foot clearance during the swing phase
- Poor stability during stance phase
- Discomfort with her orthosis

The Aims of Treatment Were to

- Correct the deformity of the foot and restore range of motion (dorsiflexion and eversion)
- Balance muscle forces; thereby prevent recurrence of deformity
- Enable the child to walk comfortably in her orthosis and relieve pain due to hyperextension of her knee
- Improve ambulation by improving the gait aberrations and relieving pain

Options for Treatment

- Correcting the deformity of the foot and restoring the range of motion
    - Nonsurgical
        - Serial casting
    - Surgical
        - Soft tissue lengthening with or without tendon transfer
        - Mid-tarsal osteotomies
        - Triple fusion
- Preventing recurrence of deformity after achieving correction
    - Tendon transfer of an invertor to the lateral side of the foot
        - Tibialis anterior transfer
            - Split tibialis anterior transfer
            - Complete transfer of the tibialis anterior
        - Tibialis posterior transfer
            - Split tibialis posterior transfer
            - Complete transfer of the tibialis posterior
- Enabling the child to walk comfortably in her orthosis and relieve pain by correcting the deformity

---

FACTORS THAT INFLUENCED THE CHOICE OF TREATMENT

- The underlying disease and its natural history
- Muscle imbalance and abnormal phasic activity of the invertors
- The age of the child
- The severity of deformity

The choice of treatment based on these factors is shown in Table 51.1.

Table 51.1 Factors That Influenced Choice of Treatment

Factors		Treatment Implications
The underlying disease and its natural history	Cerebral palsy with spasticity	The results of tendon transfers in cerebral palsy are less predictable than in conditions with lower motor neurone paralysis. In spite of this, a tendon transfer is justified as persistence of muscle imbalance will predispose to relapse of the deformity. The tendon transfer removes a deforming force and converts it into a corrective force. However, in the presence of spasticity, a complete tendon transfer may result in overcorrection, so a split tendon transfer is the preferred option.
Muscle imbalance	Observational gait analysis and instrumented motion analysis study	Continuous tibialis anterior activity through stance and swing phases of gait indicates that the tibialis anterior is contributing to the deformity. Hence a split tibialis anterior transfer is the preferred option.
The age of the child	11 and 6 months	The potential for relapse is low in older children who have little growth remaining. Data from one study on split tibialis posterior tendon transfers suggest that the risk of failure is greater in patients younger than 8 years of age at the time of surgery and in non-ambulators.[1] The age of this child is favourable for a satisfactory result after a tendon transfer.
The severity of deformity	Moderate	An important principle of tendon transfer is that adequate range of motion be restored prior to the procedure. In this child, restoration of dorsiflexion and eversion is mandatory before performing a tendon transfer. The options for restoring range of motion include soft tissue lengthening or release, osteotomies, or rarely arthrodesis. In this child, soft tissue lengthening is likely to be sufficient to restore motion prior to transfer. As the deformity is not severe, osteotomies of the midfoot and hindfoot may be avoided.

How Was This Child Treated?

- Restoration of range of motion

  o Plantar fascia release
  o Achilles tendon lengthening
  o Z-lengthening of tibialis posterior tendon
  o Intramuscular lengthening of the flexor digitorum longus and the flexor hallucis longus tendons because the dorsiflexion of all the toes was restricted after the equinus was corrected

- Balancing of muscle forces

  o Split tibialis anterior tendon transfer to the cuboid and anchored with an interference screw (Figure 51.2)

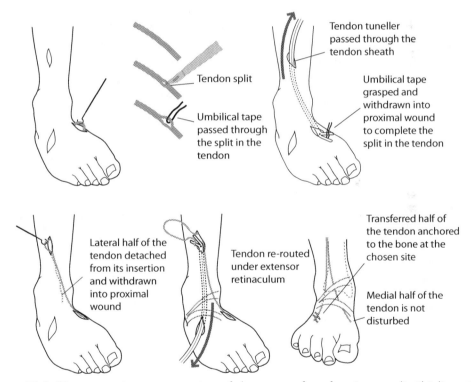

Figure 51.2 Diagrammatic representation of the steps of performing a split tibialis anterior transfer. (Reproduced from *Paediatric Orthopaedics—A system of decision-making* 2nd Edition.)

The split tibialis anterior tendon transfer was performed through three incisions,[2-4] although a two-incision technique has been reported.[5,6] One half of the tendon was harvested off the proximal first metatarsal, brought out anteriorly just above the ankle, and then tunnelled subcutaneously into a drill hole in the cuboid. After the tendon was placed into the tunnel in the cuboid, it was anchored with an interference screw.[7] Others have transferred the tendon to the peroneus tertius[4] or the fifth metatarsal base.[8] The technique of anchoring the tendon to the cuboid is most commonly achieved by using sutures over a button on the plantar surface of the foot. Since it was recognised that problems such as skin breakdown are common with this technique, and that early weight-bearing is desirable, an interference screw was used instead.

Post-Operative Management

A short leg cast was applied in the operating room and was maintained for six weeks. Weight-bearing was not permitted till the cast was removed. At eight months follow-up, the deformity was well corrected (Figure 51.3), her strength was 90% of the contralateral extremity, and she was able to maintain single limb stance on the left foot for 7 seconds. She no longer requires the use of an ankle-foot orthosis, and is able to run. She uses a 1-centimetre shoe lift to address her mild leg length discrepancy.

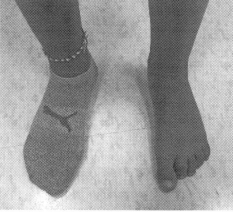
(A)

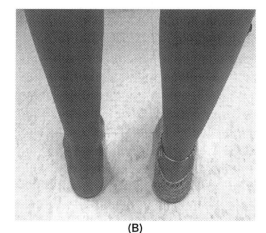
(B)

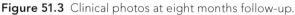
(C)

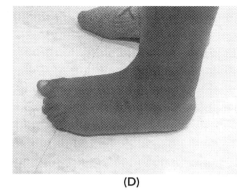
(D)

Figure 51.3 Clinical photos at eight months follow-up.

Comment

The equinovarus deformity results from muscle imbalance between strong invertors and weaker evertors. Defining whether the tibialis anterior or tibialis posterior is the cause is challenging on clinical examination and instrumented motion analysis with dynamic EMG may help to answer this question.[9,10] While the tibialis anterior can be evaluated with surface electrodes on the skin, the tibialis posterior is deeper and requires placement of a thin wire electrode in the muscle belly.

Dynamic EMG studies suggest that in one-third of children with hemiplegic cerebral palsy the tibialis anterior is responsible for the deformity, in one third the tibialis posterior is responsible, and in one third both the muscles contribute to the deformity.[10]

In the absence of dynamic EMG, indications for the split tibialis anterior tendon transfer have been based on observational gait analysis and the confusion test. The confusion test (flexor withdrawal test) is performed by asking the patient to flex the hip against resistance, and is positive when the ankle dorsiflexes during this manoeuvre (Figure 51.4).[11]

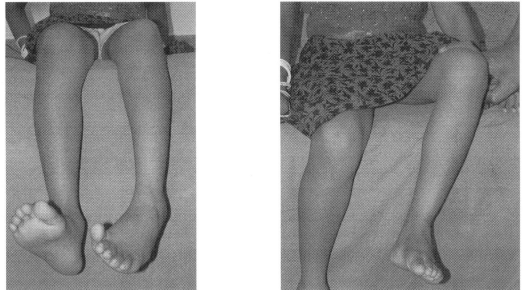

(A)   (B)

Figure 51.4 The confusion test: The child attempts to dorsiflex her ankles. The left ankle does not dorsiflex (A); when she flexes her left hip against resistance, the ankle dorsiflexes (B). (Reproduced from *Paediatric Orthopaedics—A system of decision-making* 2nd Edition.)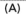

A positive confusion test indicates that the tibialis anterior is not paralysed and that dorsiflexion is possible.[11] Some surgeons consider a positive test as an indication to transfer the tibialis anterior. However, it is important to be aware that a positive confusion test does not predict how the muscle will behave during the swing phase of gait.[11]

Clinical indications for a split tibialis anterior tendon transfer with lengthening of tibialis posterior as done in this child (also referred to as the Rancho procedure) include:

- Hindfoot varus with forefoot adduction in both swing and stance phases of gait,
- Functioning tibialis anterior muscle defined by voluntary power or a positive confusion test.[5]

However, Michlitsch et al. suggest that the presence of hindfoot varus during different phases of gait was not an accurate predictor of which muscle was responsible for dynamic equinovarus deformity.[10]

Although many patients may need to continue with an AFO over the long term following this procedure, a subset are able to become brace-free as in this case. It is likely that after the range of passive dorsiflexion was restored, with therapy and hard work her pretibial muscles were strengthened sufficiently to facilitate clearance during swing phase. The child needs to be followed up till she is skeletally mature.

References

1. Chang CH, Albarracin JP, Lipton GE, Miller F. Long-term follow-up of surgery for equinovarus foot deformity in children with cerebral palsy. *J Pediatr Ortho*. 2002;22:792–9.
2. Hoffer MM, Reiswig JA, Garrett AM, Perry J. The split anterior tibial tendon transfer in the treatment of spastic varus hindfoot of childhood. *Orthop Clin North Am*. 1974;5:31–8.
3. Hoffer MM, Barakat G, Koffman M. 10-year follow-up of split anterior tibial tendon transfer in cerebral palsied patients with spastic equinovarus deformity. *J Pediatr Orthop*. 1985;5:432–4.
4. Sarıkaya İA, Birsel SE, Şeker A, Erdal OA, Görgün B, İnan M. The split transfer of tibialis anterior tendon to peroneus tertius tendon for equinovarus foot in children with cerebral palsy. *Acta Orthop Traumatol Turc*. 2020;54:262–8.
5. Barnes MJ, Herring JA. Combined split anterior tibial-tendon transfer and intramuscular lengthening of the posterior tibial tendon: Results in patients who have a varus deformity of the foot due to spastic cerebral palsy. *J Bone Joint Surg Am*. 1991;73:734–8.
6. Limpaphayom N, Chantarasongsuk B, Osateerakun P, Prasongchin P. The split anterior tibialis tendon transfer procedure for spastic equinovarus foot in children with cerebral palsy: Results and factors associated with a failed outcome. *Int Orthop*. 2015;39:1593–8.
7. Wu KW, Huang SC, Kuo KN, et al. The use of bioabsorbable screw in a split anterior tibial tendon transfer: A preliminary result. *J Pediatr Ortho B*. 2009;18:69–72.
8. Gasse N, Luth T, Loisel F, Serre A, Obert L, Parratte B, Lepage D. Fixation of split anterior tibialis tendon transfer by anchorage to the base of the 5th metatarsal bone. *Orthop Traumatol Surg Res*. 2012;98:829–33.
9. Perry J, Hoffer MM. Preoperative and postoperative dynamic electromyography as an aid in planning tendon transfers in children with cerebral palsy. *J Bone Joint Surg Am*. 1977;59:531–7.
10. Michlitsch MG, Rethlefsen SA, Kay RM. The contributions of anterior and posterior tibialis dysfunction to varus foot deformity in patients with cerebral palsy. *J Bone Joint Surg Am*. 2006;88:1764–8.
11. Davids JR, Holland WC, Sutherland DH. Significance of the confusion test in cerebral palsy. *J Pediatr Orthop*. 1993;13:717–21.

David A Spiegel

Case

A 12-year-old girl with spastic diplegia (GMFCS 3) presented complaining of progressive flexion and "rubbing together" of her knees with pain at the inferior pole of the patella. Her endurance had decreased. She was previously treated with injections of BOTOX to her adductors, gastrocnemius and hamstrings on two occasions, and also lengthening of her medial hamstrings with a non-selective recession of the gastrocnemius and soleus at the level of the mid-calf. She ambulated with forearm crutches most of the time but occasionally used a walker, and relied on a wheelchair for long distances. She was doing well in school and wished to return to her previous level of function without pain.

She had hyperreflexia and clonus, generalised lower extremity muscle weakness, poor distal motor control and poor balance when unsupported. She had mild spasticity in the gastrocnemius, rectus femoris and hamstrings. She had flexion contractures of the hips (20° right, 15° left), bilateral internal femoral torsion (80° medial rotation right, 70° medial rotation left), hamstring contractures with popliteal angles of 80° bilaterally, and fixed knee flexion deformities of 22° on the right and 27° on the left. She had no significant tibial torsion. On the Silfverskiold test, she had an isolated contracture of the gastrocnemius. Observational gait analysis demonstrated severe flexion of both knees with very limited joint excursion throughout the gait cycle, scissoring, flexion at the pelvis and hip, with a forward lean of the trunk (Figure 52.1, a–c). She made initial contact with the forefoot on the right, and with the midfoot on the left. Her right heel did not reach the ground while her left foot collapsed into planovalgus. Radiographs of her knees showed patella alta and stress fractures at the inferior pole of the patella (Figure 52.1, d, e).

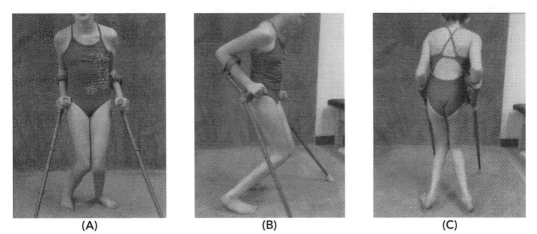

| (A) | (B) | (C) |

Figure 52.1 Standing images from the front (A), side (B) and back (C) taken from her gait video illustrate the position of her body segments during ambulation, with flexion of the hips and knees, with equinus at the ankles. Radiographs of the knees, right side illustrated here, demonstrate patella alta and a stress reaction/fracture at the inferior pole of the patella (D, E).

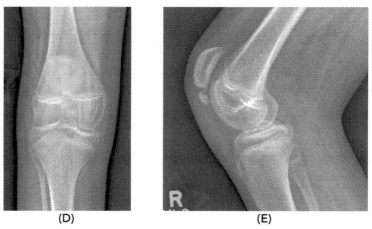

(D)   (E)

Figure 52.1 (Continued)

Questions

- What are the problems that need to be addressed in this girl?
- What are the aims of treatment?
- What are the commonly available options for treatment?
- What are the factors that may influence your choice of treatment?
- What treatment would you recommend for this girl?
- How long would you follow-up this girl after treatment?

The Problems That Need to Be Addressed Are
- Flexed-knee gait that has the propensity to progress
- Anterior knee pain
- In-toeing gait

She has both neurologic and musculoskeletal impairments at multiple levels contributing to the abnormal gait; the neurologic impairments which cannot be improved by orthopaedic intervention include:

- Increased muscle tone from spasticity
- Weakness
- Impaired selective motor control distally
- Abnormal balance

Musculoskeletal impairments that can be altered include:
- Internal femoral torsion
- Hamstring contracture
- Fixed knee flexion contracture
- Patella alta resulting in marked quadriceps insufficiency
- Ankle equinus on the right and equino-planovalgus on the left

The Aims of Treatment in This Girl Are to
- Improve the flexed knee gait and prevent progressive deterioration
- Improve the power of knee extension
- Eliminate anterior knee pain
- Eliminate the in-toeing gait and rubbing of the knees together
- Improve the base of support during ambulation

Options for Treatment of the Flexed Knee
- Physical therapy with or without dynamic splinting, serial casting[1,2]
- Soft tissue lengthening of hamstrings, posterior knee capsule[2,3]
- Guided growth of the distal femur (reversible anterior hemi-epiphyseodesis)[4]
- Distal femoral extension osteotomy (DFEO) with shortening[5-10]

Options for Improving Power of Knee Extension
- Patellar tendon plication
- Patellar tendon advancement

  - Bone block distal advancement
  - Soft tissue (tendon) advancement

FACTORS THAT INFLUENCED THE CHOICE OF TREATMENT
- Age of the girl
- Previous treatment
- Effects of specific surgical procedures
- Magnitude of deformity

The factors that influenced treatment are shown in Table 52.1.

Table 52.1 Factors That Influenced the Choice of Surgery

Factors		Treatment Implications
Age of the girl	12 years	Limited growth remaining, so less likely to respond to guided growth as a means to correct fixed flexion of the knee given magnitude of deformity and typical rate of correction around 1° per month. Recently completed growth spurt so less likely to have re-contracture.
Previous treatment	Already had hamstring recession	Revision hamstring lengthening likely to be ineffective.
Effects of specific surgical procedures	Hamstring lengthening	Hamstrings are important hip extensors in early stance, and overlengthening can result in anterior pelvic tilt which can increase crouch. Hamstrings do not usually need to be lengthened if performing a distal femoral shortening osteotomy.
	Posterior capsular release	Capsular release probably has greater risk of nerve stretch injury and relapse of deformity.
	Extension osteotomy	Extension osteotomy creates a deformity to treat a deformity, although this is rarely a clinically noticeable deformity; ideally, serial casts can be used to reduce contracture to 20° or less before osteotomy.
	Femoral shortening	Shortening of the femur reduces the risk of stretch of the sciatic nerve while correcting flexion deformity of the knee.
Magnitude	Severe deformity	Mild deformity may respond to serial casting. Severe deformities require serial casting and either guided growth or osteotomy, depending on correction achieved with casts and growth remaining.

How Was This Child Treated?

After induction of general anaesthesia, an epidural catheter was placed for post-operative analgesia. She was examined under anaesthesia as shown in Figure 52.2, and then she underwent single-event multiple lower extremity surgery (SEMLS), with the goal of addressing all of the relevant musculo-skeletal impairments under a single anaesthetic. Bilateral distal femoral extension osteotomies (with external rotation and shortening) with patellar ligament advancements, bilateral Strayer procedures (Gastrocnemius recession) and a lateral column lengthening on the left foot were performed.

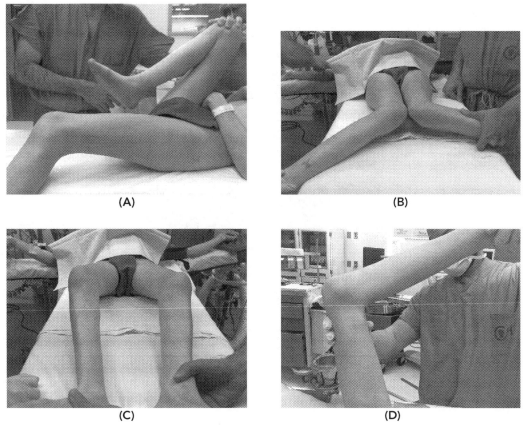

Figure 52.2 Selected physical findings on her exam under anaesthesia. She had minimal flexion contracture at the hip (A). On supine examination with her hip extended, one can see excessive medial rotation (B) and limited lateral rotation (C). Both her popliteal angle (D) and her degree of fixed knee flexion contracture (E) were similar to values measured preoperatively. Her ankle dorsiflexion was in an acceptable range when examined with her knee flexed (F), but less than neutral when the knee was extended (G).

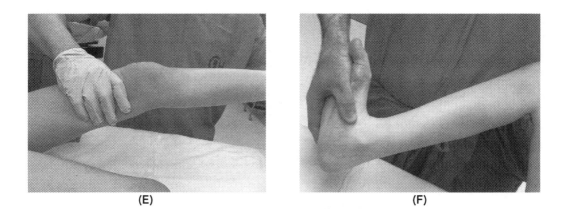

(E)　　　　　　　　　　　　　　　(F)

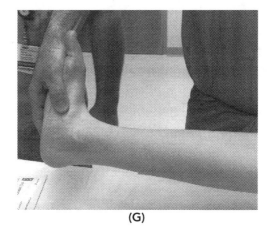

(G)

Figure 52.2 (Continued)

Post-Operative Management

She was placed in a posterior splint with her knees flexed 30° during the immediate post-operative period while limiting the degree of flexion at her hips to less than 50° to avoid a stretch injury to the sciatic nerve. The restrictions were relaxed once she was fully awake and the epidural catheter removed. She was seen in the outpatient clinic in a week to place long leg casts with her knees extended. She was admitted for inpatient rehabilitation after six weeks after radiographs revealed healing of the osteotomies and the patellar stress fractures (Figure 52.3).

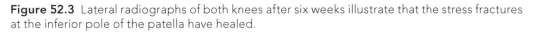

Figure 52.3 Lateral radiographs of both knees after six weeks illustrate that the stress fractures at the inferior pole of the patella have healed.

At three years follow-up, she ambulated at community level with forearm crutches and supra-malleolar orthoses (SMOs), with a neutral line of foot progression, a normal heel strike, fully extended knees during stance and much less flexion at the hips with minimal forward trunk lean. She had no knee pain. Her findings on bench examination at three years follow-up are shown in Figure 52.4, and these were maintained at more than seven years follow-up, at which time she was a college student. She still requires a wheelchair for long distances.

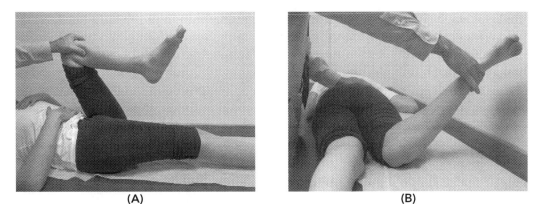

Figure 52.4 These clinical images were obtained at more than three years of follow-up. Her hip flexion contracture was less than at the time of her surgery (A). While we utilised a guidewire up the femoral neck to evaluate femoral version intraoperatively, she had slightly more internal versus external rotation on both sides (B-F), her trochanteric prominence test estimated about 20° of anteversion, shown here on the right side (D). On gait assessment, her patellae were facing towards the line of progression. Her popliteal angles were considerably improved despite not performing a hamstring lengthening (G), and her fixed knee flexion deformities remained well corrected (H). Her ankle dorsiflexion was just above neutral with the knees flexed and extended (I, J), indicating some mild residual equinus which was probably helpful given that she chose to walk with SMOs rather than AFOs. Prone exam suggested no tibial torsion (K).

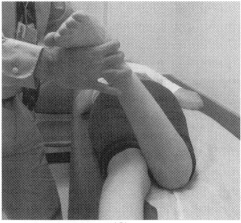

(C)

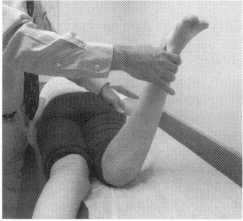

(D)

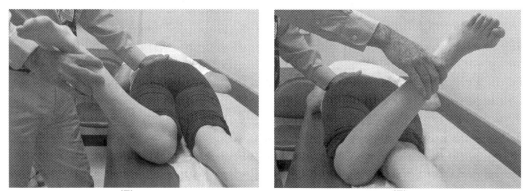

(E)

(F)

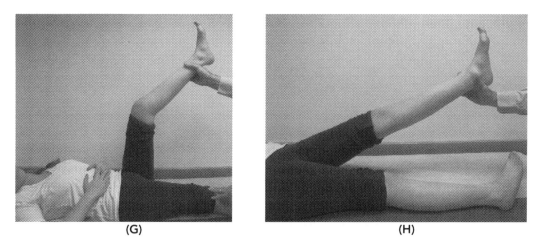

(G)

(H)

Figure 52.4 (Continued)

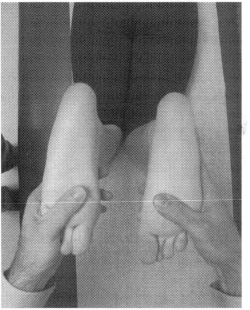

(I)　　　　　　　　　　　　　(J)

(K)

Figure 52.4 (Continued)

Comment

A flexed knee gait is often due to spasticity or contracture of the hamstrings with or without a fixed knee flexion contracture. Surgical care should be directed to the source of the loss of knee extension. The hamstrings are important hip extensors during early stance phase, and they decelerate knee extension during swing phase. Overlengthening the hamstrings may result in hip flexion and anterior pelvic tilt which, in turn, would require flexion at the knees as compensation. For this reason, only the medial hamstrings are lengthened in ambulators with hamstring contracture.

The knee flexion contracture can be addressed by serial stretch casting when mild. We utilise stretch casting for moderate to severe deformities with the goal of correcting the deformity to around −15 to −20° before osteotomy. We have no experience with posterior capsulotomy, but would anticipate that the risks of both nerve stretch injury and relapse would be higher than with osteotomy. Sciatic nerve injury is a risk with acute correction by capsulotomy or osteotomy.[3] Most authors perform a distal femoral extension osteotomy often with shortening,[3,5–9] and others have reported adequate correction with a shortening osteotomy alone.[10] An increase in anterior pelvic tilt (4–10°) is a common finding after osteotomy[7,8,10] even when an intramuscular lengthening of the iliopsoas was performed concomitantly.[8]

An important component of the distal femoral extension osteotomy procedure involves re-tensioning the extensor mechanism by patellar ligament advancement or plication.[9]

Children who undergo treatment for a flexed knee gait must be followed to adulthood.

References

1. Westberry DE, Davids JR, Jacobs JM, et al. Effectiveness of serial stretch casting for resistant or recurrent knee flexion contractures following hamstring lengthening in cerebral palsy. *J Pediatr Ortho.* 2006;26:109–14.
2. Long JT, Cobb L, Garcia MC, McCarthy JJ. Improved clinical and functional outcomes in crouch gait following minimally invasive hamstring lengthening and serial casting in children with cerebral palsy. *J Pediatr Orthop.* 2020;40:e510–15.
3. Taylor D, Connor J, Church C, Lennon N, Henley J, Niiler T, Miller F. The effectiveness of posterior knee capsulotomies and knee extension osteotomies in crouched gait in children with cerebral palsy. *J Pediatr Orthop B.* 2016;25:543–50.
4. Long JT, Laron D, Garcia MC, McCarthy JJ. Screw anterior distal femoral hemiepiphysiodesis in children with cerebral palsy and knee flexion contractures: A retrospective case-control study. *J Pediatr Orthop.* 2020;40:e873–9.
5. Stout JL, Gage JR, Schwartz MH, Novacheck TF. Distal femoral extension osteotomy and patellar tendon advancement to treat persistent crouch gait in cerebral palsy. *J Bone Joint Surg Am.* 2008;90:2470–84.
6. Boyer ER, Stout JL, Laine JC, Gutknecht SM, Araujo de Oliveira LH, Munger ME, Schwartz MH, Novacheck TF. Long-term outcomes of distal femoral extension osteotomy and patellar tendon advancement in individuals with cerebral palsy. *J Bone Joint Surg Am.* 2018;100:31–41.
7. Klotz MCM, Hirsch K, Heitzmann D, Maier MW, Hagmann S, Dreher T. Distal femoral extension and shortening osteotomy as a part of multilevel surgery in children with cerebral palsy. *World J Pediatr.* 2017;13:353–9.
8. de Morais Filho MC, Blumetti FC, Kawamura CM, Leite JBR, Lopes JAF, Fujino MH, Neves DL. The increase of anterior pelvic tilt after crouch gait treatment in patients with cerebral palsy. *Gait & Posture.* 2018;63:165–70.
9. Sossai R, Vavken P, Brunner R, Camathias C, Graham HK, Rutz E. Patellar tendon shortening for flexed knee gait in spastic diplegia. *Gait Posture.* 2015;41:658–65.
10. Park H, Park BK, Park KB, Abdel-Baki SW, Rhee I, Kim CW, Kim HW. Distal femoral shortening osteotomy for severe knee flexion contracture and crouch gait in cerebral palsy. *J Clin Med.* 2019;8:1354.

David A Spiegel

Case

An 8-year-old boy with a history of spastic triplegia presented with progressive gait disturbance and loss of endurance. He had previously been treated with physical therapy, serial casting, and BOTOX injections. He used a hinged ankle-foot orthosis and required a posterior walker for support, and at night he wore dynamic knee extension orthoses. Despite all of this, he developed progressive knee flexion and walked on his toes. He had occasional anterior knee pain, and got tired very quickly. While he had functioned at the GMFCS 3 level previously, his function had deteriorated to GMFCS 4.

On observational gait analysis with a rear walker, he walked with flexion at both the hips and the knees throughout the gait cycle, with minimal excursion at these joints (Figure 53.1). He was up on his toes and had toe-drag during swing phase, and mild scissoring. He had a neutral progression angle.

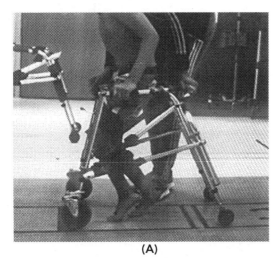
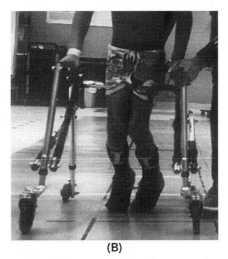

(A)   (B)

Figure 53.1 A snapshot of this patient's gait from the side (A) and front (B). He has flexion at the hips and knees throughout the gait cycle, and is also in equinus. He has very mild scissoring, left greater than right.

On bench examination, he had 10° passive hip abduction on the right and 15° on the left and hip flexion contractures of 20° on the left and 30° on the right (Figure 53.2). Hip rotation was approximately 70° medial and 20° lateral bilaterally. His popliteal angles were 60° bilaterally with fixed knee flexion contractures of 20°. His feet dorsiflexed about 10° degrees beyond neutral with his knees flexed, and 10° short of neutral with his knees extended. There was bilateral patella alta. He had elevated muscle tone in his adductors, hamstrings, and gastrocnemius-soleus. He had poor selective motor control and had generalised weakness of both lower extremities.

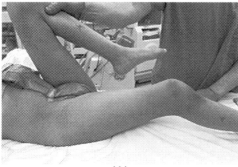

(A)

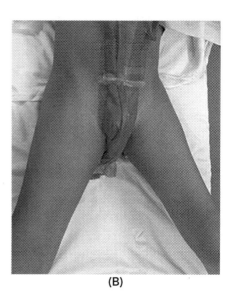

(B)

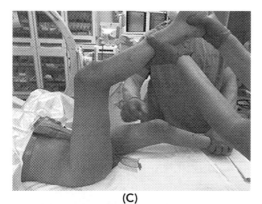

(C)

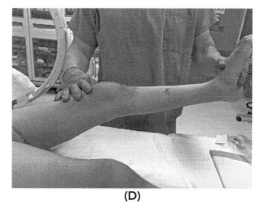

(D)

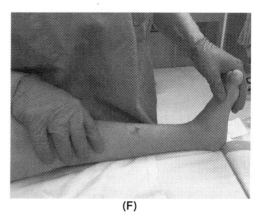

(E)

(F)

Figure 53.2 Bench examination while under anaesthesia at the time of surgery. Both hips had a flexion contracture measured at approximately 30° (A), with passive abduction of approximately 15° bilaterally (B), popliteal angles of approximately 60°, fixed knee flexion deformities of approximately 20° (C), and his feet dorsiflexed 10° with the knee flexed and −10° with the knee extended.

Questions

- What are the problems that need to be addressed in this boy?
- What are the aims of treatment?
- What are the commonly available options for treatment?
- What are the factors that may influence your choice of treatment?
- What treatment would you recommend for this boy?
- How long would you follow-up this boy after treatment?

The Problems That Need to Be Addressed Are

- He has both neurologic and musculoskeletal impairments at multiple levels.
- Neurologic impairments beyond the scope of orthopaedic intervention

    o Elevated muscle tone
    o Significant underlying muscle weakness
    o Lack of selective motor control
    o Problems with balance

- Musculoskeletal impairments

    o ***Bilateral hip flexion contractures***
    o Bilateral hip adduction contracture
    o Bilateral hamstring contracture
    o Bilateral fixed knee flexion contracture
    o Bilateral patella alta with incompetent quadriceps
    o Bilateral internal femoral torsion (mild)

The Aims of Treatment in This Boy Were to

- Correct the orthopaedic impairments with the hope of restoring his previous level of function as a limited ambulator with an assistive device.
- Address all of the musculoskeletal impairments under a single anaesthetic

Options for Treatment for the Hip Flexion Contracture

- Physical therapy
- Soft tissue lengthening or release of the iliopsoas tendon
- Extension osteotomy of the proximal femur

FACTORS THAT INFLUENCED THE CHOICE OF TREATMENT

- Deterioration in gait
- Need to address flexion deformities at the knee
- Loss of hip extension during stance phase of gait
- Severity of hip flexion contracture

The choice of treatment based on these factors is shown in Table 53.1.

Table 53.1 Choice of Treatment Based on Factors Influencing Treatment of Flexion Deformity in This Boy with Cerebral Palsy

Factors		Treatment Implications
Deterioration in gait	Deterioration has been observed	Intervention at this point to reverse some impairments and prevent further deterioration of ambulatory ability is justified.
Need to address flexion deformity of the knee	Knee deformity is significant and requires correction	The strategies to get the knee straight may result in an increase in anterior pelvic tilt, as the hamstrings will be weakened and bring the centre of gravity forward. Reducing the hip flexion contracture should help to mitigate these concerns and improve muscle balance at the hip.
Loss of hip extension during stance phase of gait	Fixed flexion contractures of the hips are present	Lengthening of the iliopsoas tendons is required as there are myostatic contractures. The downstream problems, including knee flexion and ankle equinus, also need to be addressed as they contribute to the flexed posture of the hips.
Severity of hip flexion contracture	Moderately severe deformity (20° and 30° respectively)	Lengthening of the iliopsoas should suffice.
Ambulatory status of the boy	Household ambulator	In an ambulant, the iliopsoas is released at the pelvic brim, while in non-ambulant children the iliopsoas tendon may be released from the lesser trochanter.

How Was This Boy Treated?

The boy was treated by serial casting at the knee. Long leg casts in maximum knee extension were applied and wedged a week later (Figure 53.3), and a new cast was applied the second week. The knee flexion deformities improved to approximately 15–20°.

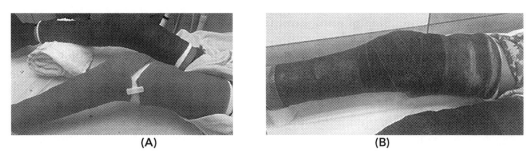

(A)   **(B)**

Figure 53.3 The fixed knee flexion contracture was addressed partially with serial casting, which involved placing a cast one week, wedging it the second week (A), and then replacing it

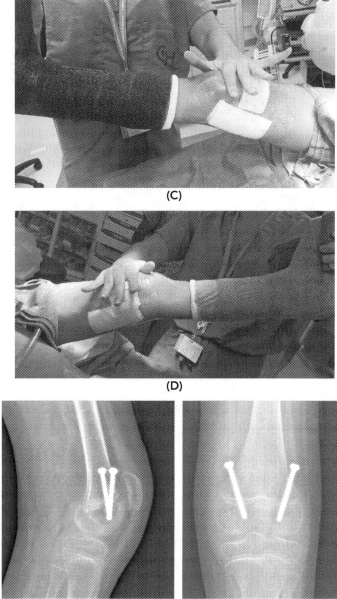

Figure 53.3 (Continued) the third week. The contractures improved more than 30° by the time of surgery, and after the hamstring lengthening the final fixed flexion deformity was in the range of 10–15° (C, D). The remaining correction will be achieved by physical therapy and guided growth of the distal femur (E, F) which essentially creates a mild deformity to treat loss of flexion. Options include placing a plate and screws across the anterior physis on both sides of the joint, and more recently cannulated screws have been utilised. The correction typically occurs at a degree or so per month.

In addition to the iliopsoas recession at the pelvic brim (Figure 53.4), he underwent bilateral adductor tenotomy, bilateral medial hamstring recession (semitendinosus and gracilis), bilateral anterior distal femoral hemi-epiphyseodesis using screws, and bilateral gastrocnemius recession (Strayer procedure).

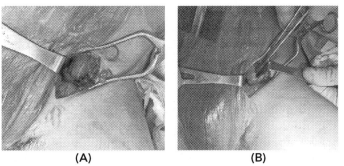

(A)   **(B)**

Figure 53.4 The intramuscular psoas lengthening is performed via the middle window of the ilio-inguinal approach (a, b). In 53.4a, the arrow on the left side just below the medial aspect of the incision overlies the femoral artery which was identified by palpation, while the circle just superior and lateral to the incision is drawn over the anterior superior iliac spine (ASIS). After opening the deep fascia, one can see the femoral nerve lying on the anterior aspect of the muscle. The nerve can be isolated and retracted laterally (b), and the underlying psoas tendon can be isolated and released from within the substance of the muscle.

Post-Operative Management

He was placed in bilateral short-leg walking casts and knee immobilisers, and was allowed to bear weight immediately. Therapy was started and included four hours a day of prone lying, as well as stretching of his adductors, hamstrings, and hip flexors. His casts were replaced with AFOs after six weeks, and we chose to utilise a ground reaction or anti-crouch brace initially, with the aim of graduating to an AFO with an ADR hinge later. The adjustable dynamic response (ADR) hinge permitted tensioning to allow fine tuning of the degree of dorsiflexion. At follow-up of more than a year, the hip flexion contractures were well corrected without signs of relapse.

Comment

Loss of hip extension during the stance phase of gait may impair forward progression of the limb. A flexed hip also contributes to internal rotation of the limb during swing due to enhanced mechanical advantage of the internal rotators of the hip when the hip is in flexion.

The indications for lengthening of the iliopsoas complex remain debated; Sutherland et al suggested "excessive anterior pelvic tilt and excessive dynamic hip flexion or hip-flexion contracture"[1,2] as indications for release, while Mallet et al suggested a hip flexion contracture of > 20°.[3]

Different techniques for lengthening of the iliopsoas complex have been reported.[1,2–4,6–8] Bleck emphasised that releasing the iliopsoas at the lesser trochanter would result in significant weakness which can impair the ability to propel the limb forward and especially for activities like climbing stairs, and recommended a recession in which the iliacus muscle and the iliopsoas tendon were cut at the level of the femoral neck and sutured each down proximally to the anterior hip capsule.[7] Our preferred technique is similar to that of Sutherland et al, but it slightly more proximal and exploits through the middle window of the ilio-inguinal approach, incising the deep fascia above the inguinal ligament.[9] The incision lies between the ASIS and the pubic tubercle, and stops just lateral to where the femoral artery is palpated. The deep dissection first goes through the fascia of the external oblique aponeurosis and then a second fascial layer of the internal oblique and transversus abdominis muscles, leaving a cuff of tissue for later repair. Avoid injuring the lateral femoral cutaneous nerve, which is often 1–2 cm medial to the ASIS. The femoral nerve is then in direct view, and can be mobilised and protected. Medially one can palpate the ilio-pectineal fascia and the femoral vessels contained within. The psoas tendon may then be identified and released.

The results of lengthening the iliopsoas per se is difficult to confirm as this procedure is typically performed in concert with a host of other procedures as part of a single-event multiple lower extremity surgery (SEMLS).[1,2–4,6–8]

References

1. Skaggs DL, Kaminsky CK, Eskander-Rickards E, Reynolds RA, Tolo VT, Bassett GS. Psoas over the brim lengthenings: Anatomic investigation and surgical technique. *Clin Orthop Relat Res.* 1997;339:174–9.
2. Sutherland DH, Zilberfarb JL, Kaufman KR, Wyatt MP, Chambers HG. Psoas release at the pelvic brim in ambulatory patients with cerebral palsy: Operative technique and functional outcome. *J Pediatr Orthop.* 1997;17:563–70.
3. Mallet C, Simon AL, Ilharreborde B, Presedo A, Mazda K, Penneçot GF. Intramuscular psoas lengthening during single-event multi-level surgery fails to improve hip dynamics in children with spastic diplegia: Clinical and kinematic outcomes in the short- and medium-terms. *Orthop Traumatol Surg Res.* 2016;102:501–6.
4. Morais Filho MC, de Godoy W, Santos CA. Effects of intramuscular psoas lengthening on pelvic and hip motion in patients with spastic diparetic cerebral palsy. *J Pediatr Orthop.* 2006;26:260–4.
5. Novacheck TF, Trost JP, Schwartz MH. Intramuscular psoas lengthening improves dynamic hip function in children with cerebral palsy. *J Pediatr Orthop.* 2002;22:158–64.
6. Rethlefsen SA, Lening C, Wren TA, Kay RM. Excessive hip flexion during gait in patients with static encephalopathy: An examination of contributing factors. *J Pediatr Orthop.* 2010;30:562–7.
7. Bleck EE. Postural and gait abnormalities caused by hip-flexion deformity in spastic cerebral palsy: Treatment by iliopsoas recession. *J Bone Joint Surg Am.* 1971;53:1468–88.
8. Bialik GM, Pierce R, Dorociak R, Lee TS, Aiona MD, Sussman MD. Iliopsoas tenotomy at the lesser trochanter versus at the pelvic brim in ambulatory children with cerebral palsy. *J Pediatr Orthop.* 2009;29:251–5.
9. Gittings DG, Dattilo JR, Fryhofer G, Donegan DJ, Baldwin KD. Treatment of hip flexion contractures with psoas recession through the middle window of the ilioinguinal approach. *J Bone Joint Surg Am.* 2017;7:e25:1–7.

Hitesh Shah and Benjamin Joseph

Case

A 10-year-old girl presented with difficulty using her right hand. She was unable to hold objects or write with her right hand. She had right-sided hemiplegic cerebral palsy and had been on regular physiotherapy. She was a bright child with an IQ of 110. She attended mainstream school, and she was coping well with her studies.

Her forearm was pronated, and the wrist was flexed and ulnar deviated (Figure 54.1). Spasticity was noted in the pronator teres, finger flexors and flexor carpi ulnaris. There were no fixed contractures of muscles of the wrist and hand; the deformities could be fully corrected passively. The supinator of the forearm and the extensors of the wrist were weak. The grasp of the right hand was achieved awkwardly with the wrist flexed (Figure 54.2a), and the grip strength was very poor. The release was good with the wrist in flexion (Figure 54.2b). When the wrist was held in dorsiflexion, the grasp of the right hand improved, as did the grip strength. When the wrist was stabilised in 10 degrees of dorsiflexion, she had no problem with release as all her fingers extended fully (Figure 54.3). The fine sensation of the hand was intact with two-point discrimination of less than 10 mm.

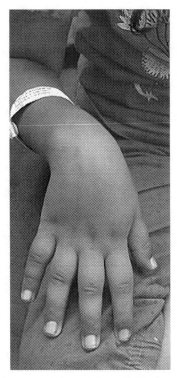

Figure 54.1 The right forearm is pronated, and the wrist is flexed and ulnar-deviated.

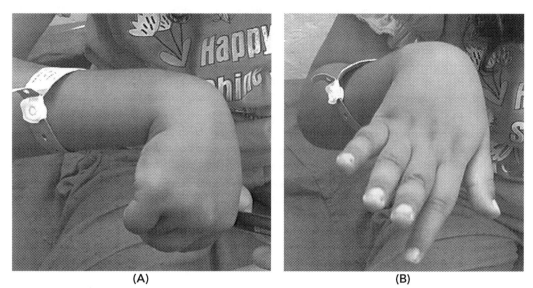

(A)   **(B)**

Figure 54.2 The child could grasp only with the wrist flexed (A), and she released also with the wrist in flexion (B).

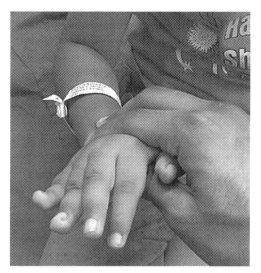

Figure 54.3 The child could release the fingers well with the wrist being held in 10 degrees of extension.

Questions

- What are the problems that need to be addressed?
- What are the aims of treatment?
- What are the available treatment options to fulfil these aims?
- What are the factors that may influence your choice of treatment?
- Based on these points, what treatment would you recommend for this child?
- How long would you follow-up this child after treatment?

The Problems That Need to Be Addressed Are

- Weak grasp
- Deformities of the forearm and wrist
    - Pronation of the forearm
    - Flexion and ulnar deviation of wrist

The Aims of Treatment in This Child Are to

- Improve grasp
- Correct deformities of the forearm and hand

Options for Treatment to Fulfil Each Aim

- Improving grasp
    - Improve the power of wrist extension
        - Tendon transfer to wrist extensors (extensor carpi radialis longus and brevis—ECRL and ECRB)
    - Weaken the power of wrist flexion
        - Release or transfer of the flexor carpi ulnaris (FCU), the main deforming force
- Correcting pronation of the forearm
    - Pronator release
    - FCU transfer to ECRB around the medial border of the ulna[1,2,3]
- Correcting wrist flexion and ulnar deviation
    - Release or transfer of FCU

FACTORS THAT INFLUENCED THE CHOICE OF TREATMENT

- Age of the patient
- Presence of contractures
- Ability of the child to grasp and release
- Intelligence of the child
- Ability to release the fingers with the wrist held in dorsiflexion
- Sensation on the palm and fingers

The choice of treatment based on these factors is outlined in Table 54.1.

Table 54.1 Factors Influencing the Choice of Treatment

Factors		Treatment Implications
Age of the child	10 years	She is old enough to co-operate during post-operative rehabilitation and tendon re-education. Treatment must not be delayed as myostatic contractures of the spastic muscles are likely to develop.
Presence of contractures	No contractures	It is appropriate to proceed with a tendon transfer without any soft tissue release.

(Continued)

Table 54.1 (Continued)

Factors		Treatment Implications
Ability of the child to grasp and release	She can grasp and release though in an awkward fashion	Functional improvement can be anticipated following treatment if the child already has the ability to grasp and release.
Intelligence of the child	Intelligent child	She should be able to co-operate with rehabilitation following a tendon transfer.
Ability to release with the wrist held in dorsiflexion	Good release possible	Transfer of the FCU to ECRB is only indicated in children who have no problem with release when the wrist is held in dorsiflexion.[1]
Sensation on the palm and fingers	Less than 10 mm two-point discrimination	Functional improvement is more likely in children who have normal sensation with two-point discrimination <10 mm.[4]

How Was This Child Treated?

She was treated with transfer of the flexor carpi ulnaris to the extensor carpi radialis brevis and longus. Through a long incision on the medial aspect of the forearm, extending proximally from the pisiform bone, the FCU tendon and the ulnar neurovascular bundle were identified.

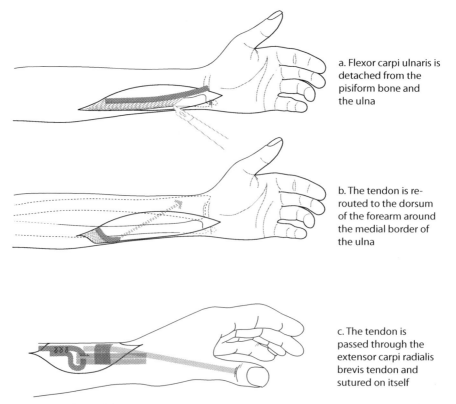

a. Flexor carpi ulnaris is detached from the pisiform bone and the ulna

b. The tendon is re-routed to the dorsum of the forearm around the medial border of the ulna

c. The tendon is passed through the extensor carpi radialis brevis tendon and sutured on itself

Figure 54.4 Diagrammatic representation of FCU transfer to the wrist extensors. (Adapted from Figure 65.4, Paediatric Orthopaedics - A system of decision-Making.)

The neurovascular bundle was protected and retracted. The FCU tendon was detached from its insertion to the pisiform bone, and the muscle fibres of the FCU taking origin from the distal half of the ulna were carefully released. A short incision was made over the dorsum of the wrist just lateral to Lister's tubercle. The ECRB and ECRL were identified by demonstrating extension of the wrist when the tendons were pulled up with a blunt hook. A tendon tunneller was passed from the second wound around the medial border of the ulna through a liberal longitudinal slit made in the medial intermuscular septum, and the free end of the FCU tendon was grasped and withdrawn into the dorsal wound. The forearm was held in supination and the wrist in extension, and the FCU tendon was passed through the ECRB and the ECRL tendons and sutured to itself under tension (Figure 54.4).

An above-elbow plaster-of-Paris cast was applied with 90 degrees elbow flexion, the forearm in the mid-prone position and 10 degrees dorsiflexion of the wrist. The cast was removed after six weeks, and muscle re-education exercises were started. The hand function improved. Three years after the surgery, the deformities remain well corrected, grasp has improved quite dramatically (Figure 54.5), and the child now uses the hand for bi-manual activity. Both the child and the parents are very pleased with the outcome.

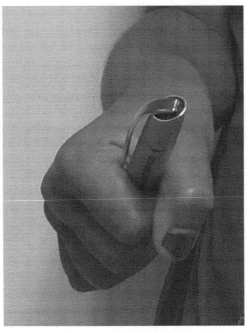

Figure 54.5 At final follow-up, the child demonstrates normal grasp with the forearm in mid-pronation.

Follow-Up

The child will be followed-up till skeletal maturity to make sure that the correction is maintained.

Comment

The FCU is a muscle that normally functions during wrist flexion and release. The FCU transfer to the ECRB is to augment ECRB and improve grasp; this should ideally involve phase conversion of the transferred muscle. However, EMG video analysis has demonstrated that phase conversion seldom occurs following this transfer despite good clinical results.[5]

A proportion of children may develop late deformities particularly following a growth spurt when growth of the transferred muscle-tendon unit does not keep pace with skeletal growth.[6] This mandates careful follow-up of children who have undergone this operation till they reach skeletal maturity.

Since cerebral palsy is characterised predominantly by motor deficits, it is often assumed that sensory deficits do not occur in cerebral palsy. Subtle deficits of fine sensations may be present in these children, which include poor stereognosis, poor recognition of texture and increase in two-point discrimination. Functional results following tendon transfers in the upper limb in cerebral palsy may be poor in children with >10 mm two-point discrimination.[4]

References

1. Thometz JG, Tachdjian M. Long-term follow-up of the flexor carpi ulnaris transfer in spastic hemiplegic children. *J Pediatr Orthop*. 1988 Jul–Aug;8(4):407–12. doi: 10.1097/01241398-198807000-00005. PMID: 3392191.
2. Bansal A, Wall LB, Goldfarb CA. Cerebral palsy tendon transfers: Flexor carpi ulnaris to extensor carpi radialis brevis and extensor pollicis longus reroutement. *Hand Clin*. 2016 Aug;32(3):423–30. doi: 10.1016/j.hcl.2016.03.010. Epub 2016 May 21. PMID: 27387086.
3. Wolf TM, Clinkscales CM, Hamlin C. Flexor carpi ulnaris tendon transfers in cerebral palsy. *J Hand Surg Br*. 1998 Jun;23(3):340–3. doi: 10.1016/s0266-7681(98)80054-5. PMID: 9665522.
4. Goldner JL, Ferlic DC. Sensory status of the hand as related to reconstructive surgery of the upper extremity in cerebral palsy. *Clin Orthop Relat Res*. 1966 May–Jun;46:87–92. PMID: 5915119.
5. Van Heest A, Stout J, Wervey R, Garcia L. Follow-up motion laboratory analysis for patients with spastic hemiplegia due to cerebral palsy: Analysis of the flexor carpi ulnaris firing pattern before and after tendon transfer surgery. *J Hand Surg Am*. 2010 Feb;35(2):284–90. doi: 10.1016/j.jhsa.2009.10.004. Epub 2009 Dec 22. PMID: 20022711.
6. Patterson JM, Wang AA, Hutchinson DT. Late deformities following the transfer of the flexor carpi ulnaris to the extensor carpi radialis brevis in children with cerebral palsy. *J Hand Surg Am*. 2010 Nov;35(11):1774–8. doi: 10.1016/j.jhsa.2010.07.014. PMID: 20888146.

EPIPHYSEAL AND PHYSEAL PROBLEMS

Randall T Loder

Case

A 4 year-1-month-old girl presented with progressive bowlegs. There was minimal pain. There were no clinical or radiologic features of rickets, and her stature and body proportions were normal. She was obese and resented contact during physical examination. A standing anteroposterior radiograph showed features of bilateral infantile tibia vara, Langenskiöld stage II on the left and stage III on the right (Figure 55.1).[1,2]

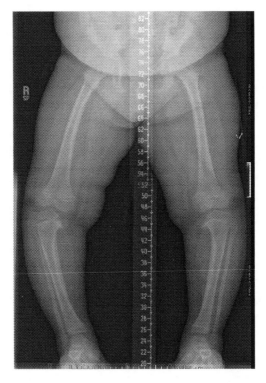

Figure 55.1 Anteroposterior radiograph demonstrating changes in the proximal tibia bilaterally suggestive of infantile tibia vara, Langenskiöld stage II on the left and stage III on the right. There are no features suggestive of metabolic bone disease or skeletal dysplasia.

Questions

- What are the problems that need to be addressed in this girl?
- What are the aims of treatment?
- What are the available treatment options to fulfil these aims?
- What are the factors that may influence your choice of treatment?
- Based on these points, what treatment would you recommend for this child?
- How long would you follow-up this child after treatment?

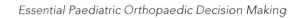

The Problems That Need to Be Addressed Are

- Progressive varus deformity of the proximal tibia of both lower limbs
- Risk of complications

  o Recurrence of deformity
  o Premature fusion of the medial aspect of the proximal tibial physis
  o Limb length inequality

The Aims of Treatment Are to

- Correct the varus deformity
- Watch for complications (namely, recurrence of the deformity, leg length inequality, and premature proximal tibial physeal closure)

The Available Treatment Options Are

- Guided growth
- Proximal tibial and fibular osteotomy with:

  o Percutaneous cross pin fixation
  o External fixation
  o Rigid internal fixation

FACTORS THAT INFLUENCED THE CHOICE OF TREATMENT

The factors that influenced the choice of treatment of the tibia vara were

- Age of the child
- The stage of the disease (Langenskiöld stage)
- The severity of the deformity
- Potential complications of the procedure being planned
- Social interaction of the child and likelihood of co-operation with the treating team
- Body habitus of the child

The choice of treatment based on these factors is shown in Table 55.1.

Table 55.1 Factors Influencing the Choice of Treatment

Factors		Treatment Implications
Age of the child	4 years	At this age, it is reasonable to try a guided growth procedure (using tension band '8' plate and screws).[3,4]
Langenskiöld stage	Stage II and III	An osteotomy of the proximal tibia is justified if guided growth fails.[5,6]
The severity of the deformity	Not severe	At this point, the deformity is amenable to a simple less invasive option like guided growth.[3]
Potential complications of the procedure being planned	Compartment syndrome	Guided growth is much less invasive and carries a lower risk of complications (especially compartment syndrome) than formal proximal tibial osteotomy.[1-4]

(Continued)

Table 55.1 (Continued)

Factors		Treatment Implications
Social interaction of the child	Unlikely to co-operate as she resents examination by the surgeon	External fixation is undesirable if the child is uncooperative.[7]
Body habitus of the child	Obese	The risk of pin tract infection following cross pinning or external fixation is greater in obese children. The body habitus made cross pin fixation of the deformity less desirable.

How Was This Child Treated?

- Initially, guided growth (temporary proximal lateral tibial hemiepiphyseodesis) with an '8' plate and screws was performed.
- The parents were unhappy that the deformity had not corrected completely after four months and were keen to obtain a more definitive correction. So, tibial and fibular osteotomy with internal fixation was performed at age 4 years 6 months (Figure 55.2) with intentional mild overcorrection. Prophylactic anterior compartment fasciotomy was performed at the same time.

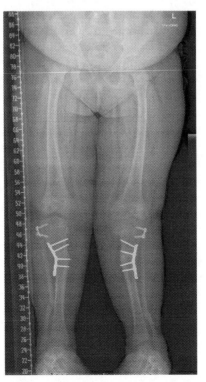

Figure 55.2 At age 4 years 11 months, five months after bilateral tibial and fibular osteotomies.

- The guided growth devices were subsequently removed, and at age 9 years 2 months there was slight persistent overcorrection on the left but excellent alignment on the right (Figure 55.3).

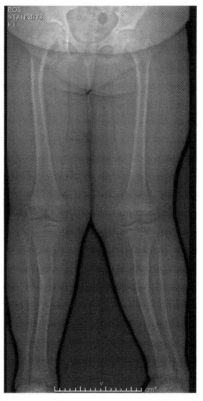

Figure 55.3 Standing AP radiograph of the lower extremities at 9 years 2 months of age. Note the excellent remodelling and filling in of the Blount's lesion of both proximal medial tibial epiphyses.

Though advised to report periodically for follow-up, the parents did not bring the child till she was 13 years 8 months old. The child had some right peripatellar knee pain, but no joint line pain. The parents were not concerned about any deformity. Final radiographs at skeletal maturity (Figure 55.4) demonstrate slight varus recurrence on the right and slight residual valgus overcorrection on the left.

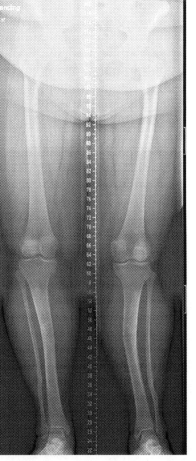

Figure 55.4 Final radiograph at 13 and ½ years of age. Note complete physeal closure, with slight varus on the right and valgus on the left.

How Long Should the Child Be Followed Up after Treatment?

- Follow-up until skeletal maturity as done in this child is necessary to monitor for

  - Recurrence or overcorrection of the deformity[8]
  - Premature proximal medial tibial physeal closure[2]
  - Leg length inequality[2]

References

1. Greene WB. Infantile tibia vara. *J Bone Joint Surg [Am]*. 1993;75-A(1):130–43.
2. Birch JG. Blount disease. *J Am Acad Orthop Surg*. 2013;21(7):408–18.
3. Heflin JA, Ford S, Stevens P. Guided growth for tibia vara (Blount's disease). *Medicine*. 2016;95(41): e4951(1–7).
4. Sabharwal S, Sabharwal S. Treatment of infantile Blount disease: An update. *J Pediatr Orthop*. 2019;37(6 S2):S26–31.
5. Loder RT, Johnston II CE. Infantile tibia vara. *J Pediatr Orthop*. 1987;7:639–46.
6. Schoenecker PL, Meade WC, Pierron RL, Sheridan JJ, Capelli AM. Blount's disease: A retrospective review and recommendations for treatment. *J Pediatr Orthop*. 1985;5:181–6.

7. Richard HM, Nguyen DC, Birch JG, Roland SD, Samchukov MK, Cherkashin AM. Clinical implications of psychosocial factors on pediatric external fixation treatment and recommendations. *Clin Orthop.* 2015;473(10):3154–62.

8. LaMont LE, McIntosh AL, Jo CH, Birch JG, Johnston CE. Recurrence after surgical intervention for infantile tibia vara: Assessment of a new modified classification. *J Pediatr Orthop.* 2019;39(2):65–70.

Benjamin Joseph and Hitesh Shah

Case

A 6.8-year-old boy presented with pain in the left groin and a limp for two months. There was no history of trauma, fever or constitutional symptoms preceding the onset of pain. On examination, he had restriction of abduction and internal rotation of the left hip joint; other movements were comparable to the opposite hip. The systemic examination was normal. An antero-posterior (AP) radiograph of the pelvis showed features of early Perthes disease of the left hip. The entire epiphysis was flattened and sclerotic. There was no evidence of fragmentation in both AP and Lauenstein lateral views, indicating that the disease was still in the latter part of the stage of avascular necrosis (Stage Ib—Modified Waldenstrom classification[1]). The medial joint space was widened, and extrusion of the femoral head was present (Figure 56.1).

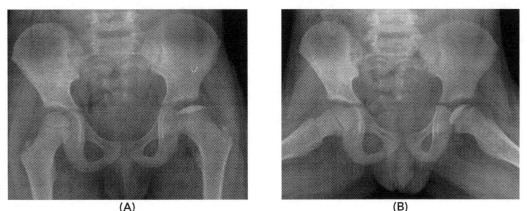

(A)   (B)

Figure 56.1 AP and Lauenstein frog-lateral radiographs of the pelvis showing sclerosis and flattening of the entire femoral epiphysis of the left hip. The medial joint space is widened, and there is extrusion of the femoral head. There is no fragmentation of the femoral epiphysis.

Questions

- What are the problems that need to be addressed?
- What are the aims of treatment?
- What are the available treatment options to fulfil these aims?
- What are the factors that may influence your choice of treatment?
- Based on these points, what treatment would you recommend for this child?
- How long would you follow-up this child after treatment?

The Problems That Need to Be Addressed Are

- Restriction of motion of the hip
- Risk of irreversible deformation of the femoral head because of:

  o Complete involvement of the femoral epiphysis
  o Extrusion of the femoral head outside the margin of the acetabulum

- Risk of premature fusion of the femoral capital growth plate and overgrowth of the greater trochanter because of complete involvement of the femoral epiphysis

The Aims of Treatment in This Boy Are to

- Restore normal motion of the hip
- Prevent deformation of the femoral head (i.e. retain the spherical shape of the femoral head and minimise enlargement of the femoral head)
- Prevent trochanteric overgrowth

Options for Treatment to Fulfil Each Aim

- To gain range of motion:

  o Physiotherapy
  o Above-knee skin traction
  o Petrie cast (abduction "broomstick" cast)
  o Soft tissue release (adductor release, medial capsulotomy)

- To prevent deformation of the femoral head:

  o Achieve containment of the femoral head by any one of the following methods:

    □ Abduction cast/brace (A-frame orthosis)[2]
    □ Femoral varus derotation osteotomy[3]
    □ Pelvic osteotomy (Salter, Triple, Shelf)[4–6]

- To prevent trochanteric overgrowth

  o Trochanteric epiphyseodesis

FACTORS THAT INFLUENCED THE CHOICE OF TREATMENT

- Age at onset of the disease
- Stage of the disease
- Extent of involvement of the femoral epiphysis
- Presence of extrusion
- Range of hip motion

The choice of treatment taking into consideration these factors is shown in Table 56.1.

Table 56.1 Factors Influencing the Choice of Treatment

Factors		Treatment Implications
Age at onset of the disease	6.8 years	In children under the age of 7 years at the onset of the disease, containment is not indicated unless femoral head extrusion develops. Since in this boy extrusion is present, he is a candidate for containment.[7]
Stage of the disease	Stage Ib	If containment is to succeed in preventing femoral head deformation, it should be achieved by Stage IIa (i.e. early in the course of the disease). Since this boy is in Stage Ib, he is a candidate for early containment.[8]
Extent of involvement of the femoral epiphysis	Entire femoral epiphysis is avascular	If half or more of the femoral epiphysis is rendered avascular, containment must be considered. In this boy, the entire epiphysis is avascular and hence containment is justified.[9]
Presence of extrusion	Extrusion is present	One of the most important factors that influences the decision to contain hips of children with Perthes disease is the presence of extrusion.[9] This boy has extrusion and containment which reverses femoral head extrusion is warranted.
Range of hip motion	The range of motion is not normal— abduction and internal rotation are limited	If containment is to work, the motion of the hip must be restored prior to containment and maintained after containment. Restoration of normal hip motion takes precedence over containment in this boy.

How Was This Boy Treated?

The boy was treated initially with bed rest and above-knee skin traction for a week. All movements of the left hip were restored to normal by the end of the week. He then underwent a sub-trochanteric, open-wedge femoral osteotomy and trochanteric epiphyseodesis. The distal fragment of the femur was fixed in 20 degrees of varus and 20 degrees of external rotation with a pre-bent dynamic compression plate. The most proximal screw crossed the trochanteric growth plate (Figure 56.2).

Post-Operative Management

No external immobilisation was used. Non-weight-bearing crutch walking was continued till the disease had progressed to the latter part of the stage of reconstruction (Stage IIIb).

Follow-Up

The boy was followed up regularly till the disease healed, at which time the implants were removed (Figure 56.3). He was then followed up till skeletal maturity and evaluated in detail. He was totally asymptomatic. He walked normally without a limp, the range of hip motion was normal,

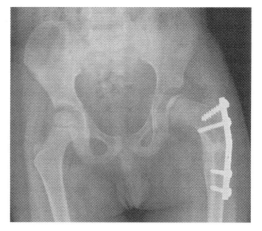

Figure 56.2 AP radiograph of the pelvis taken six weeks following proximal femoral varus derotation osteotomy. Adequate containment has been achieved. The osteotomy is uniting well.

and his hip abductor power was normal. He could squat and sit cross-legged. Radiographs of the hips and a full-length standing film showed that the femoral head was spherical and congruent with the acetabulum. Overgrowth of the trochanter had been prevented. The mechanical axis of the limb was normal, and the limb lengths were equal (Figure 56.4).

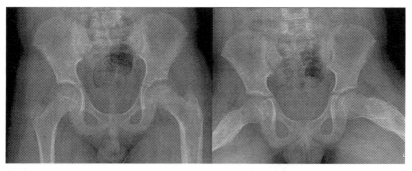

Figure 56.3 The disease has healed completely, and the implants have been removed.

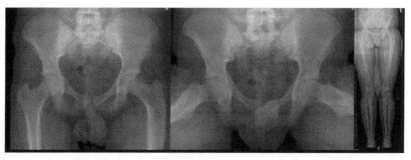

Figure 56.4 At skeletal maturity, the femoral head is spherical, the tip of the trochanter is not elevated, and the limb lengths are equal.

Comment

All the aims of treatment were fulfilled, and that can be attributed to containment early in the disease.

References

1. Hyman JE, Trupia EP, Wright ML, et al. Interobserver and intraobserver reliability of the modified Waldenström classification system for staging of Legg-Calvé-Perthes disease. *J Bone Joint Surg Am.* 2015;97(8):643–50. doi: 10.2106/JBJS.N.00887.
2. Rich MM, Schoenecker PL. Management of Legg-Calvé-Perthes disease using an A-frame orthosis and hip range of motion: A 25-year experience. *J Pediatr Orthop.* 2013;33(2):112–19. doi: 10.1097/BPO.0b013e318281ab44.
3. Copeliovitch L. Femoral varus osteotomy in Legg-Calve-Perthes disease. *J Pediatr Orthop.* 2011;31(2 Suppl):S189–91. doi: 10.1097/BPO.0b013e318223b55c.
4. Salter RB. The present status of surgical treatment for Legg-Perthes disease. *J Bone Joint Surg Am.* 1984;66:961–6.
5. Sponseller PD, Desai SS, Millis MB. Comparison of femoral and innominate osteotomies for the treatment of Legg-Calve-Perthes disease. *J Bone Joint Surg Am.* 1988;70:1131–9.
6. Yoo WJ, Choi IH, Cho TJ, Chung CY, Shin YW, Shin SJ. Shelf acetabuloplasty for children with Perthes' disease and reducible subluxation of the hip: Prognostic factors related to hip remodelling. *J Bone Joint Surg Br.* 2009;91:1383–7.
7. Joseph B, Price CT. Principles of containment treatment aimed at preventing femoral head deformation in Perthes disease. *Orthop Clin North Am.* 2011;42:317–27.
8. Joseph B, Nair NS, Rao NLK, Mulpuri K, Varghese G. Optimal timing for containment surgery for Perthes' disease. *J Pediatr Orthop.* 2003;23:601–6.
9. Catterall A. Perthes's disease. *Br Med J.* 1977;1(6069):1145–9. doi: 10.1136/bmj.1.6069.1145.

Randall T Loder

Case 57a

An 11-year-and-5-month-old girl presented with left thigh pain and a limp after a fall one month ago. Radiographs were appropriately obtained by the child's primary care physician (Figure 57.1).[1] Unfortunately, the radiographs were interpreted as normal.[2] Approximately one month later, the child slipped on an eraser on the floor at school and was immediately unable to get up and walk. Radiographs (Figure 57.2) were obtained which demonstrated a displaced slipped capital femoral epiphysis (SCFE). Clinically this was an unstable type of SCFE as the girl was unable to bear any weight on the limb.[3]

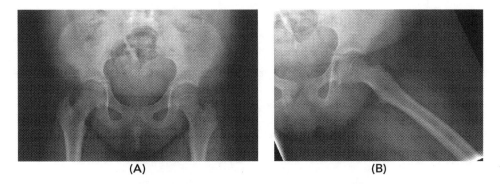

(A)　　　　　　　　　　　　(B)

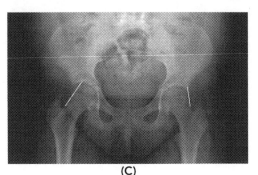

(C)

Figure 57.1 An anteroposterior (A) and frog-lateral (B) radiograph demonstrating a very mild SCFE of the left hip. Note that the Klein's line (C) does not intersect with the epiphysis on the AP view on the left hip, and that there is a very slight posterior step off of the epiphysis relative to the metaphysis on the lateral view (B).

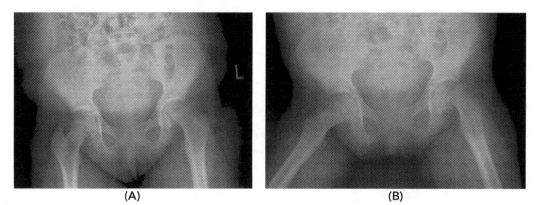

(A)   (B)

Figure 57.2 An AP (A) and lateral (B) radiograph demonstrating the displaced unstable SCFE.

Questions

- What are the problems that need to be addressed in this girl?
- What are the aims of treatment?
- What are the available treatment options to fulfil these aims?
- What are the factors that may influence your choice of treatment?
- Based on these points, what treatment would you recommend for this child?
- How long would you follow-up this girl after treatment?

The Problems That Need to Be Addressed Are

- Moderately severe, unstable SCFE
- Deformity of the proximal femur
- High risk of avascular necrosis

The Aims of Treatment Were

- Stabilization of the SCFE
- Correction of the deformity
- Reduction of the risk of avascular necrosis

The Available Treatment Options Are

- In-situ fixation of the SCFE
- Gentle closed reduction, stabilisation, and decompression of the joint
- Gentle open reduction, stabilisation, and joint decompression
- Modified Dunn procedure via a surgical hip dislocation approach with correction of the deformity and stabilisation

---

FACTORS THAT INFLUENCED THE CHOICE OF TREATMENT

- Stability of the SCFE
- Severity of the SCFE
- Risk of avascular necrosis associated with each procedure
- Complexity of surgical option
- Timing of surgery

The choice of treatment based on these factors is shown in Table 57.1.

Table 57.1 Factors Influencing the Choice of Treatment

Factors		Treatment Implications
Stability of the SCFE	Unstable slip	High risk of progression of the slip. Hence, needs adequate stabilisation with two screws to minimise risk of further progression of the slip.[4] As there is a high risk of avascular necrosis, joint decompression is recommended to relieve the tamponade effect of the effusion.[4,5]
Severity of the SCFE	Moderate deformity	If the deformity is not addressed, secondary femoro-acetabular impingement due to the cam deformity may result in progressive joint damage and deterioration of function. For this reason, in-situ fixation may not be recommended.[6]
Risk of avascular necrosis associated with each procedure	Varies with procedure	Forceful manipulative reduction runs a very high risk of further damage to the tenuous blood supply to the epiphysis, but gentle repositioning is justifiable.[4]
Complexity of surgical option	Varies with the option	The modified Dunn osteotomy of the neck through a safe surgical dislocation of the hip is a complex and technically demanding operation and should only be attempted by surgeons adequately trained in the technique.[7] Not every centre has such capabilities.
Timing of surgery (emergency versus elective)	Delay is likely to increase the risk of avascular necrosis	Emergency decompression of the joint and gentle repositioning of the slipped epiphysis is needed.[4,5,8]

How Was This Child Treated?

This child underwent an emergent gentle repositioning and fixation of the epiphysis with two screws (Figures 57.3a, b). Joint decompression was achieved by opening the hip capsule with a large haemostat (Figure 57.3c).

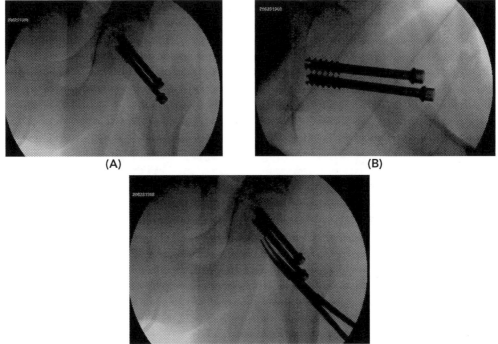

(A)   (B)

(C)

Figure 57.3 The slipped epiphysis was repositioned and fixed with two screws (a, b), and the joint was decompressed by opening the hip capsule with a large haemostat (c).

The child had immediate relief of pain. She was kept non–weight bearing with bed-to-wheelchair transfers for eight weeks, and then gradual progressive weight bearing was allowed. Five months later, the child developed early radiographic changes of avascular necrosis (Figure 57.4).

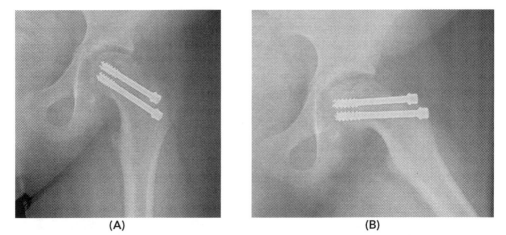

(A)   (B)

Figure 57.4 Early sclerosis in the epiphysis indicating avascular necrosis.

By age 19, the patient was having some mild discomfort, and final radiographs are shown (Figure 57.5). When the patient becomes symptomatic enough to warrant further surgical intervention, the options will include total hip replacement, femoral head reshaping, and rarely arthrodesis.[9,10]

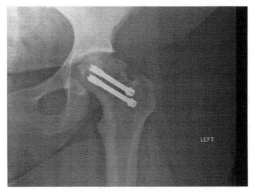

Figure 57.5 Final anteroposterior radiograph of the left hip.

Case 57b

A 13-year-old boy presented with left thigh pain over the past several months. He was very active in basketball. The left lower limb was externally rotated. Hip range of motion demonstrated reduced internal rotation of 10 degrees with obligatory external rotation of the lower extremity with hip flexion in the supine position, and a mild reduction in hip abduction compared to the opposite extremity. Radiographs demonstrated a left SCFE (Figure 57.6).

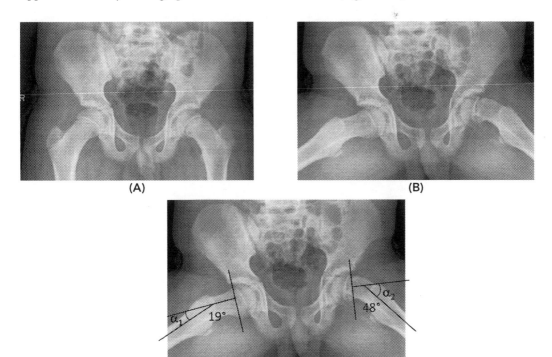

Figure 57.6 An anteroposterior (A) and frog-lateral (B) radiograph demonstrating a very mild SCFE of the left hip. The Southwick lateral epiphyseal shaft angle (c) ($\alpha_2-\alpha_1$) measures 29 degrees, indicating a mild SCFE.

Questions

- What are the problems that need to be addressed in this adolescent boy?
- What are the aims of treatment?
- What are the available treatment options to fulfil these aims?
- What are the factors that may influence your choice of treatment?
- Based on these points, what treatment would you recommend for this boy?
- How long would you follow-up this boy after treatment?

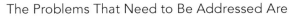

The Problems That Need to Be Addressed Are

- Stable SCFE which runs the risk of progression
- Deformity of the femoral neck that could result in cam femoro-acetabular impingement
- Risk of avascular necrosis

The Aims of Treatment Are to

- Prevent progression of the slip
- Allow for remodelling of deformity of the femoral neck and treat cam impingement if it develops
- Minimise the risk of avascular necrosis

The Available Treatment Options Are[11,12]

- In-situ screw fixation of the SCFE
- Proximal femoral realignment osteotomy with screw fixation of the SCFE
- In-situ fixation of the SCFE and osteochondroplasty if needed, at a later date

---

FACTORS THAT INFLUENCED THE CHOICE OF TREATMENT

- Stability of the SCFE
- Severity of the SCFE
- Risk of avascular necrosis associated with each procedure
- Timing of surgery

The choice of treatment based on these factors is shown in Table 57.2.

Table 57.2 Factors Influencing the Choice of Treatment

Factors		Treatment Implications
Stability of the SCFE	Stable slip	Fixation with a single screw placed in the centre of the epiphysis works very well to stabilise the SCFE.
Severity of the SCFE	Mild	A mild SCFE can be stabilised in situ with an excellent long-term outcome.
Risk of avascular necrosis associated with each procedure	Percutaneous in-situ screw fixation versus re-alignment of the epiphysis and fixation	The risk of producing avascular necrosis is least with in-situ fixation.[13]
Timing of surgery	Elective versus emergency for stabilising the slip	Emergency fixation is not required. However, it should be performed without undue delay[14] to prevent it from becoming an unstable SCFE or progressing.
	Surgery to correct femoral neck deformity	In an asymptomatic adolescent who is skeletally immature, there is potential for remodelling of the neck.[15,16] If sufficient remodelling does not occur and symptoms of impingement develop, surgery may be undertaken.[17]

How Was This Child Treated?

The patient underwent single central screw fixation (Figure 57.7).

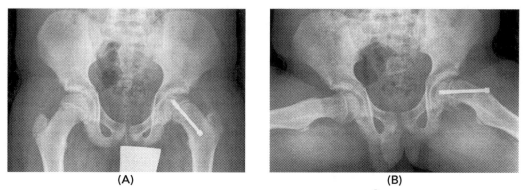

(A)   **(B)**

Figure 57.7 An AP (A) and lateral (B) radiograph demonstrating SCFE single central screw fixation. Note that the screw head is far away from the acetabular rim; more proximal screw heads can result in cam type impingement.

The boy had immediate relief of pain, and he was allowed to return to full weight bearing at four weeks post-surgery. He gradually resumed playing basketball. There was some mild limitation of internal rotation in extension at −10 degrees. At the age of 15 years and 7 months, he began to complain of left groin pain while playing basketball. Physical examination demonstrated pain with internal rotation, flexion, and adduction of the hip, indicative of cam impingement. Radiographs confirmed impingement (Figure 57.8).

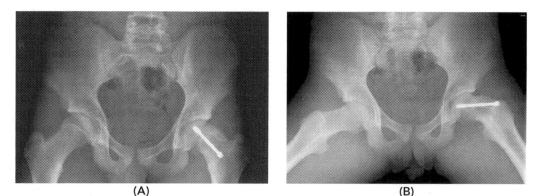

(A)   **(B)**

Figure 57.8 AP (A) and frog-lateral (B) radiographs demonstrating anterior cam impingement.

After discussion with the family, it was elected to proceed with an arthroscopic osteochondroplasty[18,19] which would allow the patient to return to sporting activities sooner than would a flexion intertrochanteric osteotomy or osteoplasty via an open surgical hip dislocation approach. The patient's symptoms were immediately relieved, and he subsequently returned to basketball activities with no discomfort. The most recent radiographs are shown in Figure 57.9.

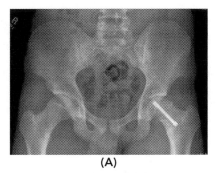
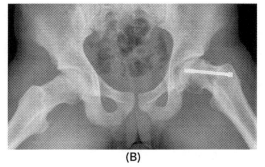

(A)   (B)

Figure 57.9 AP (A) and frog-lateral (B) radiographs at age 16 years 10 months, 10 months after arthroscopic osteochondroplasty of the cam impingement lesion.

How Long Should the Child Be Followed Up after Treatment

- All patients with a unilateral SCFE should be followed every three to four months with both AP and lateral radiographs until physeal closure to ensure that a SCFE does not develop in the opposite hip.
- In both unilateral and bilateral cases, regular (every three to four months) follow-up is needed to ensure that progression of the SCFE does not occur even though stabilised.
- Follow-up is also necessary to monitor for the development of chondrolysis.[20]
- At least one year follow-up is necessary in the unstable case to monitor for the development of avascular necrosis.

Comment

- Case 57a underscores the need to diagnose SCFE immediately. The initial radiograph demonstrated a very mild, stable SCFE. Unfortunately, it was interpreted as normal by the radiologist. After a fall, the SCFE became unstable with the subsequent development of avascular necrosis.
- The prognosis for a SCFE that develops avascular necrosis is variable; some patients have rapid deterioration and development of osteoarthritis, while others have some femoral head deformity and may not need intervention for some time.[9]
- Prophylactic fixation of the opposite hip in unilateral SCFE cases is controversial.[21] It is recommended in the younger patient and children with endocrine dysfunction.
- Treatment of cam impingement depends upon the severity of the impingement; milder cases can be addressed via an arthroscopic osteochondroplasty, although the correction may not be as good as that using an open surgical hip dislocation approach.[19,22]
- The long-term results of osteochondroplasty for cam impingement associated with SCFE are still unknown. The overall natural history for a stable SCFE is one of gradual deterioration and development of osteoarthritis.[23,24]
- Any treatment which results in avascular necrosis is far worse than those that don't develop avascular necrosis, even though the natural history of SCFE is gradual deterioration into secondary osteoarthritis.
- Modified Dunn osteotomy via a surgical dislocation approach should be undertaken with caution in the severe, stable SCFE.[25]

References

1. Lam A, Boenerjous SA, Lo Y, Abzug JM, Kurian J, Liszewski MC, et al. Diagnosing slipped capital femoral epiphysis amongst various medical specialists. *J Child Orthop.* 2018;12:160–6.
2. Hosseinzadeh P, Iwinski HJ, Salava J, Oeffinger D. Delay in the diagnosis of stable slipped capital femoral epiphysis. *J Pediatr Orthop.* 2017;37(1):e19–322.
3. Loder RT, Richards BS, Shapiro PS, Reznick LR, Aronson DD. Acute slipped capital femoral epiphysis: The importance of physeal stability. *J Bone Joint Surg [Am].* 1993;75-A(8):1134–40.
4. Chen RC, Schoenecker PL, Dobbs MB, Luhmann SJ, Szymanski DA, Gordon JE. Urgent reduction, fixation, and arthrotomy for unstable slipped capital femoral epiphysis. *J Pediatr Orthop.* 2009;29(7):687–94.
5. Parsch K, Weller S, Parsch D. Open reduction and smooth Kirschner wire fixation for unstable slipped capital femoral epiphysis. *J Pediatr Orthop.* 2009;29(1):1–8.
6. Lang P, Panchal H, Delfoss EM, Silva M. The outcome of in-situ fixation of unstable slipped capital femoral epiphysis. *Journal of Pediatrics Orthopaedics B.* 2019;28(5):452–7.
7. Sankar WN, Vanderhave KL, Matheney T, Herrera-Soto JA, Karlen JW. The modified Dunn procedure for unstable slipped capital femoral epiphysis: A multicenter perspective. *J Bone Joint Surg [Am].* 2013;95-A(7):585–91.
8. Kaushal N, Chen C, Agarwal KN, Schrader T, Kelly D, Dodwell ER. Capsulotomy in unstable slipped capital femoral epiphysis and the odds of AVN: A meta-analysis of retrospective studies. *J Pediatr Orthop.* 2019;39(6):e406–11.
9. Krahn TH, Canale ST, Beaty JH, Warner WC, Lourenco P. Long-term follow-up of patients with avascular necrosis after treatment of slipped capital femoral epiphysis. *J Pediatr Orthop.* 1993;13:154–8.
10. Larson AN, McIntosh AL, Trousdale RT, Lewallen DG. Avascular necrosis most common indication for hip arthroplasty in patients with slipped capital femoral epiphysis. *J Pediatr Orthop.* 2010;30(8):767–73.
11. Sucato DJ. Approach to the hip for SCFE: The North American perspective. *J Pediatr Orthop.* 2018;38(6S1):S5–S12.
12. Thawrani DP, Feldman DS, Sala DA. Current practice in the management of slipped capital femoral epiphysis. *J Pediatr Orthop.* 2016;36(3):e27–37.
13. Loder RT, Dietz FR. What is the best evidence for the treatment of slipped capital femoral epiphysis? *J Pediatr Orthop.* 2012;32(Supplement 1):S158–65.
14. Birch JG. Slipped capital femoral epiphysis: Still an emergency. *J Pediatr Orthop.* 1987;7:334–7.
15. Örtegren J, Björklund-Sand L, Engbom M, Tiderius CJ. Continued growth of the femoral neck leads to improved remodeling after in situ fixation of slipped capital femoral epiphysis. *J Pediatr Orthop.* 2018 Mar;38(3):170–5. doi: 10.1097/BPO.0000000000000797. PMID: 27261961.
16. Reihnardt M, Stauner K, Schuh A, Steger W, Schraml A. Slipped capital femoral epiphysis: Long-term outcome and remodeling after in situ fixation. *Hip International.* 2016;26(1):25–30.
17. Leunig M, Horowitz K, Ganz R. Femoroacetabular impingement after slipped capital femoral epiphysis: Does slip severity predict clinical symptoms? *J Pediatr Orthop.* 2011;31(1):e6.
18. Accadbled F, May O, Thévenin-Lemoine C, Sales de Gauzy J. SCFE management and the arthroscope. *J Child Orthop.* 2017;11:128–30.
19. Basheer SZ, Cooper AP, Maheshwari R, Balakumar B, Madan S. Arthroscopic treatment of femoroacetabular impingement following slipped capital femoral epiphysis. *Bone Joint J.* 2016;980B(1): 21–7.
20. Lubicky JP. Chondrolysis and avascular necrosis: Complications of slipped capital femoral epiphysis. *J Pediatr Orthop B.* 1996;5:162–77.
21. Swarup I, Goodbody C, Goto R, Sankar WN, Fabricant PD. Risk factors for contralateral slipped capital femoral epiphysis: A meta-analysis of cohort and case-control studies. *J Pediatr Orthop.* 2020;40(6):e446–53.
22. Leunig M, Manner HM, Turchetto L, Ganz R. Femoral and acetabular re-alignment in slipped capital femoral epiphysis. *J Child Orthop.* 2017;11:131–7.

23. Carney BT, Weinstein SW, Noble J. Long-term follow-up of slipped capital femoral epiphysis. *J Bone Joint Surg [Am]*. 1991;73-A(5):667–74.
24. Mathew SE, Larson AN. Natural history of slipped capital femoral epiphysis. *J Pediatr Orthop*. 2019; 39(6S1):S23–37.
25. Davis II RL, Samora III WP, Persinger F, Klingele KE. Treatment of unstable versus stable slipped capital femoral epiphysis using the modified Dunn procedure. *J Pediatr Orthop*. 2019;39(8):411–15.

Nicholas Peterson, Christopher Prior, Selvadurai Nayagam

Case

An 11-year-old boy presented with a limb length discrepancy from a short right femur. There was a previous history of septicaemia as a neonate and subsequent left hip septic arthritis resulting in growth inhibition. This had needed a proximal femoral valgus osteotomy and lengthening of his left femur to achieve limb length equality at age 6 years. In the course of follow-up, a new progressive length discrepancy involving the opposite limb developed. Radiographs taken at age 12 years showed that the right femur was 4 cm shorter. The CT scan confirmed the presence of a central physeal bar in the distal right femur involving less than 25% of the area of the physis (Figure 58.1, 58.2).

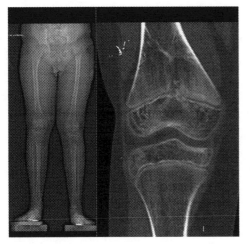

Figure 58.1 Right femoral shortening due to a central bar in the distal physis after neonatal septicaemia.

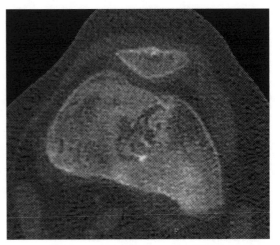

Figure 58.2 Axial slice from a CT scan showing a central physeal bar in the right distal femur.

Questions

- What are the problems that need to be addressed in this boy?
- What are the aims of treatment?
- What are the commonly available options for treatment?
- What are the factors that may influence your choice of treatment?
- What treatment would you recommend for this boy?
- How long would you follow-up this boy after treatment?

The Problems That Need to Be Addressed Are

- Progressive limb length discrepancy (LLD)
- Growth arrest from the physeal bar on the right side

The Aims of Treatment Are to

- Arrest progression of the LLD
- Allow resumption of growth of the arrested physis
- Achieve limb length equalisation by skeletal maturity

Options for Treatment to Fulfil Each Aim

- Arresting progression of LLD:

  o Physeal bar resection with interposition graft

- Allowing resumption of growth of the arrested physis

  o Physeal bar resection and interposition graft

- Achieving limb length equalisation

  o Contralateral epiphyseodesis
  o Limb lengthening

FACTORS THAT INFLUENCED THE CHOICE OF TREATMENT

- Age and gender of the child and growth remaining
- Size and location of the bar
- Preferences of the child and his parents

The choice of treatment based on these factors is shown in Table 58.1.

Table 58.1 Factors that influenced the choice of treatment

Factors		Treatment Implications
Age, gender and remaining growth	11-year-old boy with four years of growth remaining	With four years of growth remaining, the projected discrepancy at maturity was 7.6 cm. An attempt at resection of the physeal bar is a reasonable option.
Size and location of the bar	Central bar involving < 25% of the physis	A bar of this size and location is amenable to resection.[1–3]
Preferences of the child and his parents		This child had had a left femoral lengthening aged 6. He and his family did not wish to consider right femoral lengthening if this was possible to avoid.

How Was This Boy Treated?

Using a sterile tourniquet around the proximal thigh and following a regional nerve block, through medial and lateral sub-vastus approaches the extra-periosteal surface of right distal femur was exposed on both sides. A low-energy De Bastiani–type osteotomy was made in the femoral metaphysis (Figure 58.3), and the distal femoral segment was 'delivered' into the lateral wound (Figure 58.4).[4]

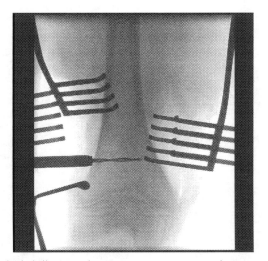

Figure 58.3 Saline-cooled drilling and an osteotome are used to create a metaphyseal osteotomy in the distal femur.

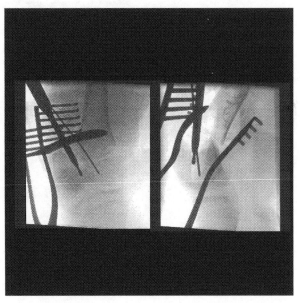

Figure 58.4 The exposed metaphysis of the femur is 'delivered' into the lateral wound to provide access to the central bar.

A K-wire was used with fluoroscopy to help locate the limits of the central bar based on the preoperative planning. It was retained to guide the resection. A saline-cooled burr was used to gradually remove the physeal bar until normal physis was seen around the periphery of the resection area. An arthroscope was used to confirm adequate resection of the bar.

A dermo-fascial graft was prepared by excising an ellipse of skin from a 'bikini-line' incision in the ipsilateral groin. The epidermal layer was removed, and an ellipse of dermis and underlying fat was harvested. The wound was closed using subcuticular sutures. The apices of the harvested ellipse were then folded inwards and sutured so as to create a cylinder with the fat within (Figure 58.5); this was inserted into the area of bar resection, and the femur was then reduced.[5–7] Medial and lateral L-shaped locking plates were used to fix the osteotomy (Figure 58.6).

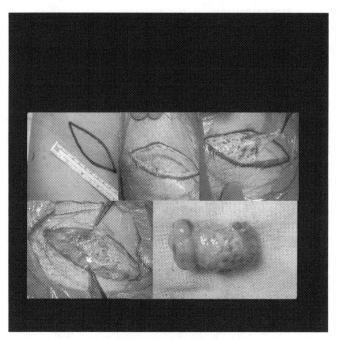

Figure 58.5 A dermal interposition graft is fashioned by removing the epidermal layer from an ellipse in the groin, and then excising the dermis with a small amount of subdermal fat and folding this into a cylindrical shape with the dermis outermost. The original elliptical wound can then be closed.

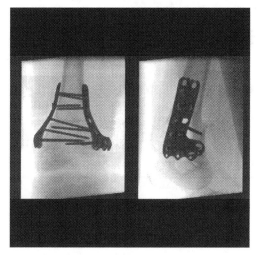

Figure 58.6 Medial and lateral plate fixation of the distal femoral osteotomy proximal to the physis.

Post-Operative Management

The patient was allowed to partially bear weight on the operated limb at 30% for the first two weeks. This was increased to 'as tolerated' over the subsequent six weeks.

In the interim period after this surgery, the left limb was noted to be in genu valgum. The deformity arose from both distal femur and proximal tibia. Corrective surgery by guided growth was proposed and undertaken.

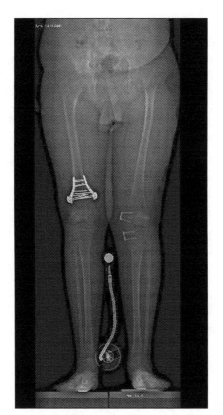

Figure 58.7 Full leg length measurement films demonstrating resumption of growth of the right distal femoral physis.

At clinical review three years following surgery, long leg radiographs were obtained (Figure 58.7).

Correction of genu valgum on the left side was complete with normalisation of the mechanical axis. Length measurements and the position of the locking L-plates indicated successful restoration of distal femoral physeal growth. At this time, the limb length discrepancy was clinically and radiologically less than 2 cm, and it was agreed that this was to be managed non-operatively.

The boy will be followed until he is skeletally mature.

Comment

An alternative approach to this central bar that avoided an osteotomy would have been to create a metaphyseal window and a 'tunnel' down to the area of growth arrest. Dental mirrors or an arthroscope or both may be used to visualise the bar resection using this technique. In practice, visualisation and confirmation that adequate resection has been accomplished are difficult. In the femur, a thigh tourniquet is less able to control bleeding from the medullary cavity than is possible in the tibia. In certain cases, the direct visualisation afforded by the metaphyseal osteotomy facilitates a more reliable bar resection.[8,9] The use of bilateral plates was to offset the reduced working length in internal fixation imposed by having to avoid the physis and the metaphyseal osteotomy being distal enough to reach the bar. This double fixation provided sufficient stability to enable partial weight-bearing soon after surgery.

This case illustrates the potential for septicaemia to cause physeal injury that presents after many years. It was not necessary to lengthen the right femur nor perform epiphyseodesis on the left side to achieve limb length equalisation acceptable to the patient and his family. This may have been due to 'rebound' growth of the right distal femur after the osteotomy and the successful untethering but may also be due to the pathology in the left femur leading to an earlier closure of the proximal capital physis.

References

1. Birch JG. Technique of partial physeal bar resection. *Oper Tech Orthop*. 1993 Apr;3(2):166–73.
2. Langenskiöld A. Surgical treatment of partial closure of the growth plate. *J Pediatr Orthop*. 1981;1(1):3–11.
3. Khoshhal KI, Kiefer GN. Physeal bridge resection. *J Am Acad Orthop Surg*. 2005 Jan;13(1):47–58.
4. Kim HT, Lim KP, Jang JH, Ahn TY. Resection of a physeal bar with complete transverse osteotomy at the metaphysis and Ilizarov external fixation. *Bone Jt J*. 2015 Dec;97-B(12):1726–31.
5. Bueche MJ, Phillips WA, Gordon J, Best R, Goldstein SA. Effect of interposition material on mechanical behavior in partial physeal resection: A canine model. *J Pediatr Orthop*. 1990 Aug;10(4):459–62.
6. Langenskiöld A, Osterman K, Valle M. Growth of fat grafts after operation for partial bone growth arrest: Demonstration by computed tomography scanning. *J Pediatr Orthop*. 1987 Aug;7(4):389–94.
7. Williamson RV, Staheli LT. Partial physeal growth arrest: Treatment by bridge resection and fat interposition. *J Pediatr Orthop*. 1990 Dec;10(6):769–76.
8. Marsh JS, Polzhofer GK. Arthroscopically assisted central physeal bar resection. *J Pediatr Orthop*. 2006 Apr;26(2):255–9.
9. Jackson AM. Excision of the central physeal bar: A modification of Langenskiöld's procedure. *J Bone Joint Surg Br*. 1993 Jul;75(4):664–5.

INFECTIONS

Hitesh Shah

Case

A 4-year-old boy presented with an inability to bear weight on the right lower limb and high-grade fever for three days. The boy was febrile and looked ill. Tenderness was present over the proximal tibial metaphysis. Haematological investigations showed an elevated ESR and C-reactive protein (CRP). Plain radiographs of the tibia were normal (Figure 59.1). Ultrasound scan of the proximal tibia showed a sub-periosteal abscess in the metaphyseal region with normal overlying soft tissue. He was diagnosed to have acute osteomyelitis of the proximal tibia.

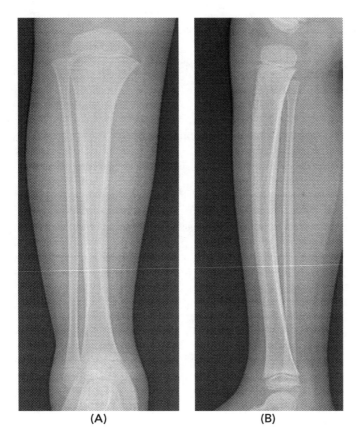

(A)   (B)

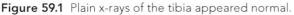

Figure 59.1 Plain x-rays of the tibia appeared normal.

Questions

- What are the problems that need to be addressed?
- What are the aims of treatment?
- What are the available treatment options to fulfil these aims?
- What are the factors that may influence your choice of treatment?
- Based on these points, what treatment would you recommend for this child?
- How long would you follow-up this child after treatment?

The Problems That Need to Be Addressed Are

- Infection of the proximal tibia
- Potential for local spread of the infection and progression to chronic osteomyelitis
- Potential for systemic spread and septicaemia

The Aims of Treatment in This Boy Are

- Control and eradicate infection of the tibia
- Prevent the spread of infection
- Prevent complications (like chronic osteomyelitis, pathological fracture)

Options for Treatment to Fulfil Each Aim

- To control and eradicate infection of the tibia

    o Intravenous antibiotics
    o Drainage of sub-periosteal abscess
    o Decompression of the bone

- Prevent the spread of infection

    o Intravenous antibiotics

- Prevent chronic osteomyelitis

    o Urgent treatment of acute infection

- Prevent pathological fracture of the tibia

    o Protect the limb in a cast
    o Defer weight-bearing

FACTORS THAT INFLUENCED THE CHOICE OF TREATMENT

The factors that influenced the choice of treatment are:

- The age of the child
- Duration of symptoms
- Presence of sub-periosteal abscess
- Probable source of infection (community-acquired versus hospital-acquired)

The choice of treatment based on these factors is shown in Table 59.1.

Table 59.1 Factors Influencing the Choice of Treatment

Factors		Treatment Implications
The age of the child	4 years	The damage to the bone due to infection tends to be more severe in neonates and infants.[1,2]
Duration of symptoms	3 days	Children with acute osteomyelitis who present within 48 hours can often be treated with IV antibiotics alone under close supervision. Children who have had symptoms for more than two days may have developed extra-osseous spread with a sub-periosteal abscess.[3]

Table 59.1 (Continued)

Factors		Treatment Implications
Presence of sub-periosteal abscess	Present	Urgent drainage of the sub-periosteal abscess is mandatory to prevent permanent and irreversible complications.[4,5]
Probable source of infection	Community-acquired infection	The antibiotics that are effective against Methicillin-resistant Staphylococcus aureus (MRSA) need not be administered pending culture as community-acquired MRSA infections are not frequently encountered.[6]

How Was This Boy Treated?

The boy was treated with emergency drainage of sub-periosteal abscess and decompression of the proximal tibia. Ten millilitres of pus were drained from the sub-periosteal plane. The proximal tibia was drilled, and a lot more pus was drained. Through a small metaphyseal window, the remaining pus was drained, and the metaphysis was irrigated with saline. Pus was sent for culture and sensitivity. The surgical wound was closed, and the limb was protected with an above-knee splint.

Post-Operative Management

The boy was treated with intravenous Cloxacillin and Gentamycin to cover Gram-positive and Gram-negative organisms pending the pus culture report. Blood culture and pus cultures grew Methicillin-sensitive *Staphylococcus aureus*. The CRP level was restored to normal, and ESR reduced to within normal limits in seven days. Parenteral antibiotics were discontinued, and oral antibiotics were started and continued for six weeks. The above-knee splint was converted to an above-knee cast after a week and retained for six weeks. Weight bearing was deferred till the cast was removed.

Follow-Up

The boy was followed up regularly, and eight years following the acute illness he was normally active without any symptoms related to the tibia. No deformity or limb length discrepancy was noted, and the radiographs of the tibia were normal (Figure 59.2). As he is 12 years old and has not shown any suggestion of growth disturbance in the tibia over the last eight years, it is highly unlikely that growth arrest or stimulation will occur in future. Further follow-up may not be required.

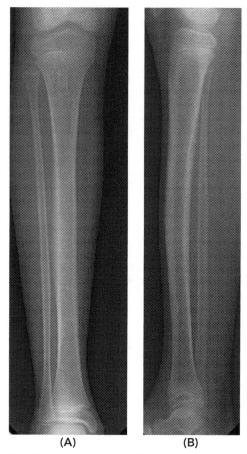

(A)   **(B)**

Figure 59.2 Eight years after the acute episode, the tibia appears normal.

References

1. Castellazzi L, Mantero M, Esposito S. Update on the management of pediatric acute osteomyelitis and septic arthritis. *Int J Mol Sci.* 2016;17(6):855. Published 2016 Jun 1. doi: 10.3390/ijms17060855.
2. Gillespie WJ, Mayo KM. The management of acute haematogenous osteomyelitis in the antibiotic era: A study of the outcome. *J Bone Joint Surg Br.* 1981;63:126–31.
3. Sukswai P, Kovitvanitcha D, Thumkunanon V, Chotpitayasunondh T, Sangtawesin V, Jeerathanyasakun Y. Acute hematogenous osteomyelitis and septic arthritis in children: Clinical characteristics and outcomes study. *J Med Assoc Thai.* 2011;94(Suppl 3):S209–S216.
4. Howard CB, Einhorn M, Dagan R, Nyska M. Ultrasound in the diagnosis and management of acute haematogenous osteomyelitis in children. *J Bone Joint Surg Br.* 1993;75:79–82.
5. Cole WG, Dalziel RE, Leitl S. Treatment of acute osteomyelitis in childhood. *J Bone Joint Surg Br.* 1982;64:218–23.
6. Arnold SR, Elias D, Buckingham SC, Thomas ED, Novais E, Arkader A, Howard C. Changing patterns of acute hematogenous osteomyelitis and septic arthritis: Emergence of community-associated Methicillin-resistant Staphylococcus aureus. *J Pediatr Orthop.* 2006;26:703–8.

CASE 60: ACUTE SEPTIC ARTHRITIS

Hitesh Shah

Case

A 3-month-old infant was brought with paucity of spontaneous movements of the right lower limb, excessive crying while the diaper was changed and refusing feeds for two days. The baby was not febrile but was irritable. The right hip was abducted, and externally rotated. Any attempt at passively moving the hip made the baby cry.

The ESR and CRP were markedly elevated. Ultrasound of the right hip revealed an effusion with subluxation. The radiograph of the pelvis confirmed that the hip was subluxated (Figure 60.1).

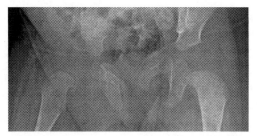

Figure 60.1 Radiograph of the pelvis showing subluxation of the right hip. The hip is abducted, flexed and externally rotated.

Questions

- What are the problems that need to be addressed?
- What are the aims of treatment?
- What are the available treatment options to fulfil these aims?
- What are the factors that may influence your choice of treatment?
- Based on these points, what treatment would you recommend for this child?
- How long would you follow-up this child after treatment?

The Problems That Need to Be Addressed Are

- Probable septic focus in the right hip
- Subluxation of the hip
- Risk of damage to the articular surface, to the epiphyseal cartilage and to the blood supply of the femoral head

The Aims of Treatment in This Infant Are to

- Eradicate infection
- Reduce the subluxation of the hip and restore stability of the hip
- Prevent other complications of sepsis in the hip

Options for Treatment to Fulfil Each Aim

- Eradicating infection
  - Adequate drainage of the joint
    - Repeated joint aspiration and irrigation
    - Arthroscopic lavage
    - Arthrotomy and washout
  - Antibiotics
    - Intravenous antibiotics
    - Oral antibiotics
- Reducing hip subluxation and restoring stability of the hip
  - Drainage of joint—resolve distension of the capsule Immobilisation of the hip
    - Hip spica
    - Pavlik harness
- Preventing complications of infection
  - Urgent drainage of joint and lavage

FACTORS THAT INFLUENCED THE CHOICE OF TREATMENT
• Age of the child • Duration of symptoms • Source of infection (community-acquired versus hospital-acquired)

The choice of treatment based on these factors is shown in Table 60.1.

Table 60.1 Factors Influencing the Choice of Treatment

Factors		Treatment Implications
The age of the child	3 months old	The propensity for cartilage destruction is higher in neonates and infants than in older children. Consequently, there is a greater urgency to perform an arthrotomy in this child.[1,2]

Table 60.1 (Continued)

Factors		Treatment Implications
Duration of symptoms	Over two days	The likelihood of onset of cartilage destruction is greater after 2 days. Hence an immediate joint decompression is warranted.[2]
Source of infection	Community-acquired infection	The antibiotics that are effective against MRSA need not be administered pending culture and antibiotic sensitivity reports as community-acquired MRSA is less frequently encountered.[3,4]

How Was This Baby Treated?

An emergency arthrotomy was performed under general anaesthesia through a short incision in the groin crease. Thick pus exuded from the joint as soon as the distended capsule was incised (Figure 60.2). A copious saline wash-out of the joint was performed after obtaining swabs from the joint. The articular cartilage of the femoral head was inspected and found to be intact and glistening. The wound was closed in layers without suturing the capsule. A hip spica was applied with the hip abducted and flexed by 30 degrees.

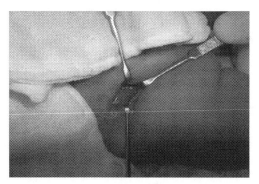

Figure 60.2 Intra-operative photograph shows pus draining from the joint.

Post-Operative Management

The infant was treated with intravenous Cloxacillin and Gentamycin to cover Gram-positive and Gram-negative organisms pending the pus culture report. Methicillin-sensitive *Staphylococcus aureus* was cultured from the pus and was sensitive to the chosen antibiotic.

The CRP level was restored to normal and ESR reduced to within normal limits in seven days. Parenteral antibiotics were discontinued, and oral antibiotics were started and continued for four weeks.

Follow-Up

The hip spica was removed after four weeks, and Pavlik harness was worn for a further period of four weeks.[5,6]

The child was followed up regularly, and at the four-year follow-up, the child was active without any symptoms related to the hip and the hip examination was normal. Radiographs of the pelvis showed a well-centred femoral head and acetabular development that was identical to the contralateral side. Minimal coxa magna and mild changes of avascular necrosis were present on the right side (Figure 60.3a, 60.3b).

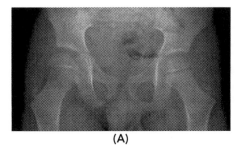
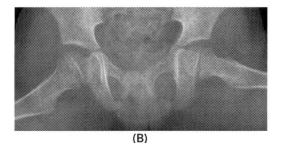

(A)   **(B)**

Figure 60.3 (A) Antero-posterior radiograph of the pelvis four years later shows mild coxa magna. (B) Frog-lateral view shows mild avascular changes in the femoral epiphysis.

Comment

The child needs to be followed up till skeletal maturity to see how the hip develops.

References

1. Agarwal A, Aggarwal AN. Bone and joint infections in children: Septic arthritis. *Indian J Pediatr.* 2016;83(8):825–33.
2. Castellazzi L, Mantero M, Esposito S. Update on the management of pediatric acute osteomyelitis and septic arthritis. *Int J Mol Sci.* 2016;17(6):855.
3. Swarup I, LaValva S, Shah R, Sankar WN. Septic arthritis of the hip in children: A critical analysis review. *JBJS Rev.* 2020;8(2):e0103. doi: 10.2106/JBJS.RVW.19.00103.
4. Arnold, SA, Elias D, Buckingham SC, et al. Changing patterns of acute hematogenous osteomyelitis and septic arthritis: Emergence of community-associated Methicillin-resistant Staphylococcus aureus. *J Pediatr Orthop.* 2006;26:703–8.
5. Vinod MB, Matussek J, Curtis N, Graham HK, Carapetis JR. Duration of antibiotics in children with osteomyelitis and septic arthritis. *J Pediatr Child Health.* 2002;38:363–7.
6. Kim HK, Alman B, Cole WG. A shortened course of parenteral antibiotic therapy in the management of acute septic arthritis of the hip. *J Pediatr Orthop.* 2000;20:44–7.

INDEX

Printed in the United States
by Baker & Taylor Publisher Services